ROUTLEDGE LIBRARY EDITIONS: CHILDREN AND DISABILITY

Volume 3

THE CHILD WITH SPINA BIFIDA

THE CHILD WITH SPINA BIFIDA

ELIZABETH M. ANDERSON &
BERNIE SPAIN

Routledge
Taylor & Francis Group
LONDON AND NEW YORK

First published in 1977 by Methuen & Co. Ltd

This edition first published in 2016
by Routledge
2 Park Square, Milton Park, Abingdon, Oxon OX14 4RN

and by Routledge
605 Third Avenue, New York, NY 10017

Routledge is an imprint of the Taylor & Francis Group, an informa business

British Library Cataloguing in Publication Data
A catalogue record for this book is available from the British Library

ISBN: 978-1-138-96230-9 (Set)
ISBN: 978-1-315-64761-6 (Set) (ebk)
ISBN: 978-1-138-10148-7 (Volume 3) (hbk)
ISBN: 978-1-315-65686-1 (Volume 3) (ebk)

Publisher's Note
The publisher has gone to great lengths to ensure the quality of this reprint but points out that some imperfections in the original copies may be apparent.

Disclaimer
The publisher has made every effort to trace copyright holders and would welcome correspondence from those they have been unable to trace.

The publishers would like to make it clear that the views and opinions expressed, and language used in the book are the author's own and a reflection of the times in which it was published. No offence is intended in this edition.

The child with SPINA BIFIDA

Elizabeth M. Anderson
& Bernie Spain

METHUEN & CO LTD

First published 1977
by Methuen & Co. Ltd
11 New Fetter Lane, London EC4P 4EE
Reprinted 1980

Typeset by Linocomp Ltd, Abingdon, Oxon
and printed in Great Britain by
Richard Clay Ltd, Bungay

ISBN 0 416 55910 7

Contents

Acknowledgements vii

Authors' acknowledgements ix

Introduction 1

1 Medical aspects

1 *Physical and medical problems* 11

2 *Incidence, causation and future trends* 46

2 Families with a spina bifida child

3 *Family problems* 67

4 *Help for families* 88

3 Abilities, attainments and schooling

5 *Intellectual development* 117

6 *The pre-school years* 145

7 *Choosing a school* 177

8 *Teaching children with spina bifida* 202

4 The child and the adolescent in society

9 *Behavioural, emotional and social problems of children and adolescents with spina bifida* 239

10 *After school: prospects for further education, training and employment* 275

Main findings and conclusions 299

Appendices

A *Glossary of medical terms* 315

B *Example of hyperverbal behaviour in a child with spina bifida and hydrocephalus* 322

C *WPPSI and WISC findings* 324

D *Extract from an intervention programme for use with spina bifida infants* 325

E *Extract from parental involvement project* 327

F *Behavioural problems in 6-year-old spina bifida children* 330
G *List of publications about aids and toys* 331
H *Residential courses available for physically handicapped school-leavers* 334
I *Useful addresses* 335

Author Index 338
General Index 344

Acknowledgements

The authors and publishers are grateful for permission to reproduce the following material:

Figure 1.2 from *Developmental Disorders of Mentation and Cerebral Palsies* (1952) by C. E. Benda, published by Grune & Stratton, Inc.

Figure 1.5 from *Your Child with Spina Bifida* (1974) by J. Lorber; Figures 1.7 and 1.8 from *Your Child with Hydrocephalus* (1974) by J. Lorber, published by Association for Spina Bifida and Hydrocephalus, with acknowledgements to Mr A. F. Foster, Medical Artist, Sheffield United Hospitals and Mr A. Tunstill, Head of Photographic Department.

Figure 1.6 from *Physically Handicapped Children. A Medical Atlas for Teachers* (1975) edited by E. Bleck and D. A. Nagel, published by Grune & Stratton, Inc.

Figure 2.2 from 'National statistics' by A. M. Adelstein in *Paediatrics and the Environment* (1975), report of the Second Unigate Paediatric Workshop, edited by Donald Barltrop, Fellowship of Postgraduate Medicine.

Table 7.3 from 'Implications of the treatment of myelomeningocele for the child and his family' by G. Hunt, *Lancet* ii, (1973), 1308.

Table 6.5 from *Social Implications of Spina Bifida – a study in South East Scotland* (1973) by M. Woodburn, published by the Eastern Branch of the Scottish Spina Bifida Association.

Table 5.2 from 'Results of treatment of myelomeningocele' by J. Lorber, *Developmental Medicine and Child Neurology* 13 (3), (1971).

Table 8.1 from 'The effects of hydrocephalus on intelligence, visual perception and school attainment' by B. J. Tew and K. M. Laurence, *DMCN* Supplement 35 (1975).

Appendix D from 'A developmental intervention programme designed to overcome the effects of impaired movement in spina bifida infants' by P. Rosenbaum, R. Barnitt and H. C. Brand in K. S. Holt (ed.) *Movement and Child Development*, Clinics in Developmental Medicine, 55, (1975).

Appendix Ea and Eb from *Parental Involvement Project Development Charts* (1976) by D. M. Jeffree and R. McConkey, published by Hodder & Stoughton.

Authors' acknowledgements

The funding for the GLC survey was provided jointly by the Department of Health and Social Security and the Inner London Education Authority, and for the other study on cognitive and motor problems in 7- to 10-year-old children with spina bifida and hydrocephalus by the Department of Health and Social Security, and we are greatly indebted to both bodies for their support, although all the views expressed here are our own.

We are particularly grateful to Professor Jack Tizard for reading through and commenting so helpfully on the whole of the manuscript, and to him and Dr Guy Wigley for their unfailing interest, help and encouragement at all times.

We would also like to thank Professor C. O. Carter, Mr H. Eckstein and Mr D. Forrest who kindly read the first two chapters, although any errors in them are our own. Brian Tew, Margaret Clark, Stephen Dorner, Roger Glanville, Miles Halliwell, Chris Kiernan and Judith Stollard read and commented on various parts of the text, and Alan Brown provided much of the material on games and PE for spina bifida, and we are grateful to all of them for their help.

A great deal of practical help was given by Gloria Martin and Miles Halliwell who assisted in collecting and analysing the data for the GLC study, and we must also thank Margaret Winkle who was largely responsible for computing the GLC data, Jean Hailes who helped in coding and analysing it and Ian Plewis for his help with the computing and analysis of the data obtained from the 7- to 10-year-old children.

Ruth Davis put many hours of hard work into typing several drafts of the manuscript, as well as helping in many other ways, and we are very appreciative of her patience and cheerfulness throughout.

Finally our great thanks go to the parents and children involved in our research studies, together with the health visitors, doctors, teachers and medical records officers who gave us their co-operation.

Introduction

Spina bifida is not a new condition: it has been described as far back as 2,000 B.C. However, until very recently the majority of children born with spina bifida died within weeks of birth, either as a result of infection to the central nervous system or of the effects of hydrocephalus, which is commonly associated with this condition, and it is only during the last fifteen years that substantial numbers of such children have survived. In 1956, as a result of co-operation between a surgeon and an engineer, himself the father of a hydrocephalic child, a valve was developed to control the circulation of the fluids surrounding the brain, and from that time it became feasible to treat spina bifida. The development of antibiotics during the previous decade was also an important factor, since their use helped to reduce or prevent infection to exposed nervous tissue. Better obstetric services and post-natal care have also played their part in improving the chances of survival. The incidence of this condition in Britain is quite high (2 in every 1,000 births) and the result of changing treatment patterns has been that over the last decade spina bifida has become, after cerebral palsy, the second of the two major physically handicapping conditions in childhood.

To someone meeting a spina bifida child for the first time the complexity and range of problems arising from this condition will not be immediately apparent. The impression given is likely to be that of a child who is essentially 'normal' both in appearance and in behaviour but whose legs are paralysed so that he has to rely on crutches and calipers or a wheelchair for getting around. Research on social attitudes towards disability suggests that a stranger may find it much easier to relate to such a child than, for example, to a cerebral-palsied child, whose appearance and speech may both have been markedly affected by brain damage. This normal appearance will help the spina bifida child to adjust to his handicap and to acquire normal social skills.

Unfortunately the problems associated with spina bifida are very rarely simply those of impaired mobility. There are nearly always many other medical and physical problems, incontinence being a major one, as well as, in many cases, some intellectual impairment. The physical problems, especially incontinence, impose heavy strains on the children's families, in particular the mother, while intellectual impairment coupled with the severity of the physical handicap gives rise to problems connected with the child's education and later may limit opportunities for further education and employment.

Similarities with children handicapped in other ways

Although this book is about spina bifida and hydrocephalus many of the physical, intellectual and family problems described in it are shared by children handicapped in other ways and the suggestions made here about how these problems can be met will also be relevant to them.

The effects of restricted mobility and of incontinence, for example, upon the social and emotional development of a primary school child or a teenager are likely to be similar in many ways, whether that child is handicapped by congenital spina bifida or by paraplegia of some other origin, and there will be similarities too with teenagers who become paraplegic later in life as a result of some trauma such as a road accident. Parents of spina bifida children frequently have anxieties about their children's health, especially in the early years: severe damage to the kidneys caused by urinary infections and blockage of the shunt which controls the hydrocephalus may have extremely serious consequences. Similar chronic anxiety is faced by parents of many other handicapped children, for example those with cystic fibrosis, or haemophilia. Even where the child's health is not at risk many of the stresses imposed on families by the presence of a handicapped child will be similar, whether that child has spina bifida, cerebral palsy, a severe mental handicap or a sensory handicap such as blindness, and families will share a need for advice and help in coping with these stresses.

Intellectual problems of varying degree are likely to result from hydrocephalus even when this has been controlled from an early age. Children with congenital hydrocephalus which is not associated with spina bifida or with hydrocephalus acquired in early childhood, perhaps from meningitis, are likely to have very similar learning difficulties. Another group whose learning difficulties are often very similar are cerebral-palsied children, although a much larger proportion of them than of spina bifida children are likely to be severely retarded. Even 'normal' children, that is those showing no measurable signs of neurological abnormalities, may sometimes have the same sorts of problems although to a lesser degree (for example marked visuo-motor difficulties). The existence of these intellectual problems means that many handicapped children will benefit, as will spina bifida children, from early intervention in the home aimed at helping parents to develop their children's skills in those areas where the impairment is greatest. It will also mean that most parents of handicapped children will face very similar sorts of problems in choosing the right school setting for their child.

These are only a few examples of the sorts of problems which spina bifida children share with those whose handicaps may, at first sight, seem very different and indeed with those who are not overtly handicapped at all, and many other parallels could be drawn.

Aims and contents of the book

Our aim in writing this book has been two-fold. First it has been to provide comprehensive information about the different aspects of this condition based primarily upon our own and other people's research findings but also on clinical and classroom experience. It is hoped that this information will make it easier for administrators, teachers, social workers, psychologists, researchers and other professionals, and also parents, to understand better the sorts of problems spina bifida gives rise to, not only those problems which they themselves are called on to meet but also those raised for professionals working in different disciplines. Where a child's handicaps are multiple it is particularly important for professionals to take a 'global' look at his condition if they are going to provide the best possible help, since different problems will interact with one another. School placement, for example, will be affected by incontinence management; the success of physiotherapy by the mother's ability to be firm with the child; intellectual progress generally by the total family situation.

Second, we have tried to couple this information on different aspects of the functioning of the child and family with practical suggestions about how problems could be reduced or alleviated. Other publications on spina bifida have been largely limited to books with a clear medical orientation, for example, *Spina Bifida for the Clinician* (Brocklehurst, 1976), although excellent booklets written specifically for parents are regularly published by the Association for Spina Bifida and Hydrocephalus and parents should also find Nancy Allum's book *Spina Bifida* (1975) useful. Little is available for those professionals who want to look in detail at all the main aspects of this condition and it is hoped that this account will help to fill that gap.

The book is arranged in four main parts. Part I (chapters 1 and 2) concentrates upon the medical and physical aspects of the condition. Chapter 1 begins with a discussion of how spina bifida develops and then deals in turn with locomotor problems, loss of sensation, bladder and bowel incontinence, sexual functioning, hydrocephalus and its consequences and the Arnold-Chiari malformation. Wherever possible the focus is not simply on describing the problem but also on discussing its management. Incidence and causation, the role of genetic counselling and the vexed question of selection for treatment are discussed in chapter 2.

Part II is concerned with the child in his family, chapter 3 being an account of the sorts of problems which arise for families with spina bifida children and chapter 4 of the ways in which the services available to these families could be improved. Problems discussed in these chapters include the crisis precipitated by the birth of a handicapped child, the question of the support and information given to parents during the early months, the relationship of the parents to the handicapped child and the effects of the handicapped child's presence upon the siblings, upon marital relationships and upon the mother's health.

In Part III (chapters 5–8) the focus is upon the child's intellectual development. Chapter 5 is an account of research findings on various aspects of intellectual development in spina bifida children (for example verbal skills, perceptual functioning and visuo-motor ability) while the three chapters which follow lay the main emphasis on what can be done to help children with such problems. The earlier the child is given appropriate help the better, and chapter 6 is an account of what can be done during the pre-school years to foster both intellectual and social development. Chapter 7 deals with the important and currently controversial question of choosing a school: the needs of the children and how these can be met by different types of schools are discussed, and the actual placement of spina bifida children is reviewed. Research findings on the attainments of spina bifida children coupled with suggestions about what can be done to help the child in school, particularly if this is an ordinary school, form the subject-matter of chapter 8.

Part IV is concerned mainly with older spina bifida children, with adolescents and with school-leavers. Chapter 9 begins with a discussion of the behavioural and emotional problems of pre-adolescent spina bifida children and this is followed by a discussion of the problems of spina bifida teenagers, especially the question of social isolation, while chapter 10 considers prospects for further education, training and employment. The book ends with a summary of conclusions and recommendations. Appendices include a glossary of technical terms.

The research basis of the book

In this book we have tried to base our analysis of the problems faced by spina bifida children and their families as firmly as possible upon research findings. The importance of research for development of services has been discussed by Tizard (1966) and is stressed in the Seebohm Report (1968) where it is stated: 'We cannot emphasize too strongly the part which research must play in the creation and maintenance of an effective service. Social planning is an illusion without adequate facts; and the adequacy of services mere speculation without evaluation.'

Whatever kind of service we are talking about, whether it is services provided by a hospital during the neonatal period to parents of a handicapped child, or social services, or the pros and cons of different types of educational provision, or employment services, this principle still applies.

Research in this country on the consequences of spina bifida can be categorized in three main ways, although research studies do not always fit neatly into one particular category. First, in a small number of centres, longitudinal studies of spina bifida children are being carried out, that is, the same children are being followed up over a number of years. Examples of such studies are the GLC survey which has been carried out by one of us (Spain), and is described in greater detail below, and the studies of spina bifida children in South Wales set up by Michael Laurence, Brian Tew and their colleagues at the Welsh National School of Medicine. Other centres have concentrated on monitoring the physical problems of the children over long periods and in this respect reference is made to Lorber's work in Sheffield. A second kind of study is the survey made at a particular point in time of selected aspects of the development of spina bifida children. Good examples of this kind of study are Margaret Woodburn's survey (1973) of the social implications of spina bifida for 86 families with spina bifida children living in a carefully defined area of south-east Scotland, and Steven Dorner's study (1976a and b) of the problems of adolescents with spina bifida. In the third kind of research a particular aspect of cognitive or behavioural functioning (for example, visual perception or writing ability) is selected and a small-scale but intensive research study carried out in which both standardized tests and specially designed experimental measures may be used. Anderson's recent study (1975), also described briefly below, would fall into this category.

In writing this book we have drawn extensively on the research findings of others; however we have also made considerable use of our own findings, particularly those provided by the GLC survey, and to end this chapter a short account is given of our own research studies.

The GLC survey (Bernie Spain)

This study was begun in 1967 at the request of the Medical Adviser's Department of the Inner London Education Authority, as a result of the realization that more and more children with spina bifida were surviving to school age, because of improved methods of treatment. At that time the proportion of children surviving was not known precisely, nor was it clear to what extent survivors were handicapped physically and intellectually. In particular, little work had been done on the intelligence of children given early surgical treatment to control hydrocephalus. The study aimed to provide this information and also to suggest ways of improving educational and social services. The project was financed in part by the DHSS.

All the children born within the Greater London area between April 1967 and March 1969 were included in the study. They were found through borough medical records, Office of Population, Censuses and Surveys, certificates of deaths and stillbirths and the admission registers of the twenty London hospitals known to treat this condition.* With the co-operation of the Medical Officers of Health, families of all children surviving to the age of one year were contacted through the health visitors and of 195 available families 183 agreed to be seen at least on one occasion and over 80 per cent of these co-operated fully. The children were seen regularly from one year till just before their sixth birthday, i.e. when they had been in school for at least two terms. On each visit to the home the child's development was assessed and the mother interviewed to discover her experience of services and what

* This part of the study was conducted in conjunction with Dr Cedric Carter and Mrs Kathleen Evans from the MRC Medical Genetics Unit at the Institute of Child Health, who were interested in determining the recurrence rate for couples who had already produced one child with a neural tube defect.

problems were arising for the family, if any. Between the age of 5 and 6 years the child was seen in school and given an extensive battery of tests and, following this, the mother was interviewed at home. At this time a control group was also included for each spina bifida child who attended normal school. The next child in the class register was selected who most closely matched the index child on sex, age and social class. Accounts of this project are available in several published papers quoted in the text. The study is referred to in this book as the GLC survey.

Cognitive problems and writing difficulties in children with spina bifida and hydrocephalus (Elizabeth Anderson)

This study, which was financed by the DHSS, was carried out in two phases between 1973 and 1975. Phase I comprised an investigation of cognitive and motor deficits in twenty-nine children aged 6½–9½ years with spina bifida and hydrocephalus, the majority of whom were attending special schools. Each child was matched for age, sex and reasoning ability with a non-handicapped child, and for age and reasoning ability only with a cerebral-palsied child. The children were tested individually on a battery selected to elicit information about overall intellectual ability and sub-test performance patterning; verbal ability; visuo-motor and visuo-perceptual ability; and hand function. Measures of reading attainment and behavioural and personality factors were included.

In Phase II twenty of the original spina bifida group (ten boys and ten girls) and their non-handicapped controls took part. The main aim was to investigate the extent and nature of copying and writing difficulties and to identify possible underlying deficits. The groups were compared on three main types of tasks: (a) clinical tasks for which developmental norms were available, including tests of handedness, left-right awareness, finger agnosia, associated movements, repetitive and successive finger-movements and kinaesthetic ability; (b) paper and pencil tests of speed and accuracy of dotting, tracing and crossing; (c) copying and writing tasks proper, including copying single digits, letters and words, and copying a series of unfamiliar symbols and a series of sentences under different experimental conditions. A detailed account of this study is available in an unpublished University of London Ph.D. dissertation (1975) but some of the main findings are reported in this book, the study being referred to as Anderson's study (1975).

References

Anderson, E. M. (1975), 'Cognitive and motor deficits in children with spina bifida and hydrocephalus with special reference to writing difficulties', unpublished Ph.D. thesis, University of London.

Brocklehurst, G. (ed.) (1976), *Spina Bifida for the Clinician*, Clinics in Developmental Medicine, 57, Spastics International Medical Publications/Heinemann, London.

Dorner, S. (1976), 'Adolescents with spina bifida – how they see their situation', *Archives of Diseases in Childhood*, 51, 439–44.

Seebohm Report (1968), *Report of the Committee on Local Authority and Allied Personal Social Services*, HMSO, London.

Tizard, J. (1966), 'The experimental approach to the upbringing of handicapped children', *Developmental Medicine and Child Neurology*, 8 (3), pp. 310–21.

Woodburn, M. (1973), *Social Implications of Spina Bifida – a Study in S.E. Scotland*, Eastern Branch Scottish Spina Bifida Association, Edinburgh.

1 Medical aspects

1 Physical and medical problems

Introduction

The term spina bifida refers, strictly speaking, to a developmental defect of the spinal column in which the arches of one or more of the spinal vertebrae have failed to fuse together so that the spine is 'bifid', a Latin term meaning split in two. Through this gap in the spine either the spinal cord itself or its surrounding membranes protrude, depending upon which of several types of spina bifida the child is suffering from. A great deal of publicity has been given to this condition during the last decade and most people to whom the term means anything at all probably associate it with a severely disabled child with paralysed legs and incontinence of the bladder and bowel. It is important to point out from the start that the general term 'spina bifida' embraces a *group* of developmental defects of the spinal column ranging from a condition called spina bifida occulta which is very common but usually has no effect on function, to the far more complex and serious condition which the term 'spina bifida' has come to mean to most of the public, i.e. myelomeningocele. (Medical terms summarized in Glossary, p. 313.)

How the condition develops

In the normally developing human embryo the central nervous system, including the brain and the spinal cord, begins as a single sheet of cells: this sheet of cells develops during the second week of pregnancy into what is called the neural plate (Fig. 1.1a). During the third week of pregnancy the neural plate enlarges and forms a symmetric longitudinal groove (Fig. 1.1b). In the fourth week the neural groove deepens and folds develop on either side, which eventually fuse so that instead of an open groove a closed tube is formed (Fig. 1.1c and d). This elongated hollow cylinder is called the neural tube and it eventually differentiates into the brain and the spinal cord. Following this, supportive and protective tissues develop to enclose the spinal cord and the brain (for example, the meninges), and finally a bony covering is formed, the vertebrae of the spinal column (which enclose and protect the spinal cord) and the cranium (the skull).

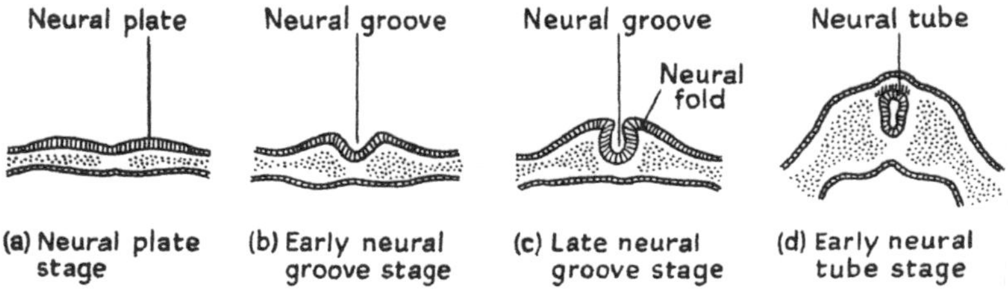

Figure 1.1 *Diagram of transverse section of embryos at different ages to show development of the spinal cord.*

In spina bifida or any other neural tube defect, some part of the nerve cord fails to close or fuse and the nerve cord at that point remains immature and improperly formed. If the nerve cord has failed to form properly then the supporting tissues, including the vertebrae or the cranium, will also be abnormal.

From the cavities within the brain (the ventricles), around which the nerve tissue is folded, a fluid is produced called cerebro-spinal fluid (CSF) which bathes and protects the nerves cells. In the normally developing foetus, the CSF circulates freely, flowing down into the spinal column through a small hole in the base of the skull, the foramen magnum, through which the spinal nerves ascend and descend from the brain (see Fig. 1.6, p. 32). Commonly associated with spina bifida is a second abnormality found at the base of the brain, called the Arnold-Chiari malformation. This is a herniation (protrusion) of the lower brain downwards through the foramen magnum and a general dis-arrangement of the lower brain structures. When this abnormality occurs it is usually accompanied by hydrocephalus, that is, a build-up of CSF within the brain, due to an obstruction in the normal circulation of the fluid. If the build-up of CSF is not checked, it causes the nerve cells to become stretched and crushed, and stretches the infant skull so that it enlarges to accommodate the additional fluid.

Interference with the normal growth and development of the neural tube and in particular with the closure of the neural tube during the early weeks of pregnancy may result in any of the disorders described in this chapter. The reasons for this interference with normal development appear to be very complex and are not yet fully understood: probably both genetic and a variety of environmental factors are involved, and these are discussed more fully in chapter 2. The exact nature of the neural tube disorder, however, will depend both upon which part of the neural tube fails to develop normally and on the extent of the interference with normal growth. If there is a failure of closure in the midline or lower end of the neural tube, then spina bifida will result. If the failure is at the upper end, the head end of the tube, this will result in either cranium bifidum or anencephaly.

Spina bifida

Much of the terminology used about spina bifida is still confusing. However, the classification used by Smith (1965) is the generally accepted one, the two main divisions being into (a) spina bifida occulta and (b) spina bifida cystica, this being subdivided into two main conditions, (i) meningocele and (ii) myelomeningocele.

In spina bifida occulta (Latin=hidden) the vertebral arches do not fuse: there is not, however, any distension of the meninges and the spinal cord and its membranes are generally (although not always) normal. The site of the spinal defect is sometimes marked by a slight swelling, a dimple in the skin, or a tuft of hairs but there is often no external evidence of the defect. This condition is very common and rarely has any consequences on function.

The other main type of spina bifida, spina bifida aperta (Latin= open) or cystica (cyst-like) is a condition in which some of the spinal cord tissue herniates into a sac-like cyst filled with cerebro-spinal fluid. There are two major sub-types of spina bifida cystica, meningocele (Fig. 1.2b) and myelomeningocele (Fig. 1.2c).

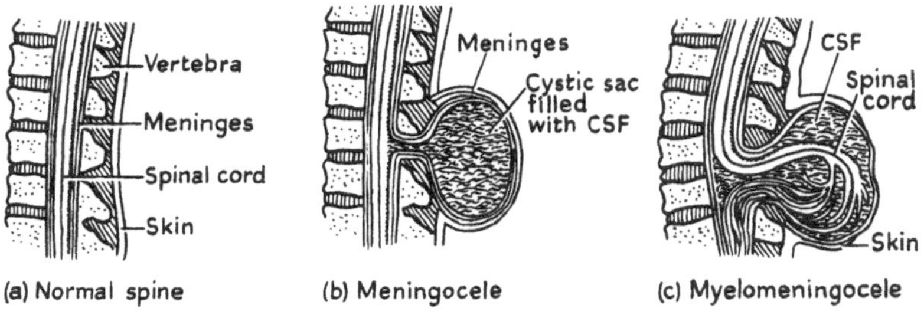

Figure 1.2 *Diagram showing section through normal spine (a) meningocele (b) and myelomeningocele (c)* (Adapted from Benda, C. E. *Developmental Disorders of Mentation and Cerebral Palsies*, 1952, courtesy of Grune and Stratton, Inc., New York).

Spina bifida meningocele is the less serious and the less common type, affecting between approximately 15 per cent and 25 per cent of all children with spina bifida cystica. In this type (Fig. 1.2b) the meninges bulge through the gap in the spine to form a smooth cystic sac usually covered by normal skin. This sac usually contains only meninges and cerebro-spinal fluid. The nerve cord functions normally, however, so that in cases of spina bifida meningocele there will be no significant degree of impairment.

The other major type is myelomeningocele (Fig. 1.2c). Again, there is failure of the vertebrae to fuse and distension of the meninges, but this condition differs from meningocele in that the spinal cord not only protrudes into the sac but is itself abnormal, the result being permanent and irreversible neurological disability. Within this type of spina bifida many variations in the structure of the spinal cord are found and different terms are used to describe these.

The changes in the spinal cord are not confined to the level of the main mass of the lesion; if any cord does continue below the level of the lesion it is usually abnormal. Again, above the main mass the cord is also frequently abnormal for several spinal segments, and indeed autonomic abnormalities may occur at any point in the upper spine (Emery and Lendon, 1973).

Cranium bifidum and anencephaly

The other major neural tube defects occur when there is a failure to fuse at the head end of the nerve cord. The term cranium bifidum refers to a defect in the fusion of the bones of the skull (cranium), usually at the back of the head, which allows soft tissues to herniate. Some of the lesions contain only meninges and some actual brain tissue but the term encephalocele is commonly applied to the various lesions associated with cranium bifidum. Encephaloceles may be quite small and covered with skin in which case the outlook is good: often, however, the swelling is large and only covered by a thin membrane and here the outlook is very poor.

In anencephaly there is an actual defect of development of the entire anterior part of the brain, not simply a cranial defect, with a failure of the formation of the vertex of the skull and incomplete formation and degeneration of the cerebral lobes of the brain; the basal parts of the brain then lie exposed on the surface (Carter, 1969). Anencephalics are commonly stillborn and those born alive do not survive.

Clinical aspects of spina bifida myelomeningocele

When the baby is born the spinal defect, whether it is a meningocele (containing only cerebro-spinal fluid and the meninges) or a myelomeningocele (containing also the spinal cord tissue) may have a variety of appearances. Most commonly there is a raised swelling or 'sac' which may be located at any point along the spinal column, and which varies greatly in size, extent and contents (Plate 1).

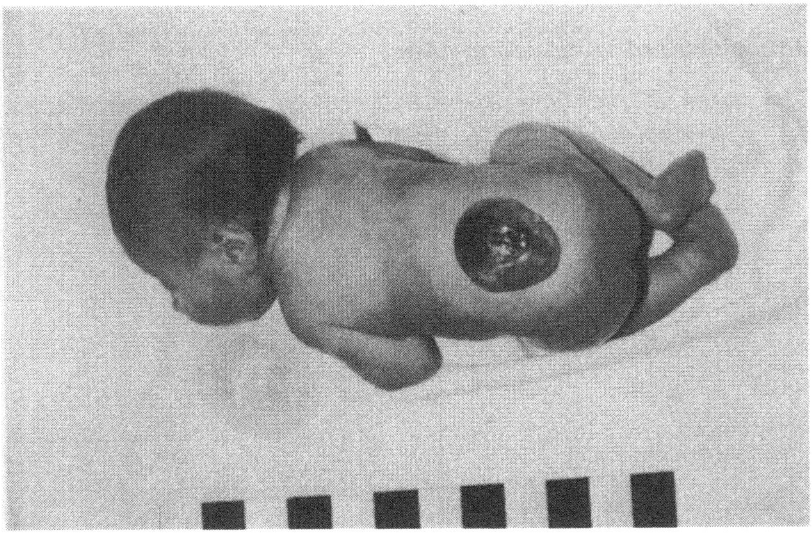

It looks rather like a large blister on the surface of the back through which can be seen the cerebro-spinal fluid, and, in myelomeningocele, the abnormal or primitive nerve cord can also be seen, often adhering to the tissue covering the sac. The sac may be covered by normal skin. Most commonly it is covered by a very flimsy membrane, the arachnoid, at the centre of the defect, with normal skin towards the outer edges.

Because the skin covering the lesion is defective, the area is exposed to injury and infection, the greatest danger being the development of meningitis. In addition, if the cystic sac is allowed to expand there may be stretching of the nerve roots leading to an increase in the paralysis and weakness of the legs or abdominal muscles. If the lesion is not protected, the exposed nerves may dry out and further deteriorate.

Consequently it has been common practise in this country since the early 1960s to 'repair' the spinal lesion by covering it with skin flaps where possible within twenty-four hours of birth. In this operation the spinal cord is put into its normal place within the spinal cavity and is covered with skin and other tissues to save the exposed tissue from infection and other damage and to reduce the risk of meningitis. However, if the lesion is a very bad one and little movement has been preserved, it may not be necessary to operate immediately, provided that effective measures can be taken to prevent infection or further damage to the nerve cord.

Locomotor and associated problems

The extent of lower limb paralysis depends on where the spinal lesion is, its severity and its extent, the location of the main areas of the vertebral column (spine) being shown in Fig. 1.3 below.

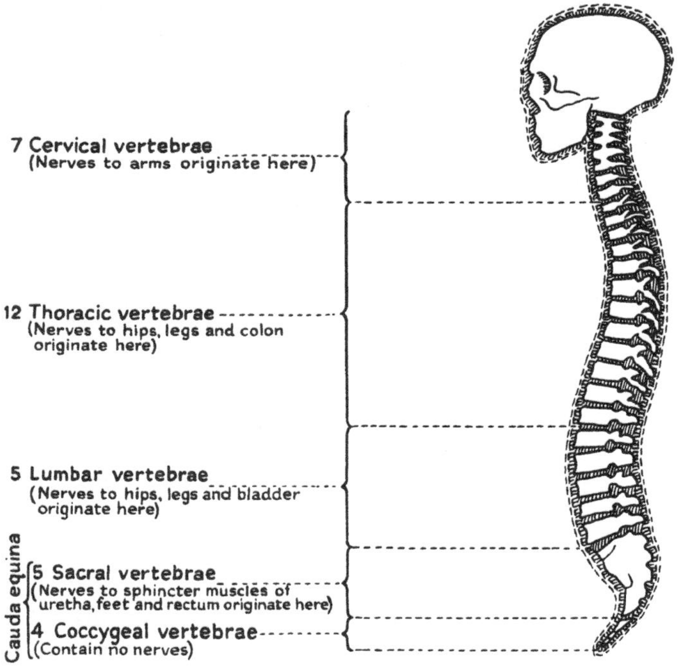

Figure 1.3 *The vertebral column.* The vertebral column consists of thirty-three vertebrae, a series of bony rings forming a hollow canal enclosing and protecting the spinal cord. Thirty-one pairs of spinal nerves originate from the cord. The main parts of the trunk and limbs with which the spinal nerves connect are indicated above together with the main internal organs controlled by the autonomic nerves which connect with particular sections of the spinal cord.

In general lumbar and in particular thoraco-lumbar lesions are likely to produce quite severe paralysis. Survivors with cervical lesions, which are usually simple meningoceles, are rarely handicapped. Sacral lesions also result in a slight handicap, because fewer nerve roots are implicated.

Broadly speaking the child will be unable to move those muscles which receive their nerve supply from the spinal cord below the level of the lesion, although surviving children with lesions at the upper thoracic and cervical levels (rather a small proportion of all children with myelomeningoceles), are usually free from severe locomotor disabilities. The majority of children with myelomeningocele have lesions at lower levels than this, particularly in the lumbar and lumbo-sacral regions since this area of the spinal cord is the last part of the neural tube to close. Smith (1965) suggests that four main groups can be distinguished. Most severely handicapped are those children with lesions at or above the third lumbar vertebra who are totally paraplegic and will need total support to the lower limbs. The next group, with lesions at or below the fourth lumbar vertebra, will have suffered from paralysis of some (but not all) of the muscles of the hips and knees, as well as paralysis of the feet and will need support in these areas. A third group with lesions at the first and second sacral vertebrae may have just adequate function left in the hips, but the feet will need support. Least handicapped are children with lesions at or below the third sacral vertebra: their lower limb function will be normal, but they may be incontinent.

Overall, between a third and a half of children with myelomeningocele are left with a total flaccid paraplegia while most of the others will have significant locomotor problems (Gabriel, 1974). Whatever the degree of lower limb paralysis, hydrocephalus makes independent walking more difficult as it disturbs balance, and intellectual impairment, if there is any, may make it more difficult for the child to work out how to use his limbs or walking apparatus.

In addition to the direct neurological consequences of damage to the spinal cord, associated abnormalities which affect locomotion may be present from birth or may arise later. These can include abnormalities of the vertebrae producing scoliosis and kyphosis (curvature of the spine), abnormalities of the rib cage, dislocation of one or both hips, or other fixed limb deformities of the ankles or knees.

Fixed limb deformities are very common indeed in spina bifida because of the imbalance of muscles resulting from disparities in innervation (nerve supplies). The large muscles on the suface of the body which move the limbs and keep them in place normally work in pairs, by a process called reciprocal innervation. This means that as one muscle contracts to raise a limb, the opposing muscle expands to release it. The action of the biceps and triceps in raising and lowering the forearm is a very simple illustration of this process. If one member of the muscle pair has a poor nerve supply then it will not be able to exert an equally opposing power and the affected limb may be held permanently in some abnormal position, or the range of movement may be diminished.

In spina bifida the hips may dislocate, the knees may be fixed in a rigid position unable to bend voluntarily, or the feet may not be aligned correctly (talipes) because calf or ankle tendons are affected. Such contractures (joint deformities) may be present in the child at birth but others may develop as the child grows or may worsen because of shortening of the muscles and ligaments around a joint as a result of lack of movement.

Paralysed children also frequently develop spontaneous fractures of the femur and other bones, especially after a period of immobilization in plaster; some of the children in Lorber's study (1971) had fractured a femur as often as eight times. Since the child feels no pain these are easy to miss, the signs being that the affected part of the limb becomes swollen and slightly warm (Sharrard, 1976).

Treatment and management

The aims of orthopaedic management and operative treatment have been summarized by Sharrard (1976) as follows: (1) to correct deformity, maintain the correction, prevent its recurrence and avoid the production of other deformities; (2) to obtain the best possible locomotor function and (3) to prevent or minimize the effects of sensory or motor deficiency. Active measures to correct deformity are usually begun when the child is about six months old and continue during the first two years. Tendons often need to be lengthened, shortened or transplanted, the main aim being to correct deformity, to allow the fitting of calipers and the development of walking, and sometimes surgery is needed by children with dislocated hips. Between the age of 2 and 5 years more surgery on the tendons and bones may be needed but between the ages of 5 and 12 surgery should only be needed for children who have developed a deformity which was not present previously but which is increasing and causing problems. After the age of 12 'the final corrective surgery may be needed either to correct deformities of the spine or to stabilize the joints of the foot' (Sharrard, 1976).

The part played by physiotherapists and occupational therapists in treatment and management is extremely important. The physiotherapist will help the child to use his limbs as effectively as possible so that he can both achieve and maintain the maximum locomotor activity, and will give regular treatment herself or teach the parents to do this to prevent new problems (such as contractures) from arising. Physiotherapy will also be needed after surgery.

Nancy Allum (1975) gives a useful account to parents of what the physiotherapist can do to help. This will include advising the mother about the handling of her baby, about seating him and about the sorts of play it is most useful to encourage; teaching the parents various passive movements of the baby's toes, feet, ankles, knees and hips which they can carry out to prevent contractures from arising and to ensure that as much movement as possible is retained by the joints, and giving advice about equipment and aids which are appropriate at the different stages. A detailed account of physiotherapy treatment for spina bifida children is given in a booklet by Leonie Holgate (1970).

As the child gets older the physiotherapist will prepare him for using calipers, their essential function being to support weak joints. Some of the exercises and games she uses are designed to help him to learn to balance; others will be aimed at strengthening his arms and shoulders, since they will have to bear his own weight and the weight of the calipers. Where possible the child will be fitted with calipers (which has to be done very carefully since they can cause pressure sores) and encouraged to stand with them at the age at which a child would normally be doing this. Since the child only has control over the upper half of his body he may need a great deal of help and encouragement to learn to balance in the standing position. An ordinary child learning to walk falls frequently; a child with spina bifida will probably have to be taught by the physiotherapist to lose his fear of falling. The younger he is when he starts learning to stand and walk the less likely he is to be afraid, and it will also help if he is not allowed to become overweight.

Depending on the severity of the handicap the child may be taught first to stand with support (e.g. a tripod), next to walk between parallel bars and then to walk with a walker, tripod or crutches. Other aids to mobility found to be helpful include baby walkers, low-wheeled trucks which the child can manipulate with his hands ('chariots') and rollators. For mobility out of doors a 'baby buggy' seems to be the best solution, though some children do use wheelchairs from an early age. Further information about the range of appliances available and useful can be found in books by Nancy Finnie (1971) and Alison Wisbeach (1974) or direct from the appliance officer at ASBAH headquarters.

Many schools and hospital departments now find it useful to employ an occupational therapist (OT) to work in conjunction with physiotherapists or teachers. She can help improve upper and lower limb dysfunction by suggesting toys or games which will encourage children to stand, walk or use their hands. She can also advise on commercially produced aids and appliances, adaptations to ordinary furniture and on the most suitable toys for children with specific problems or of particular ages, and in general has a fund of practical knowledge and advice to share with both parents and professionals on how to help the child develop as normally as possible within the limits of his handicap.

Loss of sensation

Damage to the spinal cord produces not only paralysis but loss of sensation (anaesthesia) in the parts of the body receiving nerve supplies from the cord below the level of the lesion. Pressure applied to a point on a person's body for a long period will prevent the blood from circulating through the compressed area; this will cut off the oxygen as a result of which the tissue will become damaged and will then decompose and become infected, the end product being the formation of a discharging ulcer (trophic ulcer). As soon as pressure builds up, a person with normal feeling will experience discomfort and change his position but a person without sensation will have to take very careful precautions throughout his life to prevent pressure sores from arising, particularly in those parts of the body which are especially vulnerable. These are the parts where bones and bony points lie fairly near the skin in places which support the weight of the body.

When lying in bed the most susceptible areas are the backs of the heels and the lower part of the back. When sitting the child is especially vulnerable. The chair seat should be padded with a foam rubber cushion and the child taught to raise his body off the seat of the chair and maintain this position for some seconds before letting himself down again. The feet, ankles and legs can also easily develop sores if shoes or calipers, particularly new ones, fit badly and rub. A child with insensitive skin feels no discomfort when pressure or extremes of temperature are applied, so that pressure sores, burns and even frostbite can easily occur, and it is especially important to check that the child's anaesthetized limbs are never in contact with even mild heat, for example from a hot water bottle or wall heater.

If their onset is noticed early enough most pressure sores will heal if the source of pressure is removed, the damaged area kept free of pressure for some time and simple measures are taken to prevent infection, but in some cases pressure sores can take weeks to mend because poor circulation causes healing to be slow. The child or adult may be immobilized until the sore heals and may have to stay away from school or work for several weeks. All spina bifida children must therefore be taught to examine their skin regularly so that they can recognize the early stages of a pressure sore and prevent it from becoming worse. The child should be taught to do this as early as possible so that this becomes as routine a matter as brushing one's teeth. They should also be taught about the danger of burns. It is important as well to ensure that the child's legs and feet are kept warm, particularly in winter, because of poor circulation.

The problems of incontinence

Damage to the spinal cord and associated nerve roots will, for almost all children with myelomeningocele including some of those with normal locomotion, result in loss of sensation in the bladder and a loss of sphincter control, leading to dribbling or incontinence of urine and faeces. Many useful accounts of this complex problem and its management are available (e.g. Eckstein and Chir, 1972 Forrest, 1976) and only a fairly brief account is given here. Before beginning we show the way in which the urinary system functions normally in Fig. 1.4 below.

Urinary incontinence

Smith (1965) describes two main patterns of wetting in children with neurogenic (paralysed) bladders, one being constant dribbling and the other overflow incontinence. 'The most common situation is of constant dribbling, occurring every few minutes, and in small volumes at a time. There is no sensation of bladder fullness, no consciousness of a stream flowing and no control to stop the stream.' In these cases the bladder is flaccid and has little capacity for retention.

In the other main pattern of incontinence, states Smith (1965) 'dribbling is not constant, although the children are incontinent in the sense that there is little or no bladder sensation, and no control to start or stop the stream. The dribbling is an overflow incontinence and tends to be intermittent with periods of dryness up to one or two hours at a time', i.e. in this, the retentive type of bladder, there is usually sufficient outflow resistance to keep the child dry until the bladder contains a good volume of urine.

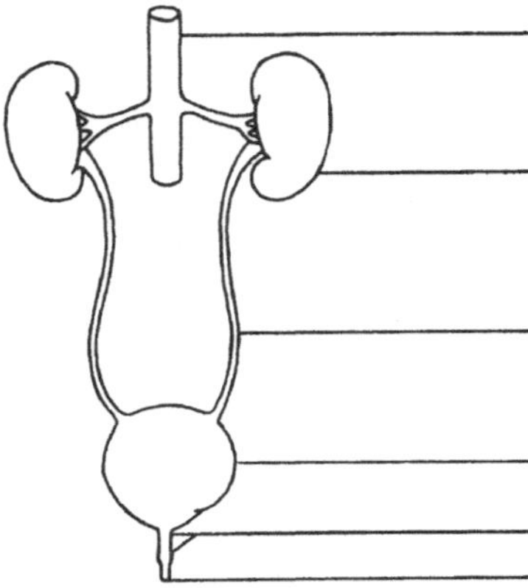

Figure 1.4 *The normal urinary system.*

Urine is formed continuously by the kidneys. It is conveyed from them to the bladder via the ureters, long muscular tubes which contract regularly. As the urine collects the bladder expands. Eventually, a sensation of fullness is felt. The smooth muscle walls of the bladder are stimulated to contract, the internal and external sphincters relax and the urine is voided through the urethra. The process is basically a reflex one carried out through nerve impluses from centres in the spinal cord, but normally, as the child grows older, a large measure of voluntary control develops and these reflex mechanisms can be restrained through control from higher centres in the brain. The parts of the spinal cord most critically involved in the reflex mechanisms are the first two lumbar nerves and the 2nd to 4th sacral nerves, these being the nerves which normally cause the bladder walls to contract. In spina bifida myelomeningocele it is frequently damage to the latter which plays the main part in urinary incontinence.

Risk of infection and kidney damage

For both of these groups the problem is not simply a social one. There are also real dangers to the child's health and life if the kidneys become damaged as a result of retention or infection of urine, and sometimes this is complicated by the existence of structural abnormalities to the renal tract. Urinary infection may occur in children with a flaccid bladder, since a small reservoir of urine is almost constantly present, but is even more likely to occur in children with the retentive type of bladder because it is normally full of urine and urine will also be present even after evacuation. The main danger with this type of bladder is the risk of infection to the upper urinary tract. This can result from any recurrent bladder infection but particularly if the ureters and kidneys fill up due to back pressure. If this process of 'ureteric reflux' is not halted the ureters will become grossly enlarged and lose their shape and elasticity and the kidneys may be progressively damaged so that their filtering mechanisms are impaired and waste products, instead of being filtered out, circulate through the body.

For all children with myelomeningocele early and regular monitoring of the kidneys and bladder is a very important part of the management programme. The state of each child's urinary tract will be kept under regular surveillance by means of a number of investigations, the most important of which is the IVP (the intravenous pyelogram). This will be given periodically from birth and is a method whereby the kidneys and ureters can be X-rayed, to check for reflux, hydronephrosis or any other damage to the upper renal tract. The child may also be investigated by cystoscopy to determine the state of the bladder and what ability it has to retain or evacuate urine. At very frequent intervals, at least every three months, the child's urine will be checked for bacteria, and any sign of infection in the child will be treated seriously and for a prolonged period with the appropriate antibiotics. Prevention is aided if the child has a large fluid intake at frequent intervals (particularly when feverish and in hot weather) thus ensuring a good flow of water through the kidneys. For some children the only answer to persistent infection may be surgery in the form of a urinary diversion which is discussed in the next section.

Management of incontinence

The method by which the child is kept dry will differ from one individual to another but three main aspects of this question can be distinguished, (i) manual expression of the urine and social training, (ii) the use of urinary appliances (without surgery) and (iii) urinary diversion procedures.

Manual expression and social training. In the case of many, although not all incontinent children, the mother will be taught how to 'express' the urine from the bladder at regular intervals by placing one or both hands on the lower part of the abdomen below the navel, and applying increasingly firm pressure in a downward and backward direction. (Forrest, 1976, states that about 40 per cent of spina bifida children have expressible bladders.) Later some children will be able to learn how to do this for themselves although initially they may need the assistance of the school nurse or welfare assistant. The frequency of bladder expression should be regulated by observing how long the child can stay dry, although the interval between expression should never be more than three hours for fear of infection (Forrest, 1976). About 30 per cent of more of children can reach an acceptable degree of continence in this way by the age of four or five years (Forrest, 1974; Nergardh *et al.*, 1974) although, as Forrest (1976) points out, many children who have achieved some control by the age of 5 years may relapse when faced by the demands of school life. In such cases mothers 'must resist the temptation to reduce fluid intake in an attempt to keep the child dry'.

Penile urinals. Probably fewer than half of spina bifida children can be taught to manage their incontinence problems satisfactorily by conservative training methods including bladder expression, and most will have to use some sort of urine collecting appliance. Urinary incontinence in most boys can be satisfactorily overcome by the use of a suitably designed flexible sheath (urinal) fitted over the penis and draining into a plastic bag which is usually strapped to the thigh. If properly managed and emptied frequently the boy can be kept dry and need wear no nappies. Generally, while a boy is wearing a urinal, it is important that he continues to express his bladder once or twice a day to reduce the residual urine and minimize the risk of urinary infection (Smith, 1965). One difficulty commonly encountered with urinals is night leakage which can usually be prevented by the use of a special additional night bag. Also, although a urinal is simple to clean the child may neglect to do this so that the urinal becomes smelly (the bags are plastic and disposable). It may also be difficult to fit a urinal on a child who is wearing cumbersome orthopaedic appliances.

Female incontinence and catheterization. For girls the problem is more difficult since there is no comparable form of external apparatus which will keep the child dry. The most common alternatives are incontinence pads and protective rubber pants or a urinary diversion, an operation to by-pass the bladder, neither solution being entirely satisfactory. It is possible to insert a catheter into the urethra connected to a collecting bag which may be strapped to the upper leg. This is often used for short periods, for example during hip operations, but until recently was never considered as a long-term measure because of the risk of infection. With the advent of non-irritating plastics it has been tried successfully for long periods with some patients and is particularly useful in cases where trunk deformities make the application of an abdominal appliance difficult, or where there is parental objection to urinary diversion. However assistance is always required in changing the catheter, so full independence can never be achieved by this method.

Urinary diversions. The age at which a diversion is carried out varies considerably but it will never be done until it has been established that control of the bladder will not be achieved naturally. If it is done early it is because renal damage makes it imperative to operate quickly and the operation may also be carried out for boys if there is a danger of damage to the kidneys. Unless there are urgent medical reasons for the operation, surgeons may prefer to wait until the child is old enough to understand the advantages of the operation and it is certainly advisable to wait until the parents are fully convinced of its necessity.

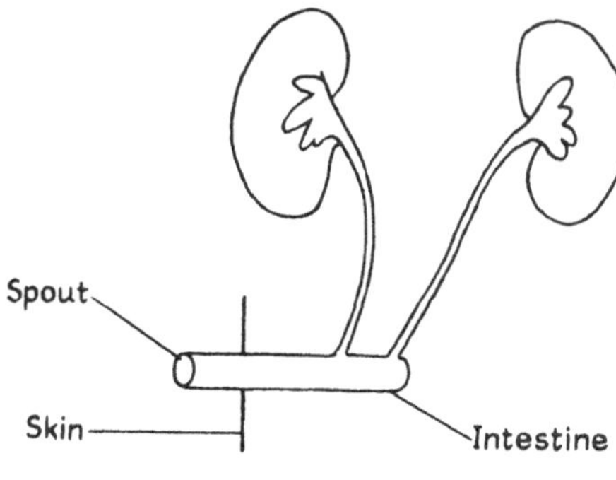

Figure 1.5 *Ileostomy spout* (From Lorber, 1974)

There are two main types of by-pass operations with many variations to suit the individual (reviewed by Eckstein, 1965) but essentially the aim is to by-pass the bladder so that the urine is brought to the surface of the abdomen. If the ureters are very dilated they may be joined together to form a spout which is brought to the surface at a point on the abdomen, or in some cases two openings are made on the abdomen, one on each side. The exact position of the spout depends, among other things, on where a collecting bag can be fitted most easily. This operation is called a ureterostomy. More commonly an ileostomy is performed in which the ureters are separated from the bladder and implanted into a spout made from a piece of ileum, or small intestine which has previously been detached (Fig. 1.5). The spout or 'stoma' is brought out onto the surface of the abdomen so that a collecting device (a rubber or preferably a plastic bag can be fitted over it (Plates 2 and 3)).

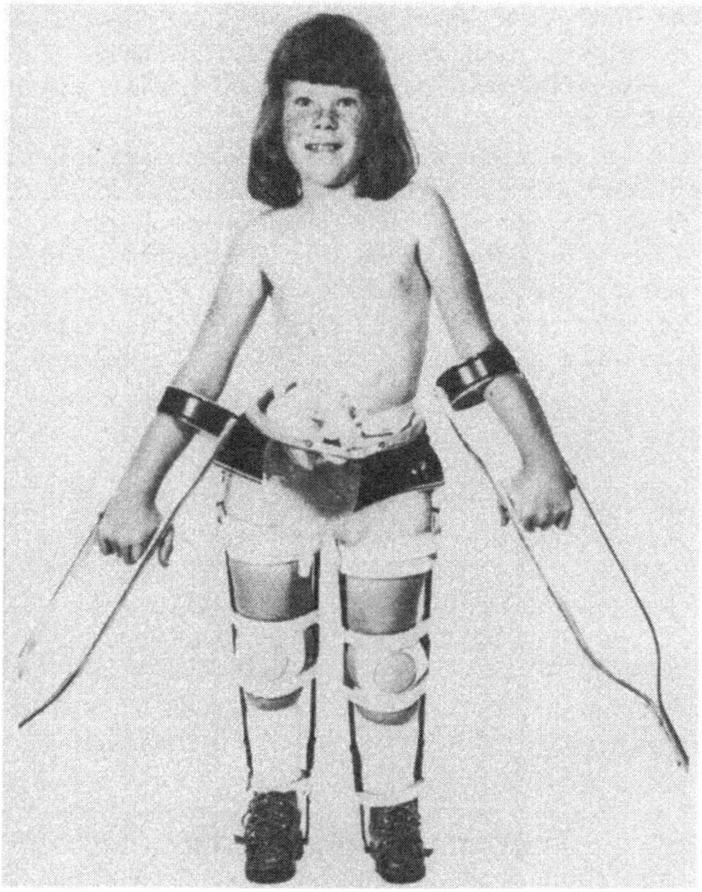

These operations are not without complications and the 'stoma' may become infected or need to be revised. There may also be difficulty in fitting the bag, particularly to a sensitive skin. However, the great majority of children on whom one of these operations has been carried out seem to find it a more satisfactory and reliable way of controlling incontinence and, in the case of the girls, one which gives them greater social freedom and confidence than reliance upon incontinence pads. The child can wear normal clothing and the bag is not visible (Plate 3).

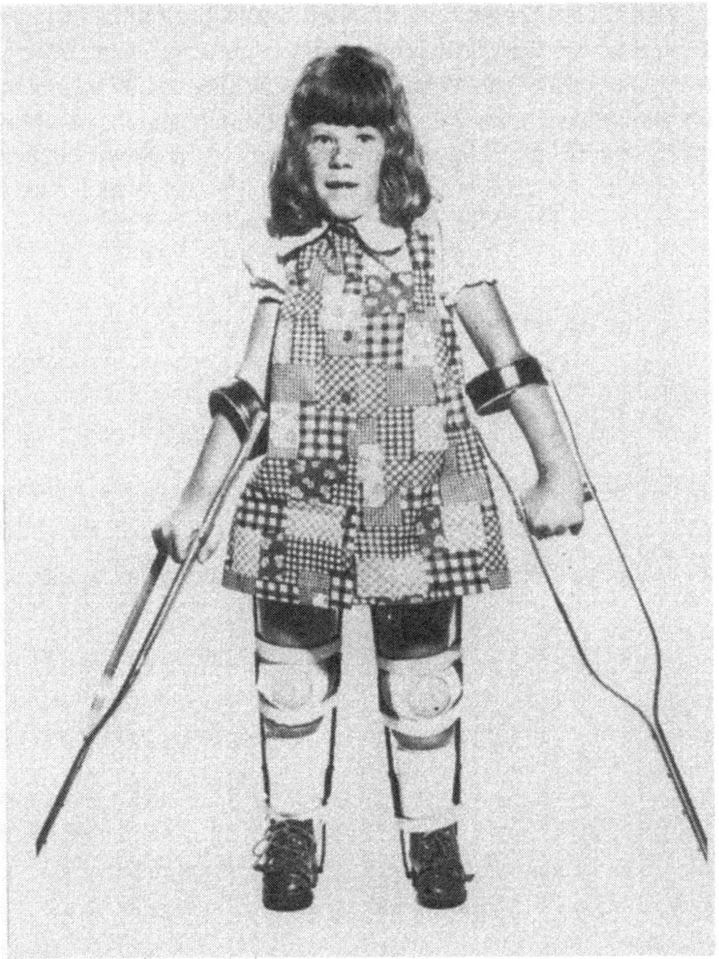

Details of the management of the spout and the use of the appliances for parents and teachers, together with details of appliances to use at night and for swimming are given by Lorber (1974). The child will need to be taught early to empty the appliance himself and will need time, space and privacy. Children in the normal range of intelligence should be able to do this by 7 years of age and often earlier and by the mid-teens the child should be completely independent (unless there are complications). Independence involves being able to empty the bag during the day, fit a larger night bag to the bag's outlet at night, and change the bag every two or three days (but not longer, since infection builds up,

Forrest, 1976)) and see to skin care. Children should also learn to drink plenty of fluids to keep the appliance well washed through.

As Lorber (1974) points out, although a well-functioning loop confers great social advantages, especially to girls, it does not solve all the problems and may create some which did not exist before. What is essential is that parents and children, if they are old enough, should have the chance to discuss very fully the pros and cons of the operation with the doctor before any decision is taken since once the ureters have been detached from the bladder the process cannot be reversed.

Bowel incontinence

Children with deficient nerve supply to the bladder will almost certainly have the same kind of deficiency of the lower bowel and are unlikely to have control over the external opening of the anus. The child may not appreciate that his rectum is full and cannot voluntarily open his lower bowel.

Fortunately infections of the bowel are not common in spina bifida children and the problem is much more a social one. Chronic constipation is very common: a minor degree of constipation does not matter as it prevents frequent soiling but occasionally severe constipation may occur with the result that the child's rectum cannot be evacuated without the help of enemas, manual removal or in extreme cases, washouts. Sometimes diarrhorea with soiling may occur, but this is rare. However, the absence of anal sphincter control may result in constant soiling which is exceedingly difficult to deal with.

It is important to try to establish a regular bowel habit from infancy and usually some kind of routine can be arrived at by which the child becomes socially continent. Many children can learn to develop an automatic evacuation of the bowel, once a day, with the help of the normal bowel action higher up which evacuates the paralysed lower bowel, but it may take several years to achieve this. Alternatively, the child may require regular treatment with medicine or suppositories in which case it may take time to discover the most effective routine, useful suggestions about this being given by Barbara Webster in the March/April 1975 issue of *Link* (the magazine of ASBAH). In either case parents need much more support than they usually get at present since a great deal of persistence is required from them to achieve an adequate regime.

Various methods of bowel training are in use in different centres: Forsythe and Kinley (1970) for example use the method which is routine practice at the Bellevue Hospital, New York, where the emphasis is on the establishment of a regular bowel evacuation after the evening meal with regular supervision until normal bowel habits are established. They point out that with careful management all children with spina bifida should eventually be able to obtain satisfactory bowel control and discuss how regular bowel habits were established in a group of children in a special school. Whatever the method of training is used it is important that it should be reliable, simple, should allow the child to become independent of adults as soon as possible and should not cause emotional disturbance which routine manual evacuation or frequent enemas is liable to do.

Research into other methods of treatment for children with severe problems includes the use of internal electrical stimulation of the rectum (e.g. Katona and Eckstein, 1974); preliminary trials suggest that this method 'may be of great benefit in the achievement of bowel function by children with paraplegia'.

The main factor in achieving effective bowel control is a systematic, planned approach. This requires patience and persistence, and discussion with other parents, both those who are experiencing similar problems and those who have successfully overcome them, can be most helpful. Behaviour modification techniques also could be used in the management of bowel incontinence as well as to help children develop routines of care for their urinary appliances. Extremely useful advice about incontinence management can be obtained from Advisory Services run by Down Brothers and Salt & Son (see Appendix G). These services are staffed by sympathetic qualified nurses who will visit the home and school and give advice on the management of appliances whatever the make, and on a wide range of technical and social problems.

Sexual functioning

It is well known that sexual functioning is likely to be affected in paraplegia but little is firmly established about precisely what functions are maintained with differing lesions in spina bifida.

The major problems for the paraplegic woman are, first, whether she is technically capable of intercourse and, second, what pregnancy will mean to her. There have been several studies of paraplegic women (reported, for example, by Talbot, 1955; Guttman, 1963; Fitzpatrick, 1974) which suggests that in paraplegics, and this includes even heavily handicapped spina bifida women, fertility seems relatively undisturbed. Fitzpatrick's conclusion after reviewing most existing studies is that 'despite increased risks of urinary tract infection, premature or abrupt delivery and anemia . . . pregnancies usually resulted in vaginal deliveries of healthy children . . . . Women with complete lesions were anorganismic but were sexually aroused by tactile stimuli above the level of the lesion'. (Loss of genital sensation will depend on the extent of the lesion.)

Although most of the women in the studies reviewed by Fitzpatrick became paraplegic as the result of an accident there is no doubt that women with paraplegia resulting from spina bifida can bear healthy children. For example Carter and Evans (1973) traced a consecutive series of 115 female patients with spina bifida who had attended Great Ormond Street or St Bartholomew's Hospital before 1954. Of the 115 women patients 38 had had children. Fifteen of those having children were severely neurologically disabled, 4 being confined to wheelchairs (one of these women was doubly incontinent and 2 had ileostomies) and all but one of the others had severe or moderately severe walking difficulties and in some cases incontinence as well. The question of genetic counselling is discussed in chapter 2 but Carter and Evans (1973) have estimated that the risk to a spina bifida parent of either sex (who is married to a partner not having spina bifida) of producing a child with neural tube malformations is about 1 in 30.

With spina bifida men it is not possible to generalize about sexual potential as this differs from one individual to another depending in particular upon the level and completeness of the lesion. Since the neuroanatomy and neurophysiology underlying erection and ejaculation differ, these functions have to be considered separately.

Fitzpatrick (1974) points out that since erection is regulated both reflexively and psychologically it is 'not vulnerable to trauma in a single segment'. Talbot (1955) reporting on two large studies of over 400 paraplegic men found that 'the closer the injury is to the lumbosacral reflex centres and the greater the consequent risk of their involvement, the more likelihood there is for interference with erection', and he goes on to point out as do Griffith and his colleagues (1973) that erection is more likely to be obtained in patients with upper motor neuron lesions than with lower motor neuron lesions, regardless of whether the lesion is complete or incomplete.

Ejaculation is much less often achieved by paraplegic men (and this includes those with spina bifida) than is erection. This is because it is a much more complex mechanism than erection and therefore much more vulnerable to trauma, as also is orgasm which is mediated through pathways similar to those in ejaculation. In a review of studies of paraplegic men Talbot (1955) concludes that overall, only between 3 per cent and 20 per cent are likely to obtain ejaculations and an even smaller proportion orgasms.

Comparatively few men with spinal cord damage are likely to be able to father children but it must again be stressed that this depends largely on the level of the lesion. In the Carter and Evans (1973) follow-up study of patients with spina bifida, 14 of the 100 of the male survivors in a consecutive series had had children. The authors note however, that some of the men in the study were impotent and others were 'almost certainly sterile'.

Hydrocephalus

Introduction

Approximately four in every five babies born with myelomeningocele are also likely to have hydrocephalus, although of course hydrocephalus is also found in children without spina bifida. The term literally means 'water on the brain' and refers to a group of conditions in which, for various reasons, an excess of cerebrospinal fluid (CSF) builds up within the brain. In this section we describe, first, the normal circulation of the CSF in the brain, second, the causes of hydrocephalus and the different types which may occur, third, the effects of hydrocephalus on the functioning of the central nervous system and, finally, its treatment. The location of the structures of the brain referred to in the following section are shown in Fig. 1.6 below.

The normal ventricular system and circulation of the CSF

As we described earlier the central nervous system in man (that is the brain and spinal cord) develops as a hollow tubular structure from which the cerebral hemispheres arise. As the brain develops the hollow cavity of the neural tube extends into it to form a series of narrow spaces deep within the brain called the cerebral ventricles. The CSF, a clear, water-like fluid is continually being formed within the ventricles, one function being to help to protect the brain from outside shocks. Normally the fluid flows from one ventricle to another through narrow connecting channels, then after leaving the ventricles the CSF passes into the subarachnoid space, this being the cavity lying between the innermost two of the three membranes (the meninges) which enclose and protect the brain. The same fluid also passes down into the spinal canal to cover and protect the spinal cord. The fluid within the subarachnoid space is constantly being absorbed into the blood stream and thus the cerebrospinal fluid is in constant circulation.

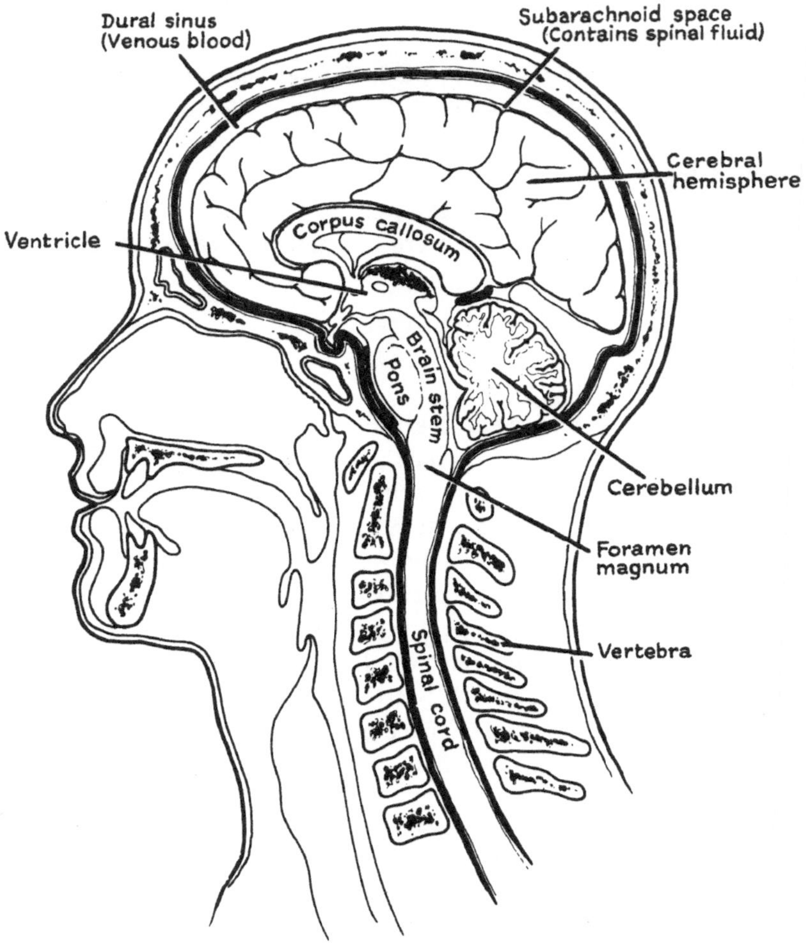

Figure 1.6 *Cross section of the head and neck showing the major portions of the brain, brain stem and spinal cord.* (Adapted from Bleck, E. and Nagel, D. A., 1975).

The causes of hydrocephalus

Hydrocephalus occurs when abnormal amounts of CSF collect in the brain. This may be caused by overproduction of CSF or, more commonly, by an obstruction to the normal circulation of the fluid. This obstruction may be congenital or it may be acquired, that is result from a disorder arising after birth such as meningitis.

If the baby's hydrocephalus is untreated his head will grow rapidly because the pressure inside it is high. The fontanelle (that part of the head where the bones of the skull join together) will usually be larger than normal because of the increased tension and if the pressure is not reduced will remain open for much longer than normal. In advanced cases, if left untreated, the baby's eyeballs may become depressed, he will develop a marked squint, and his face will look small compared to his large head. In a young baby the bones of the cranium are still soft, and can expand to accommodate the increased volume of CSF, without necessarily causing much damage to the brain itself. Once the child gets older, and the bones are set, increased pressure then inevitably causes pressure upon and damage to brain tissue.

If the hydrocephalus is very severe a diagnosis of hydrocephalus will be easy to make. In other cases a variety of means of diagnosis will be used. One important measure is the rate of head growth. The baby's head is measured with a tape at birth and at regular intervals afterwards. Charts are available to show the normal rate of growth of an infant's head and the rate of growth in the child with suspected hydrocephalus is compared with the rate of growth appropriate to a baby of a similar age and weight. In Fig. 1.7 (from Lorber, 1974) the growth rate of the head in a child with spina bifida is shown, before and after operations. Another diagnostic investigation which is very commonly carried out is the ventriculogram, a method of X-raying the head so that the ventricles clearly show up and any enlargement of these can be seen.

The effects of hydrocephalus

The symptoms shown by a child with hydrocephalus will depend mainly upon the severity of the hydrocephalus and whether and how early he was treated.

Not every child with hydrocephalus requires surgical treatment. In milder cases of hydrocephalus associated with spina bifida the disorder may not be progressive: the amount of cerebrospinal fluid formed becomes balanced with the amount which is absorbed and the child's head stops growing at an abnormal rate. In this case the child is said to have 'arrested hydrocephalus' which has been defined (Milhorat, 1972) as 'a state of chronic hydrocephalus in which the cerebrospinal pressure has returned to normal'. Children whose symptoms of hydrocephalus have been mild, and whose hydrocephalus has arrested spontaneously early on are unlikely to suffer any marked adverse effects as a result of their hydrocephalus. Their heads will be of normal size and their intelligence should be relatively unimpaired, compared with children requiring shunts (see chapter 5).

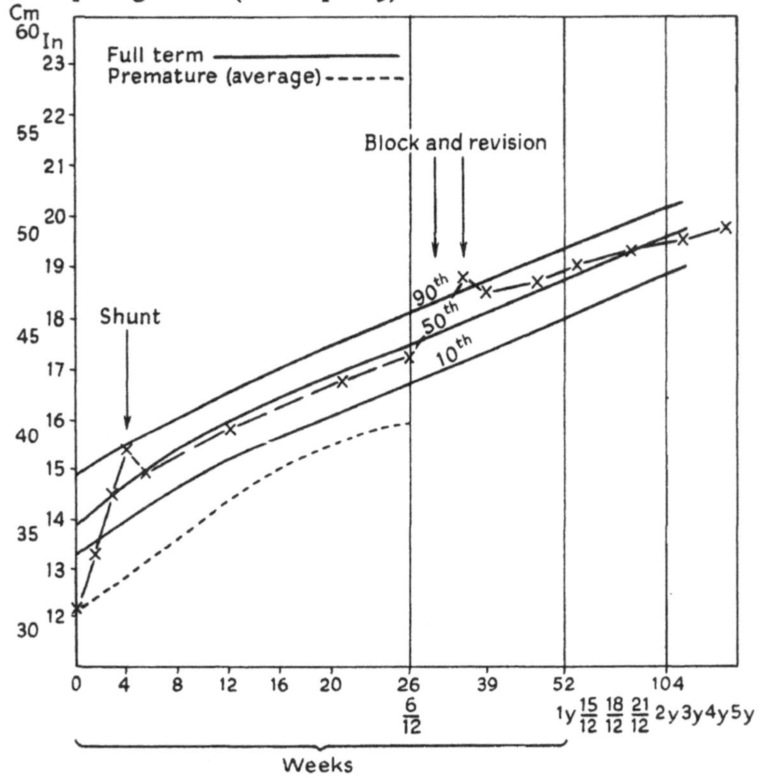

Figure 1.7 *Head circumference chart in an infant with spina bifida and hydrocephalus.*

The top continuous line shows the size and pattern of growth of a big baby's head, the middle line that of an average baby, and the bottom one that of a small baby. The lowest, dotted line represents the growth of a premature baby's head. The heavily drawn dotted line shows the infant's head circumference in an affected baby. The rapid growth is arrested by operation. Later the shunt becomes blocked and the head grows too fast again until the shunt is revised.
(From Lorber, 1973)

If the hydrocephalus is severe but is not treated, as was the case in this country before about 1958, marked symptoms are likely to develop in surviving children. By about 3 months old the child's head will be so large and heavy that he will be unable to lift it. There is likely to be damage to areas of the brain which play a major part in the control of movements of both the upper and lower limbs so that eventually the child may become entirely wheelchair-bound as a result of the hydrocephalus alone. Ocular defects are very common in untreated hydrocephalus and if nothing is done to relieve the pressure of the CSF progressive loss of sight may occur. The child may also become increasingly subject to fits and is likely to suffer from a considerable degree of intellectual retardation. If the hydrocephalus continues to progress unchecked and pressure is exerted on the life-controlling lower brain mechanisms, then death will occur.

Fortunately, the availability of modern methods of early treatment means that hydrocephalus no longer results in the gross and often progressive disorders described above. Although it is the case that a child with severe hydrocephalus will, even after treatment, probably have physical and intellectual problems which a child without hydrocephalus is much less likely to have, these are very much less severe than they would have been had the child not been treated.

What sorts of problems are children with treated hydrocephalus likely to have? Squinting is common and its incidence in spina bifida children has been discussed in some detail by Stanworth (1970) and by Clements and Kaushal (1970). The latter note that the majority of children with myelomeningocele will have ocular complications, the principal abnormality being strabismus (squint) of the convergent type. Hydrocephalus may also affect motor control in both the upper and lower limbs. There may be some weakness in the arms and some impairment of manual dexterity (see also p. 41) and as already noted the child's balance may be poor. Another effect of hydrocephalus is that the corpus callosum (one of the bundles of fibres linking the left and right side of the brain) is often stretched and thinned (Russell, 1949; Crome and Stern, 1967; Milhorat, 1972). Although little research has been done in this area there is some evidence (e.g. Miller and Sethi, 1971) that this affects the efficiency with which the corpus callosum can transfer information of many kinds from one hemisphere to another. A final very important point is that hydrocephalus of a moderate or severe degree is likely (although this does not always happen) to result in some impairment of intelligence, this whole question being fully discussed in chapter 5.

The amount of brain damage suffered by spina bifida children with hydrocephalus is likely to be less, however, than for children who develop hydrocephalus post-natally from other causes, because surgical intervention with spina bifida is normally quite prompt. Since it is known that children with myelomeningocele are very likely to develop hydrocephalus following the closure of the back, the child is normally kept in hospital for two or three weeks following closure and is kept under constant observation so that a shunt can be inserted as soon as this is considered necessary. With hydrocephalus from other causes the onset may be both gradual and less well expected and considerable damage to brain tissue may have occurred before surgery is performed.

The treatment of hydrocephalus

Whether and when surgical treatment is given depends on many circumstances, especially on the degree of hydrocephalus, the rate of its progression and the presence or absence of infection.

Where the hydrocephalus is actively and rapidly progressive, surgery will usually be necessary, the hydrocephalus being treated by one of a variety of 'shunting' procedures. These procedures are all devised (a) to reduce the abnormally high pressure of the CSF to a normal level, and (b) to keep it at a normal level. The most commonly used procedure is one in which the excess CSF is 'shunted' from one of the ventricles into either the heart (referred to as a ventriculo-vascular, ventriculo-venous or ventriculo-atrial shunt), or into the peritoneal cavity in the abdomen (ventriculo-peritoneal shunt) or, less commonly, into other body cavities. The principle involved is to drain the excess CSF away into the blood stream either directly via the heart or indirectly by absorption from the peritoneum. This is quite a satisfactory method of drainage and indeed mimics the normal process by which CSF is absorbed into the blood. Two commonly used shunt systems are the Spitz-Holter uni-directional valve, introduced in 1952 although it was not used on a large scale till the late 1950s, and the Pudenz valve, developed at about the same time. Although there are other shunt systems the Holter and the Pudenz shunts are the ones most widely used in this country. (The terms 'valve' and 'shunt' are commonly used interchangeably and we have followed this practice, although technically speaking the term shunt refers to the whole pumping system and the valve only to the valve part of the system (Fig. 1.8b).) The components of the Holter shunting system are shown in Figs 1.8a and 1.8b below.

The Holter shunting system comprises a silicone catheter (the proximal catheter) which enters the cerebral ventricle and is attached to two uni-directional valves connected by a compressible plastic tube. The latter is attached in turn to the distal (lower) catheter, leading to the heart or the peritoneal cavity. In the case of the more common ventriculo-atrial shunt (Fig. 1.8a and b above) the valve section of the system is placed under the skin, usually behind the right ear. Normally this chamber is soft and full of fluid; if it is compressed with the finger it will empty and on release can be felt to refill quickly. The distal catheter enters the jugular vein in the neck and is threaded through it into the

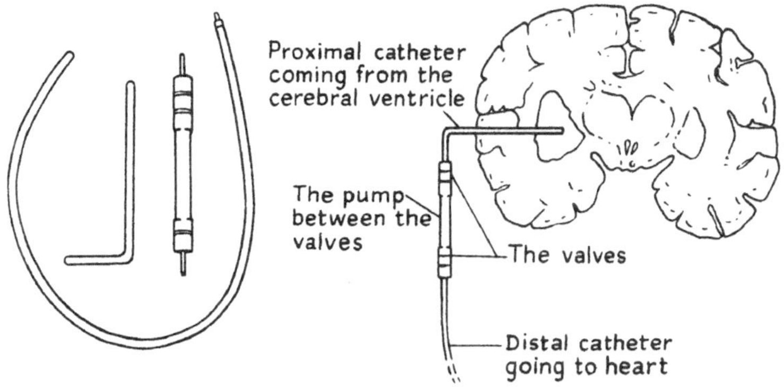

(a) Components of the Holter shunting system

(b) How the Holter shunting system works

Figure 1.8 *The Holter shunting system,* (From Lorber, 1973).

heart. In the case of the ventriculo-peritoneal shunt a much longer plastic tube is used, which is threaded under the skin of the chest wall and into the peritoneal cavity of the abdomen. The time at which the shunt is inserted varies somewhat, there being some difference of opinion about the best time to operate, but generally it is done within twenty-one days after birth.

The immediate result of the shunt operation is that the pressure in the baby's head will decrease a little at once and then the head will continue to grow but at a slower rate than usual. If the operation was carried out before the child's head was much larger than normal then in about a year or two it will be of normal size; if it was already abnormally large then it may be some years before the child's body and head are in proportion to each other. As the child grows it is frequently, although not always, necessary to replace the original distal catheter leading to the heart with a longer one and X-rays will show whether this is required. For many children this lengthening operation will only be needed once, though some may need it done twice, or, rarely, more often. The valve itself will remain permanently unless it needs replacing because it becomes blocked or infected. These surgical treatments are not without some risks and complications which will be explained more fully in the next section.

There are some drug treatments available which increase the absorption rate of CSF and control the hydrocephalus in this way (e.g. Lorber, 1972) but they are not as yet satisfactory for long-term treatment. They are useful if a shunt cannot be inserted or replaced temporarily due to infection and may also be used initially in mild cases to tide the child over, in the hope that self-arrest may occur. Possibly in the future drug treatment to reduce the formation of CSF or to increase its absorption rate may become feasible for long-term use.

Complications of shunting procedures

Any serious complications in the valve system leading to malfunctioning may threaten life and permanently impair intellectual functioning and should always be treated as a matter of urgency. If the child has symptoms of any kind which persist these should be checked with the hospital. If in doubt it is much better to be over-cautious, and the hospital staff will never consider it a waste of time to check a possible fault in the shunt system.

The four most common complications are (i) obstruction of the catheter due to growth, (ii) blocked shunts, (iii) infections of the shunt system, and (iv) disconnected shunts. The first of these may arise if, as the child grows, the lower end of the tube is retracted from its position in the right atrium of the heart, this usually being followed within a short period of time by non-function of the shunt system. The distal catheter then has to be taken out for lengthening. A check is normally kept of the position of the catheter within the heart and if it seems necessary the catheter is lengthened before any symptoms occur.

The second complication, blockage of the proximal catheter, may occur for a variety of reasons, for example the end of the tube which is within the ventricles may be obstructed by brain tissue. In such a case the pressure inside the head increases rapidly giving rise to severe headaches, vomiting and drowsiness. The child may have a fit, and become unconscious. Urgent treatment has to be given. If the proximal catheter is blocked then the pump between the valves may not refill when compressed or may take a long time to do so. The fact that the pump fills very slowly does not necessarily mean that the shunt is completely blocked. If the child is otherwise in normal health it probably means simply that the pressure inside the child's head is now normal or near normal so that the valve only needs to open occasionally to let a little fluid through. However, if the child also shows the symptoms described earlier he must be taken to his usual hospital at once. (It is not advisable to depress the pump unless the child is showing symptoms, however, and even then it should only be done by someone given instructions in how to do it.) If the blockage is in the distal catheter, then the pump will be full of fluid; it will feel tense and cannot be compressed. In this case, whether or not the child appears to be ill, medical help should be sought immediately.

Third, infection of the shunt system is a major complication, and has been estimated to occur in about 10 per cent of cases (Brocklehurst, 1976). Infection may develop within days of the operation or after several years of successful shunt function. In some cases the symptoms are severe, with fever, night sweating and vomiting. In others the illness is more gradual and the child may have feverish bouts, listlessness, irritability, progressive anaemia and a poor appetite. Sometimes antibiotics will eradicate the infection but more often the infected shunt has to be completely removed and replaced.

Finally, the shunt system may become disconnected, i.e. the proximal or distal catheters may become disconnected from the metal casings of the valves. Indications of shunt disconnection include the appearance of a lump behind the ear along the line of the shunt or of a lump below the valve, or of a swelling along the length of the tube at any point. In all such cases medical help should be sought immediately since revision may be required.

People often ask whether a child with a shunt will require this for the rest of his life. At present this is simply not known but the general opinion is that although the shunt may not appear to be in operation (i.e. the pump feels flat and the child is in good health) it may still be draining a small amount of CSF from the ventricles. Also a finely balanced equilibrium of production and absorption of the CSF may have developed over the years which removal of the shunt would disturb. For these reasons a shunt is not usually removed even though the child or young adult appears no longer to need one.

The Arnold-Chiari malformation

In most accounts of myelomeningocele the main emphasis is rightly placed upon such major problems as lower limb paralysis, incontinence and hydrocephalus. It is less well known that most if not all children with spina bifida myelomeningocele and hydrocephalus are born with an abnormality of the cerebellum (that part of the brain concerned in particular with the control of movement) and of other nearby lower brain-stem structures called the Arnold-Chiari malformation (see Fig. 1.6, p. 32).

The most striking feature of the malformation is that a tongue of tissue derived usually from the lower lobes of the cerebellum extends downwards through the foramen magnum (the opening at the upper end of the spinal canal) into the upper spinal canal. Other lower brain-stem structures are also elongated and displaced downwards. Recent work by Variend and Emery (1973, 1974) shows that the cerebellum is generally smaller and lighter in weight than normal and also that some of the tissues of the cerebellum are damaged or displaced. However, the parts of the cerebellum which have not been damaged are capable of normal growth, this being most rapid during the first two years of life, in particular during the first twelve months.

The question of the causation of the Arnold-Chiari malformation and its relationship to hydrocephalus is still a controversial one: what is more important is to consider how it may affect the child's functioning. Here the most crucial point is the part played by the cerebellum in the control of movement. It has been known for a long time that three inter-connected parts of the brain – the motor cortex, the basal ganglia and the cerebellum – act together to control movement. Until recently the role of the cerebellum was thought to be only of secondary importance: it was believed that its main role was to modify the timing of movements so that they were smooth and effective, but not to initiate them. Although the exact nature of cerebellar control is still unclear recent research quoted by Evarts and his colleagues (1971, 1973) suggests that the cerebellum is probably involved in the planning and initiating of the precise and rapid movements characteristic of the extremities, especially the arm and hand.

Damage to the cerebellum in man is known to produce (depending on the parts damaged) (a) dizziness and poor balance and (b) disturbance of voluntary movements, and errors in the direction, force and rate of movements, the latter generally being referred to as 'cerebellar ataxia' (Mackenzie, 1963). The sorts of difficulties associated with cerebellar damage noted by Dow (1969) include muscle weakness in the arms, delay in starting and stopping a movement and tremor. Cerebellar damage is usually diagnosed by means of neurological testing. The effects on function are often not obvious, and as Schutt (1963) points out 'often only detectable in finer skills such as writing'.

Since most children with myelomeningocele are born with the Arnold-Chiari malformation it is surprising that so little research has been done into the functioning of their upper limbs, a question discussed further in chapter 5 where some of our own findings on hand function are presented. One exception was a study carried out by Wallace (1973) who examined neurological functioning in the upper limbs of 225 unselected children with myelomeningocele who were at least one year old. Upper limb dysfunction was found in a total of 156 children (69 per cent), including 122 (81 per cent) of the children with hydrocephalus and 34 (45 per cent) of those with myelomeningocele, but no signs of hydrocephalus. The predominant disorders were either cerebellar ataxia or mixed cerebellar ataxia and pyramidal tract dysfunction.

It seems unlikely that disorders of movement are the only functional problems arising from the Arnold-Chiari malformation. Recent research suggests that the lower brain-stem structures which are affected by the malformation play a more important part than perhaps has been hitherto realized in the processing of visual, auditory and other kinds of input (e.g. Gordon, 1972) as well as in integrating simultaneous input (Ayres, 1975) from a variety of sensory modalities (e.g. vision, touch and sound). However, the main point to be stressed here is that this malformation is present in children with spina bifida myelomeningocele and hydrocephalus and that it is likely to lead, at least in many cases, to some impairment in a child's ability to carry out rapid and skilful actions with his hands. Practice, however, through the right kinds of play, can help considerably and in chapter 6 suggestions are made about what parents and others can do to help their children with this and other problems during the pre-school years.

Hospital admissions

The information presented in this chapter must make it clear that children with myelomeningocele spend a great deal of time as hospital in-patients in their early years. In the Sheffield study of children aged 4 years it was found that the average number of admissions per child was six (Freeston, 1971). In contrast, only 20 per cent of children aged 5 years in a national population sample (Douglas and Blomfield, 1958) were found ever to have been admitted to hospital and even for this group the average number of admissions was only 1·6. In Margaret Woodburn's study (1973) of children aged between 18 months and 17 years one quarter had been admitted to hospital between 8 and 15 times and nearly 7 per cent 16 or more times. In 28 per cent of cases admissions 'were too many to count'. Particularly in the pre-school years, therefore, but during the school years also, children are likely to spend quite long periods in hospital, for major or minor surgery, for investigations, or for the treatment of infections to the urinary tract or shunt system.

The children's reactions to admission vary and depend partly on parental reactions, partly on the amount of time the mother can spend at the hospital and partly on the child's familiarity with the hospital. For both children and parents frequent experience of hospital usually results in a reduction of apprehension and adverse reactions. On most children's wards visiting hours are now unrestricted, with facilities for mothers to live in if they so wish, but there are some units where strict visiting hours still apply and this causes great distress to both the child and the parents. Where the hospital is a great distance away from the child's home, which is often the case outside London, mothers are unable to visit frequently or for long periods even if unrestricted visiting is allowed. One in three children in Freeston's study (1971) were said to react unfavourably on returning home from hospital. However, severe reactions to admission seem rare, possibly because most often surgical procedures are carried out on parts of the body with little feeling and, in addition, the hospital is usually a familiar place. The impression gained from the GLC study was that admission was far more distressing to the rest of the family than it was to the child unless he was actually feeling ill, or the mother was unable to visit regularly, provided that the admission had been fully explained to him beforehand. Although there were some complaints about the children's treatment as in-patients, such as some children developing pressure sores or burns or being given food they disliked to eat, most parents were full of praise for the medical and particularly the nursing staff for their patience and understanding. However, parents often find it hard to get a satisfactory explanation of the child's treatment and have trouble in 'contacting staff who could or would give them information' (Woodburn, 1974).

References

Allum, N. (1975), *Spina Bifida: The Treatment and Care of Spina Bifida Children*, Allen and Unwin, London.

Ayres, A. J. (1975), 'Sensorimotor foundations of academic ability', ch. 8

in Cruickshank, W. P. and Hallahan, D. P. (eds.), *Perceptual and Learning Disabilities in Children,* vol. 2, Syracuse University Press, New York.

Bell, W. E. and McCormick, W. F. (1972), *Increased Intracranial Pressure in Children,* Saunders, Philadelphia.

Bleck, E. E. and Nagel, D. A. (eds.) (1976), *Physically Handicapped Children. A Medical Atlas for Teachers,* Grune and Stratton, New York.

Brocklehurst, G. (1976), 'Assessment and management of hydrocephalus', ch. 8 in Brocklehurst, G. (ed.), *Spina Bifida for the Clinician,* Clinics in Developmental Medicine, 57, Spastics International Medical Publications/Heinemann, London.

Carter, C. O. (1969), 'Spina bifida and anencephaly: a problem in genetic-environmental interaction', *Journal of Biosocial Science,* 1, pp. 71–83.

——, and Evans, K. (1973), 'Children of adult survivors with spina bifida cystica', *Lancet,* ii, pp. 924–6.

Clements, D. B. and Kaushal, K. (1970), 'A study of the ocular complications of hydrocephalus and meningomyelocele', *Transactions of the Opthalmic Society, UK.,* 40, pp. 383–90.

Crome, L. C. and Stern, J. (1967), *The Pathology of Mental Retardation,* Churchill, London.

Douglas, J. W. B. and Blomfield, J. M. (1958), *Children Under Five,* Allen and Unwin, London.

Dow, R. S. (1969), 'Cerebellar syndrome', ch. 15 in Vinken, P. J. and Bruyn, G. W. (eds.), *Handbook of Clinical Neurology Vol. 2,* North Holland Publishing Co., Amsterdam.

Eckstein, H. B. (1965), 'Urinary diversion in children', *Developmental Medicine and Child Neurology,* 7 (2), pp. 167–74.

——, and Chir, M. (1972), 'The management of the neurogenic bladder in children', *Pädiatrie und Pädologie,* Supplement 2, pp. 110–19.

Emery, J. L. and Lendon, R. G. (1973), 'Local cord lesions in neurospinal disraphism (meningomyelocele)', *Journal of Pathology,* 110, pp. 83–96.

Evarts, E. V. (1973), 'Brain mechanisms in movement', *Scientific American,* 229, pp. 96–103.

——, Bizzi, E., Burke, R. E., Delong, M. and Thach, W. T. (1971), 'Central control of movement', *Neurosciences Research Program Bulletin,* 9 (Whole No. 1).

Finnie, N. (1971), *Handling the Young Cerebral-palsied Child at Home,* Heinemann, London.

Fitzpatrick, W. F. (1974), 'Sexual function in the paraplegic patient', *Archives of Physical Medicine and Rehabilitation,* 55, pp. 221–7.

Forrest, D. (1974), 'The use of the Foley Catheter for long-term urine collection in girls', *Developmental Medicine and Child Neurology*, Supplement 32, p. 54.

——, (1976), 'Management of bladder and bowel in spina bifida', ch. 11 in Brocklehurst, G. (ed.), *Spina Bifida for the Clinician*, Clinics in Developmental Medicine, 57, Spastics International Medical Publications/Heinemann, London.

Forsythe, W. I. and Kinley, J. C. (1970), 'Bowel control of children with spina bifida', *Developmental Medicine and Child Neurology*, 12 (6), pp. 27–31.

Freeston, B. M. (1971), 'An enquiry into the effect of a spina bifida child upon family life', *Developmental Medicine and Child Neurology*, 13, pp. 456–61.

Gabriel, R. W. (1974) 'Malformation of the central nervous system, ch. 4 in Menkes, J. H., *Textbook of Child Neurology*, Lea and Febiger, New York; Henry Kimpton, London.

Gordon, B. (1972), 'The superior colliculus of the brain', *Scientific American*, 227, pp. 72–82.

Griffith, E. R., Tomko, M. A. and Timms, R. J. (1973), 'Sexual functions in spinal cord-injured patients, a review', *Archives of Physical Medicine and Rehabilitation*, 54 (12), pp. 539–43.

Guttman, L. (1963), 'The paraplegic patient in pregnancy and labour', *Proceedings of the Royal Society of Medicine*, 5.

Holgate, L. (1970), *Physiotherapy for Spina Bifida. Early Treatment*, Publ. Queen Mary's Hospital for Children, Carshalton.

Katona, F. and Eckstein, H. B. (1974), 'Treatment of the neuropathic bowel by electrical stimulation of the rectum', *Developmental Medicine and Child Neurology*, 16, pp. 336–9.

Lorber, J. (1971), 'Results of treatment of myelomeningocele', *Developmental Medicine and Child Neurology*, 13 (3), pp. 279–303.

——, (1972), 'The use of isosorbide in the treatment of hydrocephalus', *Developmental Medicine and Child Neurology*, Supplement 27, p. 87.

——, (1973), *Your Child with Hydrocephalus* (Revised edition), Association for Spina Bifida and Hydrocephalus, London.

——, (1974), *Your Child with Spina Bifida* (3rd edition), Association for Spina Bifida and Hydrocephalus, London.

Mackenzie, I. (1963), 'A neurologist's view of cerebellar function', pp. 63–9 in Walsh, G. (ed.), *Cerebellum, Posture and Cerebral Palsy*, Little Club Clinics in Developmental Medicine, 1–8 Spastics Society/Heinemann, London.

Milhorat, T. A. (1972), *Hydrocephalus and the Cerebro-spinal Fluid*, Williams and Wilkins, Baltimore.

Miller, E. and Sethi, L. (1971), 'Tactile matching in children with hydrocephalus', *Neuropaediatrie*, 3, pp. 191–4.

Nergardh, A., Hedenberg, C. von, Hellström, B. and Ericsson, N. O.

(1974), 'Continence training of children with neurogenic bladder dysfunction', *Developmental Medicine and Child Neurology*, 16, p. 47.

Russell, D. S. (1949), *Observations on the Pathology of Hydrocephalus*, MRC Special Report, No. 265, HMSO, London.

Schutt, W. (1963), 'Congenital cerebellar ataxia. A review of 32 cases', in Walsh, G. (ed.), *Cerebellum, Posture and Cerebral Palsy*, Little Club Clinics in Developmental Medicine, 8, pp. 83–90, Spastics Society/Heinemann, London.

Sharrard, W. J. W. (1976), 'General orthopaedic management and operative treatment', ch. 9 in Brocklehurst, G. (ed.), *Spina Bifida for the Clinician*, Clinics in Developmental Medicine, 57, Spastics International Medical Publications/Heinemann, London.

Smith, E. Durham (1965), *Spina Bifida and the Total Care of Spinal Myelomeningocele*, C. C. Thomas, Illinois.

Stanworth, A. (1970), 'Squint in hydrocephalus: an analysis of cases', in *Strabismus 69, Transactions of the Consilium Europaeum Strabismi Studio Deditum*, Henry Kimpton, London.

Talbot, H. (1955), 'The sexual function in paraplegia', *Journal of Urology*, I.

Variend, S. and Emery, J. L. (1973), 'The weight of the cerebellum in children with myelomeningocele', *Developmental Medicine and Child Neurology*, Supplement 29, pp. 77–83.

——, ——, (1974), 'The pathology of the central lobes of the cerebellum in children with myelomeningocele', *Developmental Medicine and Child Neurology*, Supplement 32, pp. 99–106.

Wallace, S. J. (1973), 'The effect of upper limb function on mobility of children with myelomeningocele', *Developmental Medicine and Child* Neurology, Supplement 29, pp. 84–91.

Webster, B. (1974), 'Health matters: bowels', *Link*, 37, pp. 5 and 7 (the magazine of ASBAH).

Wisbeach, A. (1974), 'Disabled child' in *Equipment for the Disabled, no.* 9, publication of National Fund for Research into Crippling Diseases.

Woodburn, M. (1973), *Social Implications of Spina Bifida – a Study in S.E. Scotland,* Eastern Branch Scottish Spina Bifida Association, Edinburgh.

2 Incidence, causation and future trends

Incidence

As Carter (1969) points out, anencephaly and spina bifida, the most common of the neural tube malformations, are in terms of public health 'the most important congenital malformations in Britain, and especially in the north and west of Britain'. Anencephaly is the most common single cause of stillbirth in this country, and spina bifida is the second most common cause of physical handicap in childhood.

The incidence of anencephaly in Britain (i.e. the number of new cases occurring) is about 2 per 1,000 total births, but this does vary slightly over time. Spina bifida occurs more frequently than anencephaly and the incidence is approximately 2·4 per 1,000 births. These figures are very high and in fact the British Isles record some of the highest rates of neural tube malformations in the world, particularly from some parts of Ireland and the west of Great Britain.

There are very striking regional variations in the incidence of both anencephaly and spina bifida. Variations in the regional incidence are known in more detail for anencephaly than for spina bifida and these are shown in Fig. 2.1 below. The pattern of incidence for spina bifida parallels that of anencephaly although it is always more common.

As is shown here the areas of highest incidence are Wales and Scotland and the north-west region, the incidence falling progressively as one moves south and east across Britain, with the lowest incidence in East Anglia and the south-east region. In both the north and south of Ireland the incidence is as high or higher than that in Wales and Scotland (Carter, 1969). Possible reasons for these regional variations are discussed later in this chapter.

Children with anencephaly do not survive. In the case of spina bifida however, there have been very marked changes in the mortality rate over the last fifteen years and until very recently approximately 47 per cent of all those born survived the first year of life, of whom the majority (approximately 87 per cent) are still alive at 6 years. In 1968 Lorber estimated that there were about 4,000 children with spina bifida in England and Wales and approximately 600 survive each year, although this may change in the future.

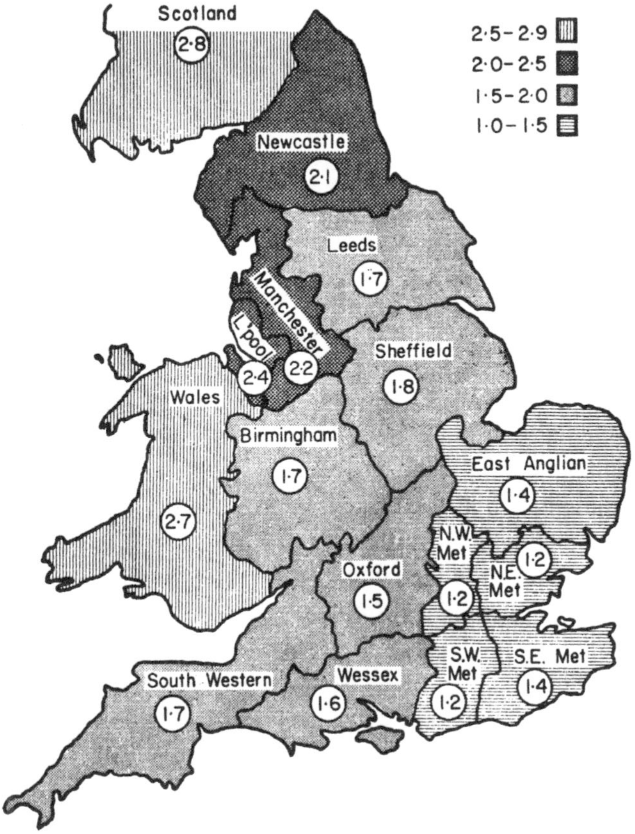

Figure 2.1 *Anencephalic stillbirths by regional hospital areas* 1963–5 (From Carter 1969).

Causation

It needs to be stressed at the outset that the causes of this condition are probably multiple and complex. Many parents will naturally wonder whether they have done anything which might have caused this condition: they can be reassured that there is no evidence whatsoever that illness or injury in pregnancy or the taking of any drug or any one specific item of diet caused the malformation; as Lorber states (1974):

'parents should feel no guilt if they have a baby with spina bifida – they could not possibly help it and they did nothing known to be wrong . . .'.

In discussing possible causes we have drawn heavily from C. O. Carter's essay 'Clues to the aetiology of neural tube malformations' (Carter, 1974) and begin by quoting from his own introduction to the problem. He points out that despite much research we have no more than clues to the aetiology (causation) of the related group of neural tube malformations to which spina bifida belongs.

'We have evidence that genetic predisposition plays some part in their aetiology as do intra-uterine environmental factors. We have indications that it is not a question of some factors being largely genetically and some environmentally determined, but rather that both types of factor play a part in all cases . . . . However, we do not know anything in detail of the mechanisms by which the genetic predisposition acts, nor of the detailed nature of the environmental factors. True prevention of the malformations is likely to be possible only when we have such detailed knowledge' (Carter, 1974).

Genetic factors

Indications for genetic factors being important in the aetiology come from a preponderance in one or other sex; ethnic differences in birth frequency which persist after migration; and family studies.

Sex differences. Evidence for genetic factors is supplied by the high ratio of females to males, especially for anencephaly, most studies showing three girls born for every one boy. For spina bifida the ratio of girls to boys is about 1·3 : 1.

Ethnic variation. There are striking ethnic variations in the incidence of spina bifida and anencephaly. For example there is a high incidence in the UK and in northern India and in northern Egypt; an intermediate frequency in much of Europe; a low frequency in Mongolian people, for example the Japanese, and a very low frequency in Negro peoples. Such differences are of course not necessarily genetic: they could reflect differences in the environment, and it is therefore important to look at the incidence following migration of racial groups to different geographical environment.

The present indications are that in general migrants retain the incidences of the areas from which they originate. This does not necessarily mean that the observed racial differences are genetic: in some cases migrants may have taken certain cultural characteristics, for example diet, with them. However, the Negro population have a low birth-frequency of neural tube malformations wherever they are, whether in West Africa, the United States, the West Indies or in Britain (Leck, 1972). The cultural and geographical environments of these populations are so different that one must assume their relative immunity is due to a genetic factor. However, there are also examples of ethnic groups in which the birth frequency of neural tube malformations changes following migration, which must imply an environmental influence. For example the incidence in Australia is much lower than in Britain even for people of British origin.

Family studies. Most geneticists find studies of twins very valuable in investigating the causation of a condition, by comparing rates for identical (monozygotic) twins, with those for fraternal (dizygotic) twins. Unfortunately, good twin studies are not available for the neural tube malformations for a variety of reasons, but other family studies do offer evidence that genetic factors are important.

The most valuable evidence has come from studies of the incidence of these malformations in the siblings (brothers and sisters) of affected children. The main finding is that the proportion of sibs affected is between 3 and 6 per 100 (i.e. around 1 in 25). This means that the brother or sister of an affected child is between 7 and 15 times more likely to be affected than is an unrelated child. It is a general finding that a child with spina bifida or anencephaly is more likely to have a sib with either type of malformation, suggesting that all neural tube malformations spring from similar causes. Very little good evidence is yet available for those less closely related. However, there is some indication that the risk to cousins is almost twice as high as it is for the general population.

Some evidence is now available about the likelihood of children of affected parents also having neural tube malformations. Data from three different studies quoted by Carter (1974) showed that a total of 106 adults with spina bifida (30 men and 76 women) had had between them 212 children: of these, 7 were affected, 5 by spina bifida and 2 by anencephaly suggesting that the proportion of children affected may be between 3 per cent and 4 per cent, that is about the same risk as for the sibs of affected children. The findings also suggested that affected men were as likely to have children with malformations as were the women.

Carter suggests that the pattern of incidence in families 'fits well with the hypothesis that the aetiology of the condition is multifactorial, depending on a genetic predisposition to develop the malformation which is polygenic (that is, depends on minor additive genetic variations at several gene loci), with a threshold beyond which individuals are at risk of developing the malformation if environmental factors also predispose'. This could mean that the time at which closure of the neural tube occurs (see p. 11) varies somewhat between individuals, but that there may well be some families who are particularly prone (genetically) to later closure. A certain amount of delay is probably tolerable, i.e. does not result in a malformation, but if the delay is too long then a malformation is inevitable. Environmental influences which act on the mother in early life or during the pregnancy may also tend to delay closure, but in this case those families already genetically prone to late closure would be most at risk, since any further delay in this group would tend to result in a malformation.

Environmental factors

Introduction. As we have already pointed out, there is evidence that an ethnic group may change its incidence pattern following migration. Evidence from a number of countries suggests that it is where the mother spent her childhood rather than where she had the pregnancy which is the important factor. For example in Israel the incidence rates of spina bifida and anencephaly are relatively high in the children of immigrants from Iran, Iraq and the Yemen compared with Israelis of East European origin. However these are reduced in the next generation when the parents are born in Israel (Naggan, 1971). The off-spring of couples of Irish stock but born in Boston have relatively high rates compared with rates for other Bostonians, but lower rates than the off-spring of first generation immigrants from Ireland (Naggan and MacMahon, 1967).

The marked difference in the frequency of neural tube malformations within a country such as Britain where there is little ethnic variation also suggests environmental factors (see Fig. 2.1). Although there are some genetic differences between the populations of the north-west and south-east of Britain it is thought unlikely that such differences could account for the large regional variations. So far attempts to find the environmental causes of these regional differences have been unsuccessful. One suggested agent is the relative softness of the water supply. While this fits the overall geographical picture the correlations appear to break down at the local level. For example, within north-west England there are areas of hard and areas of soft water but the incidence of malformations does not appear to vary accordingly, remaining high in both kinds of areas.

Social class. A negative correlation between social class and the incidence of anencephaly has been recorded in both England and Wales, and Scotland, the incidence being higher among the lower social classes. However, this clue has not led to the direct identification of any specific environmental factor. Carter suggests that it would be interesting to investigate whether it is the social class in which a mother grew up which is important rather than that into which she married.

Seasonal trends and long-term ('secular') trends. Both anencephaly and spina bifida have peak seasons of incidence, the rates being higher than average in winter births and lower in summer births. This means that the high-rate months for conception of neural tube malformations in England are March, April and May, this relationship to seasons being reversed in Australia. Again, this suggests that environmental factors are important although no specific factor has yet been identified.

The incidence of neural tube malformations also shows consistent trends for years at a time. In the decade up to 1961 the incidence of anencephaly appeared to rise, between 1961 to 1968 it decreased steadily and between 1968 and 1972 the rates again began rising. As yet no specific factors have been identified which would explain these puzzling trends.

Maternal age and birth order. Differences in incidence rates for neural tube malformations according to the age of the mother and the birth order of the child can be interpreted as indicating the effect of environmental factors including of course the intra-uterine environment. The effects of maternal age and birth order can easily be confused since late maternal age and a high birth order are likely to be associated but statistical procedures are available which make it possible to look at these effects separately.

As regards the age of the mother most studies have shown a raised incidence in the off-spring of young mothers under the age of twenty and of older mothers over thirty-five. There is also a birth order effect with a raised incidence in first-borns, a lower incidence in second-

and third-born children, and an excess again in later births, but again no specific environmental factor has been discovered to account for this.

Dietary factors. Attempts to find a specific environmental agent which would account for at least some of the associations discussed here (for example the regional variations, seasonal variations, long-term trends and social class differences) have been hitherto confined to dietary factors. One suggestion which gained wide publication was that blighted potatoes were a major cause of neural tube malformations (Renwick, 1972). Although this theory is in fair agreement with the regional variation in frequency in Britain and the seasonal variation, it does not fit with broader geographical variations.

Carter refers to two other interesting studies which may give clues well worth further study. In a study by Knox (1972) a positive correlation was found between the incidence of anencephaly and the consumption of canned cooked meats, large white loaves, canned peas and ice-cream, and he makes the point that the nitrates and nitrites used in curing cooked meat might give rise to teratogenic compounds (i.e. chemical compounds producing congenital malformations in the foetus). Another study was carried out by Fedrick (1974) who found a regional correlation between the consumption of tea and the birth frequency of anencephaly, and a higher intake of tea by the mothers of anencephalics than of control children in Britain.

However, finding a significant correlation between two variables does not prove that there is necessarily a causal relationship between them: both may be related to some crucial third factor which we do not yet know about. Crocker (1969) gives the example that the further up a mountain we climb the more likely we are to get symptoms such as headaches, dizziness or fainting. A high positive correlation could be plotted between the height of the mountain and incidence of these symptoms. However, it is not the height of the mountain which causes the symptoms. The two factors are not directly related but are linked by a third all-important factor, the availability of oxygen. In the same way both tea-drinking and a high incidence of anencephaly may not be directly related but rather be related to some third factor which we have not yet identified.

Summing up

The evidence suggests that a very complicated interaction of genetic and environmental agents is responsible for the occurrence of neural tube malformations. Animal experiments indicate that a wide variety of toxic or mechanical agents acting on the foetus at the critical time may result in this defect. The fact that no single environmental agent has yet been identified despite years of intensive research, argues that multiple factors are involved. Carter points out that 'true prevention of these malformations is likely to be achieved by the discovery of ways of recognizing couples at risk of having affected children and the protection of their children from the additional environmental triggers. If we are lucky and only one or two environmental factors play the major part in contributing to the liability to develop the malformation, then prevention should not be too difficult. If on the other hand, multiple genetic and environmental factors contribute . . . prevention is not impossible but may well take some decades. True prevention must remain the ultimate end but, in the meantime, screening of all pregnancies and selective termination of affected foetuses offers the best immediate hope of reducing the birth frequency of these malformations.'

Screening procedures

The amniotic fluid is the fluid found inside the amniotic sac (the membranes which contain the developing foetus within the womb). The fluid acts as a protective barrier for the foetus and also has an important function in helping to remove its waste products. In 1972 Brock and Sutcliffe noticed an association between anencephaly and a raised level of a chemical substance called alpha-fetoprotein (AFP) normally found in the amniotic fluid. Since then, in a number of centres amniocentesis (a procedure by which a sample of the amniotic fluid is obtained) is carried out in early pregnancy, to estimate the AFP level so as to detect neural tube malformations in the foetus. It is now well established that at 16 to 18 weeks following conception there is a considerable difference between the AFP levels in normal pregnancies and in pregnancies where the foetus is anencephalic. Cases of myelomeningocele and anencephaly seem to be consistently associated with high AFP levels, but most 'closed' lesions including encephaloceles, and meningoceles cannot be detected by this technique. It is usually carried out in conjunction with ultrasound, a technique which produces an image similar to an X-ray and will detect an anencephalic foetus quite reliably.

There are a number of clinical and ethical problems associated with this screening procedure. Amniocentesis, although not dangerous, carries a very small risk of precipitating a miscarriage. Timing is important: if carried out too early on in pregnancy AFP levels may be normal even with a malformation, if too late it may be difficult to terminate the pregnancy. Furthermore although it is known that the test will detect the very severe cases and miss the very mild, the procedure is too new for doctors to be able to say with complete certainty at which point the cut-off occurs. There is also the ethical problem involved in all terminations, and in addition, since the test may not be reliable under 16 weeks, the termination cannot be carried out as early as doctors normally recommend for the safety and health of the mother.

It is only feasible with this method to monitor the pregnancies of 'high-risk' women, that is, those who have had a previous child with a neural tube malformation or a family history suggesting they are at risk. Even if all high risk pregnancies were monitored by this method and terminated, the incidence in the community of neural tube malformations would only be reduced by about 10 per cent (Laurence, 1974) mainly because such a high proportion of children with anencephaly and spina bifida are first-borns and there is nothing to suggest the woman is at risk.

More recently, it was reported by Leek and his colleagues (Leek *et al.*, 1973) and by others that a high amniotic fluid level is associated with a raised level of AFP in the mother's serum (the thin transparent part of the blood). This finding is extremely important since it is much simpler, safer and less costly to take a sample of the maternal serum than it is to carry out amniocentesis. In theory, therefore, it should be possible to screen all pregnancies by looking at AFP levels in the maternal serum, and, where abnormally high levels are found, to follow this up by amniocentesis.

Studies using this method of screening with a large sample of pregnant women (over 1000) indicate that it is possible to identify over 90 per cent of foetuses with anencephaly or open myelomeningocele (Leighton *et al.*, 1975). One difficulty encountered was the problem, in some cases, of dating the time of conception. This must be known quite accurately since the blood sample must be taken between 16 and 25 weeks of gestation if the test is to be reliable. Before and after those dates low levels of AFP may occur in the blood serum even if the foetus is abnormal. The main problem however, is that the method of detecting the level of AFP is not yet reliable. In a special study such as this one it was possible to control the technique closely but this would not always be the case if general screening was introduced. The concentration of AFP in the serum is 500 times lower than in the amniotic fluid (Laurence, 1974) and very sensitive laboratory tests are necessary to detect the level with precision. There is a danger at present therefore that some cases might be missed or that there might be a false alarm in others, and until these difficulties have been overcome the test cannot be applied routinely.

However, there is little doubt that it will be feasible in time to offer such a test as a routine procedure in all ante-natal clinics. If this were the case, there would be a problem when a high serum AFP result was obtained for a particular mother: the obstetrician would have to explain that something might be wrong with the foetus (and this in itself would lead to considerable anxiety) and that further tests (i.e. amniocentesis) were required. Laurence (1974) suggests that before amniocentesis was carried out the parents' views on the termination of an abnormal pregnancy should be obtained since 'it would be inappropriate to confirm the diagnosis [i.e. by amniocentesis] if it were impossible to take appropriate action'.

Should nationwide screening of all pregnancies by means of maternal serum AFP estimation become a reality then it would certainly be a major step forward in reducing the incidence of spina bifida in the community, even if quite a large proportion of abnormalities remain undetected. Nevertheless, this could never be a satisfactory solution to the problem and one would still hope that a means could be found of preventing the malformation occurring in the first place, since this would be greatly preferable to termination, particularly if this cannot be done till after the sixteenth week.

Genetic Counselling

The aim of genetic counselling in spina bifida is not primarily to reduce the numbers of affected children born (since so many are first-born) but to help parents who have already had one child with a neural tube malformation, as well as other people known to be at risk. For example, those who have an affected sibling might want advice before embarking on a family, as might young adults with spina bifida who are themselves considering the possibility of having a family.

As noted earlier, the risk to parents who have already had one child with a neural tube malformation (e.g. spina bifida or anencephaly) is approximately 1 in 25. Whether parents are prepared to accept this risk will depend partly on the number of children they already have and also whether the affected child has survived and if so how handicapped he is. However, as a general rule, Carter *et al.*, (1971) describe the risk to such mothers as 'a low or moderate risk' and they have adopted the practice of telling parents with a risk of this order 'in your place I would be prepared to take this risk'. As Carter and Roberts (1967) have shown, the risk increases substantially, to about 1 in 10, in a situation where a couple has already had two children with such malformations. As already noted, where one parent has spina bifida, the chances of having an affected child are probably the same as for a 'normal' mother who already has one affected child, that is about 1 in 20, although the figures available are still small. Each couple, however, should seek individual advice since these figures can only give a general idea of the risks involved.

Carter and his colleagues (1971) have followed up 455 couples seen at the genetic clinic at The Hospital for Sick Children, Great Ormond Street, between 1952 and 1964. Most of these couples sought advice because they already had a child with a possibly inherited disorder and wanted to have more children. The largest group of parents were those who had a mentally handicapped child, and the second largest group those whose child had a disorder of the nervous system, over half of these being parents whose child had a neural tube malformation.

The object of the follow-up was to discover how far couples understood the information they were given on risks, what decisions they took about planning further pregnancies and the outcome of further pregnancies. First, it was found that on the whole parents had understood the information they had been given. Second, they tended to take responsible decisions on the basis of the information. Thus where the recurrence risk was high (equal to or greater than 1 in 10) two-thirds had been deterred from planning to have children and a number of these had adopted children instead. Where the risks were low (less than 1 in 10) only a quarter were deterred. Third, it was found that the risks given had on the whole been accurate. Of children born to high risk couples about 1 in 6 had been affected while of those born to low risk couples only 5 out of 229 children were affected (i.e. 1 in 50).

Genetic counselling is clearly of great value to all 'at risk' parents and siblings and also to young people with spina bifida who may become parents, and 'at risk' groups should be actively encouraged to seek genetic counselling and told exactly where this can be obtained. It must also be stressed that genetic counselling is a matter for specialists. The average GP, for example, is likely to see only two spina bifida children in a life-time in general practice and cannot be expected to know what the risks are for this and all the other comparatively rare conditions which he may occasionally encounter. The evidence clearly suggests that couples do understand and behave responsibly if they are given the correct advice. However, most studies show that between 30 per cent and 60 per cent of parents with a surviving spina bifida child have not been given correct genetic advice (Spain, 1973a; Richards and McIntosh, 1973). In families where the child is stillborn or dies early this information is even less likely to have been given (Evans, 1971).

In the Richards and McIntosh (1973) study eighty-six mothers with children aged between 2 and 6 years were interviewed and it was found that most 'were oblivious to the risks of subsequent pregnancies'. Some had been given incorrect advice by doctors or nurses who did not know about the genetic risks. In other areas where a special effort was made to inform parents, the situation was considerably improved and in the Sheffield study over 90 per cent of mothers understood the frequency (Freeston, 1971). This clearly demonstrates that genetic counselling can be given routinely, and that the majority of parents can be helped to understand the implications. However, the facts may be difficult to grasp on first hearing and everyone who has contact with the family has a responsibility to see both that the information has been given and that it has been understood. The need to do so has become even more urgent with the advent of amniocentesis, because it is only if parents appreciate the risks involved that they can choose whether or not to avail themselves of this service.

Selection for treatment in spina bifida cystica

Before concluding this chapter we felt it necessary to say something about the currently controversial issue of selection for early surgery. The ethical issue of whether or not a severely malformed baby should be encouraged to live is an old one, but it is only comparatively recently that the development of modern methods of treatment has turned the issue into a concrete rather than an abstract problem.

As Stark and Drummond (1973) point out, there are three possible approaches to the question of the early treatment of new-born babies with open myelomeningoceles, these being (1) conservative management (i.e. no operation at all), (2) unselective early operation (i.e. operation for all spina bifida babies) or (3) selective operation (i.e. surgical treatment for selected babies only).

(1) *Conservative management*
Until the late 1950s or, in some centres, early 1960s it was rare for children born with spina bifida and hydrocephalus to be given early surgical treatment and mortality rates were very high. Laurence and Tew (1971) followed up 381 cases of myelomeningocele born in South Wales in 1956–62. By 1968 only 15 per cent were still alive, and of these survivors 70 per cent were considered to be severely or very severely handicapped. Although a policy of non-intervention results in the early death of the most severely afflicted children, the survivors will undoubtedly be more handicapped both physically and mentally than they would have been had early active treatment been given.

Now that sophisticated modern treatment is available not only for the control of hydrocephalus but also for the child's other physical problems, the major issue is whether such treatment should be given to all neonates with open myelomeningoceles or only to selected children.

(2) *Unselected early operation* (i.e. operation in every case)
From about 1963 to 70, it became a matter of policy in many major centres to accept all spina bifida babies for early surgery and massive efforts in treatment thereafter. This policy was typified in Sheffield and Lorber in 1971 published his evaluation of the results of unselected early surgery. His findings were disappointing: as the children grew older it became clear that the majority of survivors had major physical defects and were often intellectually impaired. Not only was the quality of life of many of the children very poor but their families were living under great long-term stresses. In addition, the financial cost of the policy was enormous (Lightfowler, 1971).

(3) *Selection of children for early surgical treatment*
In some cases the decision to select for treatment has been a comparatively recent one, and sometimes (for example, in Lorber's case) a reversal of former policy. In others, such as at the Royal Hospital for Sick Children in Edinburgh and The Royal Children's Hospital in Melbourne, an active policy of selection for surgical treatment has been carried out since the early 1960s when modern methods of treatment first became available and published reports from these two centres indicate the effect of such a policy (Stark and Drummond, 1973; Smith and Smith, 1973).

The data from Stark and Drummond (1973) can be summarized as follows. Between 1965 and 1971 163 unselected infants with open myelomeningoceles were admitted to the spina bifida unit, of whom 48 per cent considered to have the most favourable prognosis were selected for early back closure and vigorous subsequent treatment. More than 70 per cent of the treated group survived to 6 years. When compared to the children in Lorber's study (Lorber, 1971) all of whom had been treated as a routine matter, 25 per cent (compared to 49 per cent) were mainly or entirely in wheelchairs, only 16 per cent (compared with 34 per cent) had upper urinary tract damage with incontinence, and a combination of mental and severe physical handicap occurred in only 20 per cent (compared to 36 per cent).

The children not selected for active treatment (52 per cent of the original group) were the more severely affected children, the major adverse criteria being severe paralysis, gross hydrocephalus and spinal deformity such as kyphosis. These children were retained in the unit where they received good nursing care, were fed normally and kept comfortable. When life-threatening situations occurred, antibiotics were withheld and therapy confined to analgesics. 80 per cent of this group had died by the age of 3 months, and by 6 years only 8 per cent were still alive. If children seemed to be thriving despite lack of active treatment a shunt was inserted where necessary to control the hydrocephalus. Like Smith and Smith (1973) who have published comparable data on the quality of life in surviving selected children, Stark and Drummond conclude that 'the overall results of selective early operations compare favourably with those of purely conservative management on the one hand, and with routine early operation on the other'.

Most doctors would concur with these conclusions and selection of some kind, not always as extensive as this, is now taking place in most centres. If selection is practised systematically it should effectively reduce the number of children surviving with severe handicaps. Indeed there is evidence that the mortality of infants with spina bifida is now increasing again after a decade of continuing decline (see Fig. 2.2).

It is hard to know precisely how far the trend towards selection for treatment will go, but Spain (1975) estimates that survival rates might be reduced by about 25 per cent if the Stark and Drummond criteria were applied widely. Those failing to survive would be mainly the most severely handicapped children, but it must be recognized that some badly handicapped children will survive even with selection, partly because of inevitable errors in the initial selection but more commonly because severe secondary complications arise which were unforseeable at birth. Also, of course, a small percentage of the children not selected for treatment do survive at least until early childhood.

No one could deny that there are still unresolved technical as well as ethical problems inherent in a policy of selection and we have tried

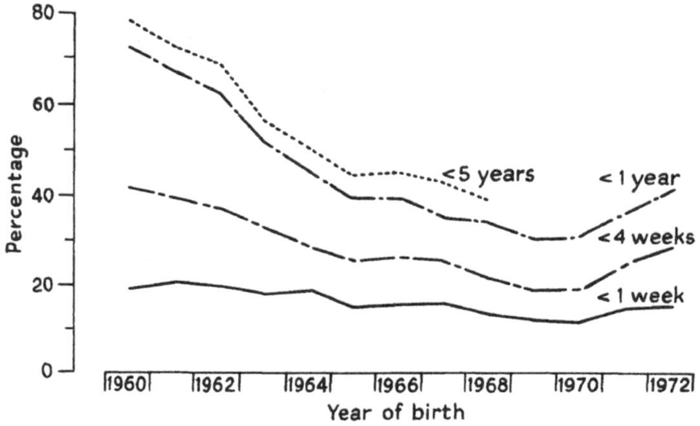

Figure 2.2 *Mortality of children born live with spina bifida, hydrocephalus or both between 1960 and 1972. England and Wales* (From Adelstein, 1975).

to summarize these here. One problem is the extent to which the parents should be involved in the decision to treat or not to treat. This is discussed in detail by Ellis (1974). He points out that at present, for a variety of reasons, most doctors think that they should make the decision about treatment. A few do not discuss the situation with the parents at all, or only briefly. He explains that while most consultants talk in depth to the parents, for good reasons they also think the decision to treat should be made by the doctor. 'They may think that only by making full use of their clinical judgement and expertise can the correct verdict be reached: they may consider it wrong for parents to be held accountable for their babies, when the choice before them is life with handicap or of eventual death after handicap; or they may believe that parents prefer the doctor to make the decision.' Many doctors and others have also pointed out that the parents may be in no state either emotionally or physically to make a rational decision. In contrast, other consultants like Ellis believe that the parents wish to be and should be involved in the decisions. Parents are likely in any case to accept the advice offered to them by the doctor but they may need time to reach a decision, and as Forrest (1974) has pointed out 'any attempt to ride rough-shod over the parent's wishes will result in permanent loss of confidence, risking more to the baby's future than possible loss of muscle power'. Various suggestions have been made about who should inform the parents of all the relevant facts before the decision is made; Ellis considers this should be done by a pædiatrician or pædiatric surgeon.

Another group of people who must be consulted are the nursing staff. Eckstein *et al.* (1973) points out that if back surgery is withheld 'then it is only reasonable to withhold other forms of treatment such as antibiotics, oxygen and tube-feeding'. To do this the co-operation of the nursing staff (whose training is, of course, focused upon saving life) is essential. Their opinion, states Eckstein, 'must be seriously considered and is often overriding'.

Much of the argument about whether it is right to select has centred around the question of whether enough is yet known about the criteria used for selection. Is it possible to assess the potential of a new-born infant with a myelomeningocele? Reasonably reliable and objective criteria for assessing future potential have been described in detail by Lorber (1971), Smith and Smith (1973), Hunt *et al.* (1973), Stark and Drummond (1973) and others and there is now fairly good agreement about what constitute adverse criteria. Despite this, selection can in some cases be difficult even for consultants with great experience in this area, and sometimes decisions have to be taken by those without such expertise.

A major criticism of a policy of selection is that the severely affected child whose back has not been repaired and who has not had a shunt inserted early on may survive with greater physical and/or intellectual disability than he would have had with early surgery. Clearly too, as Stark and Drummond point out (1973) parental acceptance of children, who have been expected to die but do not, may be prejudiced. Although most studies suggest that the number of untreated children surviving is very small indeed, this is a very real problem. Many untreated babies will die within a month, but some may live for up to a year or longer and this period, during which the child is gradually deteriorating, will clearly be an extremely difficult one for parents. The hospital staff must be prepared to give parents the support they need until the child dies: the clinician must also, as Smith and Smith point out (1973) be flexible enough to change the treatment programme with the changing status of the child. Whether the child goes home or remains in hospital during this period will vary, but terminal care in hospital must always be offered. Indeed many people would argue that parents should be positively encouraged to leave the child in hospital partly because the terminal care of a young baby is very distressing for mothers but mainly because it is very much easier for hospital staff than for mothers to carry out a consistent policy of withholding treatment. Some parents, however, want to care for the child themselves and if this is their choice then they should be supported medically and emotionally in this decision.

What must be avoided is a situation where children not selected for surgery survive many years in a grossly handicapped state because a policy of withholding treatment has not been systematically carried out. At the same time, if it seems preferable that a grossly deformed child should not survive this does not mean that he should be neglected and the parents may need to be convinced that everything possible is being done to make him comfortable. In Forrest's words (1974) 'any feeling that the child was neglected or given less than adequate treatment will leave long-lasting resentment. This does not imply that heroic surgery or resuscitation are necessary. Parents can often be shown that the operation would serve no useful purpose. What they rightly expect is concerned care and continued interest.'

In this short account we cannot cover every facet of this very difficult decision. Clearly, the ethical and religious views of some doctors, parents and others involved in the decision will stress that life should be saved at all cost. Others believe the burdens imposed on a family by a grossly handicapped child are too great to justify. The Department of Health (1973) puts the onus for a decision squarely on 'the doctor concerned'. We ourselves concur with Stark and Drummond's conclusions (1973) that a policy of selection 'offers the best prospects of independence for the less severely affected child, and the least distress and suffering for the grossly afflicted'.

References

Adelstein, A. M. (1975), 'National statistics', pp. 57–67 in Barltrop, D. (ed.), *Paediatrics and the Environment*, Publ. Fellowship of Postgraduate Medicine.

Brock, D. J. H. and Sutcliffe, R. G. (1972), 'Alpha-fetoprotein in the antenatal diagnosis of anencephaly and spina bifida', *Lancet* ii, pp. 197–9.

Carter, C. O. (1969), 'Spina bifida and anencephaly: a problem in genetic-environmental interaction', *Journal of Biosocial Science* 1, pp. 71–83.

——, (1974), 'Clues to the aetiology of neural tube malformations', *Developmental Medicine and Child Neurology*, Supplement 32, pp. 3–15.

——, and Evans, K. (1973), 'Children of adult survivors with spina bifida cystica', *Lancet* ii, pp. 924–26.

——, and Fraser Roberts, J. A. F. (1967), 'The risk of recurrence after two children with central-nervous system malformations', *Lancet* i, pp. 306–8.

——, ——, Evans, K. A., and Buck, A. R. (1971), 'Genetic clinic. A follow up', *Lancet* i, pp. 281–5.

Crocker, A. C. (1969), *Statistics for the Teacher*, Penguin Books, Harmondsworth.

DHSS (1973), *Care of the Child with Spina Bifida*, HMSO, Edinburgh.

Eckstein, H., Hatcher, G., and Slater, E. (1973), 'Severely malformed children', tape-recorded discussion published in *British Medical Journal* 2, pp. 284–9.

Ellis, H. L. (1974), 'Parental involvement in the decision to treat spina bifida cystica', *British Medical Journal* 1, pp. 369–72.

Evans, K. (1971), personal communication.

Fedrick, J. (1974), 'Anencephalus and tea drinking', *Proceedings Royal Society of Medicine*, 67, p. 356.

Forrest, D. (1974), 'Spina bifida, practical and ethical considerations in its treatment', *Modern Medicine*, 17, p. 108.

Freeston, B. (1971), 'An enquiry into the effect of a spina bifida child upon family life', *Developmental Medicine and Child Neurology*, 13, pp. 456–61.

Hunt, G. M., Walpole, L., Gleave, J., and Gairdner, D. (1973), 'Predictive factors in open myelomeningocele with special reference to sensory level', *British Medical Journal* 4, pp. 197–201.

Knox, E. C. (1972), 'Anencephalus and dietary intakes', *British Journal of Preventive and Social Medicine*, 26, p. 219.

Laurence, K. M. (1974), 'Clinical and ethical considerations on alpha-fetoprotein estimation for early prenatal diagnosis of neural tube malformations', *Developmental Medicine and Child Neurology*, Supplement 32, pp. 117–21.

——, and Tew, B. J. (1971), 'Studies in spina bifida cystica IV', *Archives of Diseases in Childhood*, 47, pp. 128–37.

Leck, I. (1972), 'The aetiology of human malformations and insights from epidemiology', *Teratology*, 5, p. 303.

Leek, A. E., Ross, C. F., Kitau, M. J., and Chard, T. (1973), 'Raised alpha-fetoprotein in maternal serum with anencephalic pregnancy', *Lancet* ii, p. 385.

Leighton, P. C., Garden, Y. B., Kitau, M. J., Leek, A. E. and Chard, T.

(1975), 'Levels of alpha-fetoprotein in maternal blood as a screening test for fetal neural-tube defects', *Lancet* ii, pp. 1012–15.

Lightfowler, C. R. D. (1971), 'Meningomyelocele: the price of treatment', *British Medical Journal* 2, pp. 385–7.

Lorber, J. (1968), 'The problem of spina bifida', *The Medical Officer*, 129 (16), pp. 213–15.

——, (1971), 'Results of treatment of myelomeningocele', *Developmental Medicine and Child Neurology*, 13 (3), pp. 279–303.

——, (1973), 'Early results of selective treatment of spina bifida cystica', *British Medical Journal*, 27 October 1973, 4, pp. 201–4.

——, (1974), *Your Child with Spina Bifida*, 3rd ed., ASBAH, London.

Naggan, L. (1971), 'Anencephaly and spina bifida in Israel', *Paediatrics*, 47, p. 577.

——, and MacMahon, B. (1967), 'Ethnic differences in the prevalence of anencephaly and spina bifida in Boston, Massachusetts', *New England Journal of Medicine*, 277, p. 1119.

Renwick, J. H. (1972), 'Hypothesis. Anencephaly and spina bifida are usually preventable by avoidance of a specific but unidentified substance present in certain potato tubers', *British Journal of Preventive and Social Medicine*, 26, p. 67.

Richards, I. D. G. and McIntosh, H. T. (1973), 'Spina bifida survivors and their parents. A study of problems and services', *Developmental Medicine and Child Neurology*, 15, pp. 293–304.

Smith, G. K. and Smith, E. D. (1973), *Selection for Treatment in Spina Bifida Cystica*, C. C. Thomas, Illinois.

Stark, G. and Drummond, M. (1973), 'Results of selective early operation in myelomeningocele', *Archives of Diseases in Childhood*, 48, pp. 676–83.

Stevenson, A. C., Johnston, H. A., Stewart, M. I. P. and Golding, D. (1966), 'Congenital malformations. A report of a study of consecutive births in 24 centres', Bulletin WHO 34 (Supplement), p. 9.

Spain, B. (1973a), 'Spina bifida: the need for community support', GLC Intell. Unit Quarterly Bulletin, 23 pp. 66–71.

——, (1975), personal communication.

2 Families with a spina bifida child

3 Family problems

In studies describing family life where there is a handicapped child, many authors have remarked that a handicapped child implies a handicapped family (McMichael, 1971; Sheridan, 1965; Younghusband *et al.*, 1970). While it is true that some families seem to adjust to the tragedy with no apparent detrimental effect on their mental health or happiness, most families are liable to suffer severe strain unless they receive adequate support of some kind, and often a coping strategy is developed only at considerable cost to their social and psychological well-being (Dorner, 1976).

Birth and the early months

Spina bifida is a condition recognizable immediately on delivery. Some other major congenital malformations are detectable on examination within the first few weeks of life, but there are few which are so obvious at birth. In contrast to the situation for many other severely handicapping conditions, therefore, where the parents have time to get to know their child before discovering the full implications of the diagnosis, the mother of a spina bifida baby must be told right away about the defect. The child is commonly taken to another unit for treatment, before she has even had the chance to hold him. Since the treatment required is very specialized it can rarely be provided in the same hospital complex, and because it may be necessary to operate quickly the child is usually sent on to a treatment centre immediately following the birth. It may not be possible to contact the father in time and so the mother is often asked to sign the consent form for operation, sometimes while she is still on the delivery table, with very little idea of what this might actually entail.

Having hoped after nine months of expectation for an uncomplicated delivery and a happy experience of motherhood which can be shared with her husband, close relatives and friends, she finds herself instead the only mother in the maternity unit with no baby to cherish. Often she has only a hazy knowledge of the reason for the child's absence or of the prognosis for his future, and she often feels also that she has failed her husband and her family. One mother said, 'It wasn't as if you'd had a baby at all' (Walker *et al.*, 1971), and another, 'When she was born it was like a dream. The nurse said she might not live and it would be a good thing if she didn't' (Fox, 1974). The father too is shocked, confused and distressed. He must try to comfort his wife and convey to her what he has learnt about the child's condition from the doctor at the treatment centre, and also face family and friends with the disconcerting news.

There is no way of removing from parents the distress of this event or of breaking the news to them in a way which will eliminate all fear and leave them feeling confident and happy. But the recurrent claim by parents that the situation at birth and during the days following is needlessly distressing is so common a feature of studies on such families that one cannot dismiss this as due simply to the trauma inherent in the circumstances (Freeston, 1971a; Walker *et al.*, 1971; Richards and McIntosh, 1973; Younghusband *et al.*, 1970). Parents complain most often that the diagnosis was insufficiently explained or that it was minimized, being described as 'only a little hole in the back' or 'just a lump on the spine'. In one survey, only a quarter of the fathers and even fewer mothers felt that they had understood the diagnosis at the point when they signed the consent for operation form (Freeston, 1971b). During the subsequent days while the mother is separated from the baby, it is rare for anyone well informed about the baby's condition to visit and discuss the prognosis with her and she has to rely on the father's recall of what he has been told at the treatment centre. Prevarication by staff in the maternity unit will often 'aggravate the mother's worst fears, add to her confusion and precipitate fantasies whose horrors often exceed the reality' (Spain and Wigley, 1975).

When the mother is allowed to visit the child at the treatment centre she may find him lying prone in an incubator with a bandaged back. Sometimes he has an enlarging head or deformed feet, but he may look surprisingly normal with a dressing concealing the operation scar. Being unable to pick him up or nurse him, the mother often finds it hard to relate to him or even to believe that he is truly her baby, and the opportunity to get to know him before his discharge from hospital is often minimal. While usually encouraged to feed him, the mother commonly has little experience of bathing or dressing him till she gets him home at 4 or 6 weeks of age. In many parts of the country, the treatment centre is far from the child's home and parents cannot visit more than once or twice a week. Many mothers say that it is not until the point when they have the baby home, where they can hold him and care for him that they begin to feel that it is actually their own child (Halliday *et al.*, 1965).

It is in this context of shock, disappointment, bewilderment and unreality surrounding the birth and the first few weeks of life that the spina bifida child enters his family. Even the most well-adjusted parents with the most stable and loving marital relationships are likely to be overwhelmed, at least temporarily. For the unmarried mother, or where the marital relationship is poor or the pregnancy unwelcome the effect may be devastating.

Approximately 40 per cent of spina bifida births are first children (Spain, 1973; Walker *et al.*, 1971) and for these mothers in particular the first months at home with the baby are very difficult ones (Hunt, 1973; Freeston, 1971a). Caring for a first baby, learning how to handle him, interpreting his needs and judging the seriousness of his ailments, has problems for any young mother. When, in addition, he suffers from a serious condition, the nature of which may still not be very clear to her, the anxiety produced can be very great indeed. In the GLC study many mothers spoke of how worried they felt about handling their babies when they first brought them home from the pædiatric hospital. In particular they were nervous of bathing or changing them, having had little or no experience of these activities before bringing the baby home. In another study, one third of mothers had never picked up their child until the day of discharge (Freeston, 1971b).

Mothers with hydrocephalic children are likely to be particularly anxious, since they are told to watch for signs of a malfunctioning valve, for example a rise in temperature, drowsiness and vomiting – symptoms likely to accompany any minor baby ailment such as a normal healthy infant might experience many times during the first few months of life. A mother with a hydrocephalic child is likely to face this problem frequently and it can become a great source of concern, especially for those with no previous experience of dealing with babies. In the GLC study 40 per cent of mothers interviewed with a child aged one year and 32 per cent with children aged two years stated that the child either had some problem with his valve or produced symptoms which might have indicated a blockage. Even at three years a quarter had shown symptoms suggestive of a blocked valve in the previous year.

Communication with the hospital and community support

In all the studies where this point has been covered, many parents have expressed dissatisfaction with the amount and quality of information given to them at the hospital not only in the early weeks but throughout the child's life (Walker *et al.*, 1971; Woodburn, 1973; Richards and McIntosh, 1973; Freeston, 1971b). In the GLC study most parents agreed that the clinical treatment received from the hospital was excellent (Spain, 1973), but when asked if they were satisfied with how much explanation they were given about the child's condition, the treatment applied or planned and the child's general prognosis, 30 per cent expressed dissatisfaction. These were usually parents who acknowledged fully the general excellence of in-patient care and expressed gratitude for all that had been done for their child. However, they did not feel that they understood the nature of the treatment the child had received or what they should be expecting of him, and consequently felt very confused. Mothers often did not understand what was involved in a catheter-lengthening operation, why a urinary diversion might be necessary, what was the purpose of the leg exercises taught by the physiotherapist or why limb deformities, such as talipes, were likely to recur in some children. Parents frequently spoke about how overawed they were by consultants and by the whole procedure in the out-patient clinic, especially if a number of doctors were present, and how questions they had intended to ask were remembered only on the way home. Others said that when explanations were given it was often difficult to understand these immediately and that questions which occurred to them on reflection usually remained unanswered because there was no one to talk to once they left the hospital.

Spina bifida is a complex condition, difficult even for a medically informed person to understand, and particularly so for lay people. But parents have additional difficulties since distress obviously limits the ability to appreciate fully medical technicalities. What parents want is a careful and sympathetic discussion of the child's medical problems, but often there is no one available to provide this. Hare *et al.* (1966) state that 'Doctors and nurses didn't seem to appreciate the worries and anxieties parents had, and didn't say the simple words of comfort which would have indicated their understanding and sympathy'.

This apparent indifference or unwillingness of hospital staff to discuss medical problems would not be so important if parents could rely on some other professional person within the community to elaborate on the information received there. However, the hospital staff, particularly the consultant, are usually the principal source of information about the child's condition and its consequences (Richards and McIntosh, 1973). Parents in the GLC study were asked about the help or information they had received from their GP, health visitor or clinic doctor. 26 per cent of health visitors were reported to visit rarely or never and only a third were regular visitors. Similar results were found in other studies (Freeston, 1971a; Walker *et al.*, 1971). In the Glasgow study (Richards and McIntosh, 1973) of children aged 2 to 6 years, it was found that only 15 out of 86 children had been visited up to five times during the previous year which suggested that 'children with spina bifida receive little or no priority in domiciliary visiting'. Few mothers in the GLC study used the clinic except for innoculations, and 40 per cent did not attend at all, innoculations being done by the GP. The reason usually given was that they already had a lot of visits to make to hospital out-patients and that in any case they felt that the clinic doctors often did not know much about their child's problems. Where the health visitor or clinic doctor did take an interest in the child this was greatly appreciated, but many presumably felt that they did not have the time to devote to the study of a condition which they would meet so rarely.

When asked about the involvement of the GP, 67 per cent of parents in the GLC study found him to be helpful if the child was ill, but few regarded him as someone they could talk to at length about their special problems or who could elaborate on information gained from the hospital, and Freeston (1971b) reports that 'some family doctors admitted that they knew little more than the parents about spina bifida'. In some instances, failure by the GP to recognize symptoms of a blocked valve early on left parents with no faith in his ability to offer real assistance, and it is a very common finding that 'if the parents were concerned about the child's condition they usually went straight to hospital without informing the general practitioner' (Richards and McIntosh, 1973). Again there were notable exceptions, some GPs offering very real expertise and sympathy, but the general trend in all these studies suggests that mothers cannot necessarily rely on anyone in the community to offer help or support (Freeston, 1971b; Richards and McIntosh, 1973; Walker *et al.*, 1971). This problem seems common to other chronically handicapping conditions in childhood (Bayley, 1973; Hewett, 1970).

Many parents comment on the failure of hospital or community staff to give instruction in how to handle the child or how best to help him.

The most common piece of advice offered on discharge from hospital was 'Go home and treat him as a normal baby'. It is obviously impossible to treat a child so handicapped as if he were normal, and the parents felt very confused by this advice. What was meant presumably was 'see that he has the same experiences as a normal baby', or 'don't over-protect him'. However, most parents with a severely handicapped child need much more concrete guidance and help than this. In particular, a sound knowledge of normal child development would be necessary if parents were to put this advice into practice, a point which is discussed in more detail in chapter 6.

Most parents see their prime task as that of accepting the child and his limitations. As the parents of a mentally handicapped child said in Bayley's study (1973) 'That was the worst thing, accepting, knowing, bringing yourself to terms with what you'd got in front of you.' In order to accept the child the parents need information about the nature of his problems and this information is often lacking. Kellmer Pringle and Fiddes (1970) put this point well; they argue that the first need of a handicapped child, as for all children, is the need for security, for 'unconditional acceptance'. However, 'to give a sense of security one needs to feel secure oneself. But this is just what many parents of a handicapped child do not feel; some are overwhelmed by their lack of knowledge and afraid that they may not be able to meet his special needs'. Without a good understanding of the child's physical and intellectual problems and what needs to be done to overcome these, or at least to minimize them, the parents are in no position to help and may even unwittingly exacerbate some problems.

The effect on the family's daily life

As the spina bifida child grows older, the limitations that his handicap imposes will become more apparent and his presence will affect the family in many ways. On a day-to-day basis, the ordinary routine of living will be disturbed and the necessity to make special arrangements to accommodate the child and his disabilities will become a major consideration.

A child who cannot stand without calipers and who has no useful walking but must be pushed in a wheelchair or buggy is difficult to take out of doors, even to do the shopping. Dealing with public transport is found to be a universal problem, particularly if there are other young children who need to be helped on and off buses. Since many spina bifida children cannot stand at all unsupported, two pairs of hands are necessary each time a bus or train is used, one to hold the child and one to fold or unfold the pushchair. A trip that is to last more than a few hours will mean that extra baggage has to be carried along to deal with the incontinent child. Over 60 per cent of the 3 year olds in the GLC study had no useful walking, and 25 per cent of mothers with a child of this age found getting out with him to be a major difficulty.

Outings for the family are necessarily limited therefore, especially if there is no car, as was true for about 50 per cent of families in Woodburn's survey (1973) and 40 per cent of those in the GLC survey. The main difficulty was taking the children out when only one adult was available; the problem was not so great at the weekend when the father was home from work. However, although about 50 per cent of families in the GLC study managed to get out together at least once a week, in two-thirds of these families the child had a minimal locomotor handicap, and families with the more severely handicapped children tended to go out less often.

Developing techniques to manage a growing child who has calipers or other appliances; discovering ways to get him up the stairs, out of the bath, into the garden; learning how to manage a urinary device so that it is applied quickly but efficiently; all these things take time to learn and can become pre-occupying problems for the family if a smooth routine cannot be readily achieved. Incontinence, particularly incontinence of faeces, may become a very dominating aspect of daily organization, since the child will then require much supervision from his parents. If a urinary diversion has been carried out, the appliance will need to be renewed every two or three days and even though the child may be able to empty his bag unassisted, it will still need daily checking by an adult. An ill-fitting or slightly perforated appliance can soak the child and his surroundings in no time at all. Faecal incontinence is an even greater problem, often solved only by a routine of suppositories every few days and the whole family schedule may have to revolve around the occasions when the child must have his bowels emptied. In the GLC study less than 30 per cent of children were clean and dry by day at the age of 3 years and over half were doubly incontinent (including 4 with a urinary diversion). By the age of 6 years 25 per cent were still incontinent of urine and had had no appliance fitted, and almost as many had no bowel control at all and no means of regulating it had been arrived at. Many parents had not been told that they were eligible for free disposable nappies and sheets, and learnt about this incidentally from friends or not until the child entered school. Even with disposables, incontinence always involves extra washing and drying.

Lifting becomes an increasing problem as the child grows older and heavier, especially when he is wearing calipers, which may weigh over 6 lbs themselves. In the GLC study many mothers complained of backache, mainly due to lifting, and sometimes both parents had back trouble. Climbing stairs was particularly difficult and older children often have to wait for their father to return home from work before they can be got upstairs to bed.

Hospital attendances cause further problems. Although in the GLC survey the distances parents had to travel to the hospital were less than in some parts of the country, journeys by public transport or by ambulance could be very awkward or long, and frequently took between one and two hours. Outside London, centres for the treatment of spina bifida are only to be found in large towns, usually in conjunction with a teaching hospital, and parents may live many miles away. In Hunt's study (1973) of children attending Addenbrooke's Hospital in Cambridge, the average distance travelled was 47 miles, and in Woodburn's study in Scotland (1973) the majority of journeys to hospital took between two and five hours and in 23 per cent of cases over six hours.

Even going for a short out-patient appointment may, therefore, take a whole day, either because of travelling time or because the family has to wait around the hospital until the ambulance is ready to take them home (a very frequent complaint). Arrangements have to be made for the other children to be taken care of, or they must be brought along as well with the necessary food, drink, nappies and toys. During childhood the majority of patients with myelomeningocele attend out-patient clinics every three months at least so this becomes a very regular problem.

Family life is greatly disrupted when the child needs to go into hospital and this is quite a common occurrence. In the GLC study, each year between 50 per cent and 60 per cent of children were admitted to hospital on at least one occasion and many needed several readmissions, each one lasting two or three weeks. In more than a third of cases mothers visited daily, but even less frequent visiting was very costly for the whole family, both financially and in terms of daily care.

Because the child needs special handling, particularly if he is incontinent, the mother is often reluctant to leave the child, even for a short while, with a neighbour or other member of the family during the day. Only a third of mothers with 3 year olds in the GLC survey left their children regularly (at least once a fortnight) with someone else during the day. It was noted in Bayley's (1973) study of families with mentally handicapped children that such parents show a 'deeply rooted reluctance to intrude on relatives or neighbours or to ask them for help'. While it is true that people outside the immediate family are often nervous of a handicapped child and parents consequently hesitate to approach them, this timidity on the one hand or fear on the other may well be quite misplaced. Parents who overcame their diffidence usually found other people helpful, but most need encouragement before they will ask for help.

Very commonly the parents themselves do not find relief from the care of the child even to the extent of going out regularly together in the evenings. In the GLC study only 40 per cent of the parents of 3 year olds went out as often as once a month and less than 20 per cent went out once a week. This was obviously most difficult where there was another young child, and over a quarter of mothers interviewed had had at least one more baby since the birth of the handicapped child. The main problem, however, was finding a baby-sitter whom the parents trusted. In 70 per cent of cases the child was only ever left with a sibling or other relative, and if the relative did not live nearby then an evening out was a rare event.

A very detailed account of the daily management problems encountered by parents with a handicapped child is given in Margaret Woodburn's study *Social Implications of Spina Bifida* (1973), and is essential reading for anyone dealing with such a family, particularly because she makes very sensible practical suggestions about the help that can be offered.

The effect on family relationships and the mother's health

Given the trauma and confusion surrounding the child's birth, the lack of community support, the uncertainty parents frequently feel about the child's state of health and inevitable fears for his future, it is hardly surprising to find that studies of the family life of spina bifida children reveal a high rate of anxiety in the mothers and disturbance among the siblings.

Despite this, however, families do cope amazingly well and rejection of the child is relatively rare. In the GLC study, out of 183 children, only 7 were in permanent residential care from birth. 4 of these were profoundly retarded and the remaining 3 were illegitimate and born to teenage mothers. In all but one case these children were visited by at least one parent. Two others who had been in care from birth were successfully fostered by six months of age.

One aspect of family life which is likely to be affected by the presence of a handicapped child is the relationship between the parents, and a number of researchers have looked at the incidence of marital breakdown in such families. In the case of families with a spina bifida child the evidence is somewhat conflicting. In most studies the rate for separation or divorce reported is the same or lower than in the general population (Walker *et al.*, 1971; Richards *et al.*, 1973; Freeston, 1971; Dorner, 1976) although a fairly high rate is quoted in the South Wales study (Tew *et al.*, 1974). In the GLC survey 16 couples had separated by the time the child had reached 6 years of age, but on the other hand, five unmarried mothers caring for their children at home had successfully married, and in over half the cases of divorce the partner retaining the child had already remarried. The Tew *et al.* study (1974) suggests that the marriages most at risk are those where the child is conceived before marriage, or where the parents are very young, and it is in these cases that social work help is most needed.

In the Newcastle study (Walker *et al.*, 1971) out of 106 families, 43 couples thought that the marital relationship had deteriorated and 72 mothers felt increased tension in the family. These were all families with very young children, under 3 years of age, where parents were still trying to come to terms with the child's handicap and its implications, and family harmony may improve with time. When asked to assess the impact of the handicap on their marriage, mothers in the GLC study were as likely to find the effect beneficial as detrimental. Many felt that although the marriage had been difficult immediately following the child's birth, it had subsequently improved and the child had brought the parents closer together. This has also been reported for parents of children with muscular dystrophy (Henley and Albam, 1955), cerebral palsy (Hewett, 1970) and cystic fibrosis (Burton, 1975).

Evidence on maternal health, however, suggests that many mothers suffer from physical or emotional problems of some kind. In the Newcastle study only 19 out of 100 mothers interviewed felt themselves to be fit and well, tiredness, worry and depression being the common complaints. In contrast only half of the fathers in the Newcastle study felt unwell and a much smaller percentage of fathers compared with mothers complained of tiredness, anxiety and depression (Walker *et al.*, 1971). This should be seen in the context of the high rate of depression (affecting about 30 per cent of women) found in mothers with non-handicapped pre-school children (Richman, 1977). None the less when maternal anxiety is measured on a standard rating scale, where comparable figures can be given for other groups, there is evidence of significantly higher levels of distress among the mothers of spina bifida children.

In the South Wales and the GLC studies, the 'Malaise Inventory' was used, a scale developed by Rutter *et al.* (1970) to obtain information about emotional and psychosomatic symptoms, including depression, irritability, worry, or physical complaints such as headaches or upset stomachs. In both studies a much higher percentage of mothers with spina bifida children showed stress symptoms than did mothers of non-handicapped children (Tew and Laurence, 1975). A similar result was found in Dorner's study (1976) of mothers with a teenage spina bifida child, where the rate of depression in mothers was much higher than for mothers with a non-handicapped child of similar age in the Isle of Wight Study (Rutter *et al.*, 1970).

It is interesting to note that both in Tew's study and in the GLC survey, there was no evidence that mothers showed less distress if their child was only mildly handicapped. In such a case parents still appear to experience much anxiety, perhaps because it is then harder to judge what to expect of the child. If there is obvious handicap, this is difficult to adjust to initially, but once over that hurdle parents know that they must modify their expectations. With a mild handicap, the child is trying to compete fully in the normal world and parents are often unsure when they should make allowances for the child or when they should, for his own sake, be very tough with him.

One factor in these studies which seemed to be related to maternal distress was incontinence; in both studies the children were aged between $5\frac{1}{2}$ and 10 years and parents were probably still trying to establish the best method of managing incontinence. In the GLC study a significant association was found between both bowel and bladder incontinence in the child and maternal distress, particularly in cases where the child had a urinary appliance (in most cases recently acquired) or where the bowel incontinence was said to be 'regulated' (i.e. a degree of social control had been achieved) or 'poor'. Management of the young child's urinary diversion imposes a very heavy burden on the mother. Sometimes a grandmother, aunt or older sister will learn how to change the appliance but it is not an easy skill to acquire, and findings from the GLC study for 6-year-olds with diversions indicate that only a small percentage even of fathers could cope with the diversion unaided. In such cases the mother is tied to the child in a very direct and compelling way: the child simply cannot function adequately without her care. The fact that no association was found in Dorner's study (1976) between maternal depression or stress and the degree or type of handicap including incontinence may have been because these were mothers of teenagers for whom management routines had probably been established for quite a long time.

Two other points must be made before concluding this section. The first is that it is not only mothers of spina bifida children who experience high levels of stress. Bradshaw (1975) has carried out a study of 303 families with handicapped children who applied to the Family Fund for help. The children were all severely handicapped, but for a great variety of reasons. The average level of stress (measured on the Malaise Inventory) was higher than in 'any other sample the scale has ever been administered to': however, mothers of children with conditions as varied as cerebral palsy, severe mental retardation, muscular dystrophy and deafness were just as likely to experience stress as were mothers of spina bifida children.

The other important point to come out of Bradshaw's study was that although the amount of stress experienced by a mother was related partly to features of her environment (including, for example, her financial resources, whether she was able to work outside the home if she so wished, the amount of help and support received from relatives and friends, the child's health, whether the child played normally, and whether he was normally active) these factors were not by themselves enough to explain why some mothers experienced comparatively little stress and others a great deal. Clearly there are other factors operating which are more difficult to quantify and to study, such as the quality of the marital relationship or the mother's personality. These must be taken into account in any attempt to understand stress in mothers with non-handicapped and handicapped children alike.

The effect on the siblings

Relatively little research has been done into the ways in which the presence of a handicapped child affects the other children in the family, although one child psychiatrist has written that she has 'frequently seen siblings of handicapped children with emotional problems more severe than those of the handicapped youngsters themselves' (Poznanski,

1973). This is not surprising since the general anxiety in the home created by the problems of the handicapped child and the fact that the attention of the parents and other adults is likely to be focused on him will almost certainly affect the other children in the family.

The severe physical problems of many spina bifida children mean that a mother has to spend a great deal of time on their care. In Woodburn's Scottish Survey (1973) about two-thirds of parents felt that more time had to be spent with the handicapped child than with the other children and about half of these thought it was a substantially larger amount of time. A younger able-bodied child in particular may be unable to understand this. He finds that he is being urged to independence, and that his mother is spending less and less time on his bodily needs while his handicapped sibling is still receiving a good deal of physical care. A child with poor balance will need help with dressing, especially with shoes, socks and trousers since it is difficult for a child to fit these onto anaesthetized feet or legs, and a child with poor hand function (see chapter 5) will find it hard to manipulate caliper straps, or fasteners. The amount of time required for the care of incontinent children can be particularly distressing for their brothers and sisters. Older siblings may be embarrassed by the prominence of this problem within the family, and the younger ones may resent the time that this requires of the parents, even when they are obviously very fond of the handicappd child.

Many mothers in the GLC survey with a 6-year-old spina bifida child felt that the other children's activities had been restricted by the presence of the handicapped child. They could not easily be taken even to the local park, or to visit friends with other small children unless within walking distance, and trips further afield to the zoo, the seaside, the countryside or a museum were usually out of the question. Indeed this was the one restriction on the family that they commented on most frequently. It was felt most strongly, of course, during school holidays when mothers would normally have tried to arrange special trips of some kind, these often being impossible if the handicapped child had to be included.

The apprehension parents feel about a handicapped child's health and progress may produce an undercurrent of heightened anxiety in the home, present much of the time, but felt particularly acutely if the child needs to be admitted to hospital, or if there is a possibility that the valve is not working well. Even if parents are able to control their anxieties on a day-to-day basis, these episodes of illness or treatment will inevitably cause tension, and during such times the whole family will suffer. During a hospital admission it is impossible to shield the other children completely from the ill effects. The whole family routine is disrupted while the parents endeavour to spend as much time as possible at the hospital; meals are hastily prepared, treats are neglected and events important to the siblings may be overlooked. At such times the parents may be tense, short-tempered and preoccupied and as Burton (1975) points out in her study of children with cystic fibrosis, the siblings tend to 'view parental preoccupation as a rejection of themselves'. In addition they may miss the handicapped child following admission, and worry over his safety and well-being (Freeston, 1971a; Hunt, 1973). In the GLC survey of 3-year-old children, half of the siblings showed anxieties of some kind when the spina bifida child was admitted to hospital and, as was pointed out earlier (p. 41), hospital admission is a frequent occurrence in the life of the young child with myelomeningocele.

Burton (1975) noted in her study that older siblings reacted to a chronically sick child differently from younger siblings. The older children tended to have a more positive reaction; they often felt very responsible for the handicapped child, helped to care for him and treated him protectively, sometimes even when he was making unreasonable demands or being aggressive. The handicapped child's younger siblings on the other hand were quite understandably much more likely to show jealousy and resentment. However, more often this took the form of cheek or defiance towards the parents, than of spiteful behaviour towards the handicapped sibling. Both Burton (1975) and Kew (1975) in his study of families with a handicapped child, point out that this jealousy is of course simply an extension of the sibling rivalry found in all families. Where there is one child who constantly demands and receives much of his parents' time and attention, at the expense of the others, it is difficult to avoid some feeling of resentment, although many parents find it possible to compensate their other children in some way.

Siblings who are distressed may show this in their behaviour at school. In the South Wales Study (Tew and Laurence, 1975) teachers were asked to complete the Bristol Social Adjustment Guide (BSAG) for the siblings of spina bifida children and for a control group of children without a handicapped sibling. Where there was a handicapped child in the family, the children were much more likely to show disturbance as measured by this scale. No simple relationship was found between BSAG scores and the degree of handicap in the child, and indeed some of the highest disturbance scores were found in children with a mildly handicapped sibling.

It is clearly helpful if siblings are given information appropriate to their ages about the handicapped child's problems and an explanation of why the child needs so much attention, but often this does not seem to be done. Burton (1975) for example found that in over half the families she studied the mother had never discussed the child's handicap with her other children, and when explanations were given these were often very limited. As she points out, this attitude 'did little to allay the anxieties and frustrations of the well siblings and may have contributed to the problem behaviours they displayed'. It is also important to remember that the siblings are going to have to come to terms with the attitudes to their handicapped brother or sister of other people, including their peers, from outside the home. They are often quick to perceive the social stigma attached to handicap and this may be reflected in their unwillingness to bring their friends into the home. It is only through frank discussion of the child's condition and how to explain it to others that the non-handicapped sibling can be helped to accept it. As Burton (1975) observed, many parents will need help 'in deciding how best to answer their well children's questions and how to give age-appropriate and anxiety allaying explanations, where no spontaneous queries had occurred'.

Although these problems do exist it must also be stressed that the great majority of siblings are said by parents to be generally helpful and understanding towards the handicapped child, and relatively few show overt jealousy or resentment (Richards and McIntosh, 1973; Walker *et al.*, 1971; Burton, 1975; Kew, 1975). This was certainly the experience of mothers in the GLC survey, where most siblings were no trouble to their parents and said to be helpful and friendly towards the handicapped child. Indeed parents sometimes comment on the positive aspects and explain how much more understanding and sympathetic the normal siblings have become as a result of their experience of handicaps (Woodburn, 1973).

Attitudes of parents to the handicapped child

It is commonly said by teachers, nurses, social workers and other professional people involved with them that mothers frequently 'over-protect' their handicapped children. This concept of over-protection has been questioned by Hewett (1970) on the grounds that 'the point at which reasonable care of children becomes over-protection is difficult to establish with any degree of justice or accuracy, even when the child is normal'. It may be very difficult for parents to judge whether it is right or even practicable to urge early independence on a child who, because of his handicap, is quite inescapably dependent. Another view commonly put forward is that parents of handicapped children often feel guilty about their child and therefore over-react to this by being extra compassionate or over-protective. Again, as Hewett points out, mothers of completely normal four-year-olds in the Nottingham study (Newson and Newson, 1968) had many misgivings about their own competence and 'frequently expressed feelings of guilt because of failure to be the sort of mother they considered to be ideal'. Guilt feelings of this kind seem to be a natural part of motherhood and not something peculiar to those with handicapped children.

It is perhaps more accurate and less judgemental to say that parents of spina bifida children often treat them as if they were younger than their chronological age. This is hardly surprising since the child himself behaves as if he were younger in terms of mobility and incontinence, while intellectual impairment may sometimes also contribute to the problem. A child who is heavily handicapped often looks younger than his age because he is rarely in an upright position and may move about on the floor like an infant. Lack of development in the lower limbs may make him short in stature even when upright. Inexperience may also make a child appear younger than he really is.

A heavily handicapped child seldom has the experience of doing things away from adults. They may indeed be in the next room or in the garden, but he is rarely if ever out of earshot or sight of grown-ups. Mothers with spina bifida children aged 6 years were asked if their child ever went outside the house or garden unaccompanied by an adult. Very few of the heavily handicapped did so compared with the more mobile children. These children have limited opportunity, therefore, to experiment in new situations without adult supervision, or to do 'forbidden' things which help normal youngsters to acquire independence and self-confidence.

Some of what is called over-protection arises from parental confusion about what to expect of a handicapped child, or from lack of information. Anxieties about the child's safety may mean that he is not given the opportunity to exploit even his limited potential for mobility. Being unclear about the extent of his sensation or muscular control, parents are reluctant to attempt to toilet train a child lest they make impossible demands on him. With the time she can spend with her other children already severely limited, it is not unreasonable for a mother to dress her handicapped child herself rather than watch patiently a clumsy, ill-balanced child's attempts to half-clothe himself, especially since she has often little idea of the age at which a child is actually capable of doing such things. Even though it may sometimes be necessary or expedient to treat the child physically as if he were a younger age, it is not necessary, but unfortunately too easy, to behave towards him as if he were younger in *every* way, and particularly as if he were emotionally younger than his chronological age. This often means that the same demands are not made on the child as on his normal siblings.

A further problem with many spina bifida children is that they are frequently 'off-colour' because of minor infections, usually urinary tract infections, but sometimes also infections of the respiratory tract. In a few cases, the valve goes through long periods of working sluggishly or 'sticking' and this also makes the child feel lethargic or unwell. At such times parents, quite reasonably, put less pressure on the child to be independent. Following a period of hospitalization, also, a child may regress somewhat and insist that the parents give him more attention or become more permissive. The fact that spina bifida children are often sick as well as handicapped makes it doubly difficult for parents to be constantly firm with them.

Not surprisingly many parents experience problems with discipline or over the routine management of such things as eating or sleeping. Difficulty in getting a child to sleep or disturbed nights were frequently experienced by the mothers of 3 year olds in the GLC survey and 20 per cent of these children had a serious sleeping problem of some kind. Many children resisted going upstairs, sometimes for several hours, and could only be put in bed when they finally fell asleep in the living-room. 14 per cent of children were taken into their parents' bed regularly because of disturbed sleep. Sleeping problems often originated when the child became fearful or clinging following hospitalization. In all these cases, parents felt at a loss to know how to alter the unacceptable habits that had developed or who to ask for assistance. The same problem occurs, of course, for parents of non-handicapped children who may also not know to whom to turn for advice. Nevertheless it was a source of grievance to some parents that when they discussed this with the doctor at the out-patient clinic they were simply assured that the child would 'grow out of it', and given no practical advice on how to speed up this process.

On the other hand very few parents (4 per cent) found their handicapped child really difficult to manage, and less than 6 per cent of children were said to have frequent temper tantrums. While the numbers experiencing these very severe management problems were quite small, the distress caused was severe in some cases. Judging from the mother's answers to questions and her attitude towards the child during testing, about 10 per cent of mothers in the GLC study were thought to have poor relationships with their children, and to need expert help. This was usually because of an excessively indulgent attitude, but a few mothers were unnecessarily strict or critical of their children.

The most common observation made of the mother–child relationship was the fact that the bond between the two was often extremely close. In some cases they were never separated even for a few hours, except perhaps when the child was an in-patient, and because of the physical dependency of the child they were constantly in close bodily proximity. This was no great problem to mother or child during the early years, except in extreme cases where the child would complain or 'grizzle' if the mother was out of sight for longer than a few minutes. Many children had difficulty in attending school initially, being very tearful or withdrawn for several weeks, but this could be dealt with by understanding teachers or welfare assistants. The real problem with the over-close parental bond comes at a later stage, during adolescence, when the young person must loosen the ties if he is ever to become an adult. This subject will be dealt with more fully in chapter 9, but it is important to realize that it is during the child's early years that these behaviour patterns develop and that tactful guidance given to parents at this stage can lay the basis for better parent–child relationships in the later years.

In discussions with parents about their handicapped children in the GLC study a striking tendency for parents to underplay their negative feelings towards the child was noticed. This is only natural of course, particularly when a mother is being interviewed by a relative stranger. However, most parents feel their children to be a nuisance at times, even when they are quite normal, and the constant attention that a handicapped child demands does in fact curtail the parents' freedom and independence far more than a non-handicapped child would do.

Parents find it hard to admit that they have feelings of resentment at times and express guilt when they do so. While it cannot be assumed that every parent feels resentful, many do, and in most cases they have never been helped to explore such feelings or told that it is perfectly natural to feel over-burdened from time to time. Many parents half hope that the child will die during periods of serious illness but each tends to think that his reaction is unique. For example, in the GLC survey, when it was pointed out to a mother that it is common for parents to hope that the child will not survive the operations performed at birth, she often expressed great relief, each mother having believed that she was alone in having had such a thought. Of course not all parents feel anger or resentment and, as Martin (1975) stresses, parental response to a handicapped child will differ from one individual to another. However, when such feelings do occur parents must be helped to admit them and accept them as justifiable, provided that the child is not made to feel responsible. Parents can then be encouraged to organize their lives in such a way that they can relinquish the care of the child to others from time to time (which can benefit the child too). They also need encouragement in trying to overcome in other ways the limiting effect that the handicap has on the family life.

This chapter perhaps paints too gloomy a scene, since it concentrates on the problems experienced by families. However it has been a consistent finding among researchers working with families who have children handicapped in various ways that many families attain a remarkable degree of harmony and satisfaction in spite of all their problems. As Dorner states in his account (1976) of families where there was a teenager with spina bifida: 'It cannot be concluded . . . that a poor quality of life is inevitable . . . since there were a number of families who, because of the resilience of some or all of the members, the supportiveness of the marriage, or for other reasons, had made a good adjustment to the problems of handicap.' The point we wish to stress, however, is that many families do need help and this help is not always forthcoming. As Walker and his colleagues have remarked 'there seems to be an imbalance between attention given to the child's physical needs and the needs of the family. . . . The social and psychological management of the family must improve to the point where it matches the high standard of clinical care available for the child' (Walker *et al.*, 1971). Suggestions about how this can be done are made in the next chapter.

References

Bayley, M. (1973), *Mental Handicap and Community Care*, Routledge and Kegan Paul, London and Boston.

Bradshaw, J. (1975), 'Tracing the cause stress in families with handicapped children', unpublished manuscript, Department of Social Administration, University of York.

Burton, L. (1975), *The Family Life of Sick Children*, Routledge and Kegan Paul, London and Boston.

Dorner, S. (1976), 'The relationship of physical handicaps to stress in families with an adolescent with spina bifida', *Archives of Diseases in Childhood*, 51, pp. 439–44.

Fox, M. (1974), 'They get this training but they don't know how you feel', Action Research for the Crippled Child.

Freeston, B. M. (1971a), 'Caring for a child with spina bifida', report to Association for Spina Bifida and Hydrocephalus.

——, (1971b), 'An enquiry into the effect of a spina bifida child upon family life', *Developmental Medicine and Child Neurology*, 13, pp. 456–61.

Halliday, J., Rawlings, H. E. and Whipp, M. A. (1965), 'The spina bifida/hydrocephalic child in the community', *The Practitioner*, 195, pp. 346–50.

Harf, E. H., Laurence, K. M., Payne Helly, Rawnsley, K., (1966), 'Spina Bifida Cystica and Family Stress'. British Medical Journal 2, pp. 757–760.

Henley, T. E. and Albam, B. (1955), 'A psychiatric study of muscular dystrophy. The role of the social worker', *American Journal of Physical Medicine*, 34, pp. 358–64.

Hewett, S. (1970), *The Family and the Handicapped Child*, Allen and Unwin, London.

Hunt, G. (1973), 'Implications of the treatment of myelomeningocele for the child and his family', *Lancet*, ii, pp. 1308–10.

Kellmer Pringle, M. L. and Fiddes, D. O. (1970), *The Challenge of Thalidomide*, Longmans, London.

Kew, S. (1975), *Handicap and Family Crisis*, Pitman, London.

McMichael, J. (1971), *A Study of Physically Handicapped Children and Their Families*, Staples Press, London.

Martin, H. P. (1975), 'Parental response to handicapped children', *Developmental Medicine and Child Neurology*, 17 (2), pp. 251–2.

Newson, J. and Newson, E. (1968), *Four Years Old in an Urban Community*, Allen and Unwin, London.

Poznanski, E. O. (1973), 'Emotional issues in raising handicapped children', *Rehabilitation Literature*, 34 (ii), pp. 322–6.

Richards, I. D. G. and McIntosh, H. T. (1973), 'Spina bifida survivors and their parents: a study of problems and services', *Developmental Medicine and Child Neurology*, 15, pp. 292–304.

Richman, N. (1977), 'Depression in mothers with young children', in preparation.

Rutter, M., Tizard, J. and Whitmore, K. (1970), *Education, Health and Behaviour*, Longmans, London.

Sheridan, M. (1965), 'The handicapped child and his home', National Children's Home, London.

Spain, B. (1973), 'Spina bifida: the need for community support', GLC Intelligence Unit Quarterly Bulletin, 23, pp. 66–71.

——, and Wigley, G. (1975), *Right From the Start*, Association for Mentally Handicapped Children.

Tew, B. and Laurence, K. (1975), 'Some sources of stress found in mothers of spina bifida children', *British Journal of Preventive Medicine*, 29, pp. 27–30.

——, Payne, H. and Laurence, K. M. (1974), 'Must a family with a handicapped child be a handicapped family?', *Developmental Medicine and Child Neurology*, Supplement 32, pp. 95–8.

Walker, J. H., Thomas, M. and Russell, I. T. (1971), 'Spina bifida and the parents', *Developmental Medicine and Child Neurology*, 13, pp. 462–76.

Woodburn, M. (1973), *Social Implications of Spina Bifida – a Study in S.E. Scotland*, Eastern Branch of Scottish Spina Bifida Association, Edinburgh.

Younghusband, E., Davie, R., Birchall, D., and Kellmer Pringle, M. L. (eds.) (1970), *Living with Handicap*, National Bureau for Co-operation in Child Care, London.

4 Help for families

The number and complexity of problems described in the previous chapter no doubt gives an impression of a depressingly heavy burden of family ills for social workers and others to shoulder. However we are quite convinced, and many parents themselves have expressed the same view, that most of these problems could be alleviated, and many could be greatly reduced if help were available to families at the appropriate time.

In this chapter we shall be considering the ways in which help could be given to families with a congenitally handicapped child through the ordinary medical, social and educational services. We will make some comments initially on the general approach to such families, and then go on to consider what help families need most at particular stages in the child's development. Lastly, we shall look at the organization of services as they exist at present and suggest some ways in which these could be made to cater more effectively for family needs.

General approach to families with handicapped children

Understanding parents' reactions to stress

Distress symptoms shown by families with a handicapped child are often considered to be as 'neurotic', in the sense of indicating permanent or long-term personality problems. There will be of course some parents or siblings who do have long-term personality problems just because such people are to be found in any population sample. The majority, however, if they show disturbance, are behaving in a way which is very natural in view of their life situation, and cannot therefore be regarded as 'sick'.

Most people are vulnerable to extreme stress and most disturbed behaviour in the families of handicapped children is usually of this nature. Wing (1966) has pointed out in relation to autistic children that 'the tensions created by a disturbed child may bring to the fore emotional difficulties of the parents or siblings which otherwise would have remained dormant'. A spina bifida child does not pose the same behavioural problems as a child with autism, but the principle holds true for all types of handicapping conditions. While there are some parents who show very abnormal or exaggerated responses to the stress of the handicap and who need expert psychiatric care, these are relatively few and they may need expert care for a short period or only intermittently. The great majority do not require help of the psychiatric or case-work type. They simply need information, practical advice or assistance, and encouragement to help overcome their natural feelings of incompetence or inadequacy when faced with a problem of this magnitude.

Having a handicapped child inevitably causes the parents grief and anxiety, indeed, the absence of such feelings would give real cause for concern. No one can remove that grief entirely but a great deal can be done to help parents and siblings accept the things that cannot be altered and to change those which can. The high levels of family problems of various kinds recounted in the previous chapter are measures of our own failure to come to terms with the problems of handicap rather than the failure of the families. As Woodburn (1973) states, 'All families with spina bifida children are at risk of developing pathological patterns of behaviour unless society recognizes the extent, the degree and the complexity of the demands made on them, and unless help is actively offered and appropriate to need.'

Increasing parental self-confidence

The main task of any professional worker involved in the care of the child or his family must be to increase the confidence of parents in their own ability to care for the child. As one parent explained, the aim should be 'to help them a bit, but not a lot – you know – to be able to do things for themselves' (Hewett, 1970). The parents' attitudes and activities will be the main influences on a child's progress and consequently nothing that professional people themselves can offer to the child will have as great an impact on him as the counselling that they give to the parents. First and foremost parents must be helped to recognize their own value as therapists or educators in the broadest sense.

Parents often feel, both initially and at later stages, unequal to the task of rearing a handicapped child. There is at present little real appreciation of this and systematic attempts to ensure that parents do develop confidence in themselves or have the necessary background knowledge are seldom made. As Richards and McIntosh (1973) have remarked about families with pre-school children, 'The overall impression gained . . . is of a group of parents who are completely bewildered and lacking in any appreciation of the nature or consequences of spina bifida, or of what the future is likely to hold for their children.' It is essential that parents be given the fullest information about their child's condition and the likely consequences, and that they be helped to develop the skills that they will need in order to observe, assess and teach him.

Parents as participants not as clients

In order to utilize fully the resources within the family, parents must be regarded as participators in treatment; as people who can both carry out instructions given *and who themselves* can offer important suggestions (Younghusband *et al.*, 1970). In order to elicit full parental co-operation and to develop the parents' abilities as therapists, professional people must treat parents as colleagues, rather than as clients or patients. This is not to imply that parents are able or should be expected to take over the functions of professionals, nor does it deny the role of the professional as one who can offer information and specialized skills. What we are suggesting is, first, that these skills can be most efficiently used if they are disseminated to those involved in the child's day-to-day care, especially to parents, rather than remaining the exclusive prerogative of any particular profession, and, second, that parenthood itself must be respected as a profession, as valid and requiring as much knowledge and skill as any other. One mother described the attitude of many professional people very accurately: 'They speak as though they know more than me . . . or better than me . . . about my own child. They won't accept what I have to say. That's what people in authority are like . . . I still have this feeling Mr G. [a surgeon] doesn't take any notice of me, there's this barrier there, and it's as though I'm just ignorant, not worth talking to . . . because I wouldn't understand what he said' (Fox, 1974). It is common to single out the medical profession for this sort of criticism, but all professionals are capable of responding to parents in this way.

Involving the father

Throughout this chapter we will speak mainly of the 'parents' rather than of the 'mothers', except where the discussion relates specifically to her. This is because we feel strongly that fathers must be more involved than is usual at present. Some fathers do participate very fully, attending out-patient clinics with the mother, helping to exercise the child or to deal with incontinence, but this is usually done on the father's own initiative, rather than because his interest has been deliberately fostered. In the GLC study only a small percentage of fathers regularly attended out-patient clinics and in Fox's study (1974) one father complained that he had never been invited to hospital visits or meetings with the school doctor, this being a common experience. The father may of course be unwilling or unable to attend but the point being made is that he must be invited. The initiative should not be left entirely with the mother since sometimes she does not encourage her husband to attend clinics in order to spare him distress. It should be made clear to the father, from the beginning, that his attendance at the clinic or the school is seen to be important. Undoubtedly the support and help that a fully participating father can give to the family far exceeds anything that can be offered by professional people. Burton (1975) for example in her study of families of a child with cystic fibrosis found that 'parents adapted best to the illness where they mutually accepted responsibilty for treatment'. Consequently, it should be one of the prime concerns of professionals to foster the father's involvement.

A related point made by Nordqvist (1972) is that sometimes the father would welcome the opportunity to talk about the child's condition and his own or his family's response to this, but is not sure how to set about this. He may also feel at a disadvantage insofar as the mother usually has more information about the child than he does. The father should, therefore, be given the opportunity of having a consultation with the doctor or other professional on his own so that he can be as well informed as the mother and has the chance to discuss his feelings about the handicap if he wishes to.

Contact with other parents

Professional people also need to accept their own limitations in helping parents in that they have not themselves experienced the pain of having a handicapped child. As one mother said in relation to social workers, 'I know they don't really know how you feel . . . I would have liked someone who had the same, or nearly the same problem . . . . A parent, someone you could have really poured out your heart to and known that they could have fully understood' (Fox, 1974). Parents give each other a different kind of help from that which can be offered by professionals. This is not necessarily *better* help but for some parents it may be as important as help from professionals. Certainly parents can learn a great deal from each other about day-to-day management. Professional people should recognize this and initiate contact between families in similar situations.

It should also be appreciated, however, that some families do not wish to discuss their feelings with others, or feel their child's combination of handicaps to be unique so that advice from others seems quite irrelevant. In the Richards and McIntosh study (1973), for example, less than half of the couples interviewed were members of ASBAH (the Association for Spina Bifida and Hydrocephalus) and some did not want to join, especially those whose children were minimally handicapped. Nevertheless, opportunities for families to meet should always be offered, especially since there are some parents who would like occasionally to discuss a particular problem with someone in a similar situation but who are 'non-joiners' and would not wish to belong to any formal association.

Accepting parental aggression

A final general point which needs to be made is that from time to time parents inevitably feel anger, perhaps against fate, perhaps because of some administrative or professional ineptitude, or they may be so tense and edgy that their patience wears thin. At such times they may well appear aggressive or demanding and even ungrateful towards those who are trying to help them. Learning how to accept parents' anger, realizing that it is not personal, and understanding and sympathizing with the underlying reasons is an essential part of a professional's role. If parents are treated with understanding at such times they are themselves likely to become more tolerant of shortcomings in the professionals.

The help needed at different stages

The birth and the first year

Breaking the news to the parents. Telling parents that their child is handicapped is a very difficult and distressing task and for these reasons it is often done rather ineptly (Woodburn, 1973; Walker *et al.*, 1971; Spain, 1973). Sometimes it is left to an inexperienced junior member of staff, even though this is a task requiring emotional maturity on the part of the medical and nursing staff as well as the allocation of considerable time. This is by no means a situation unique to spina bifida, but is reported commonly in many studies where parents' views on services have been sought (Hewett, 1970). In the GLC survey, mothers were asked to say what was the one thing which, in their experience, was most needlessly distressing or which they felt could have been handled better. Without any hesitation, 25 per cent of the mothers spoke of the way that they had been first told of the handicap, or of how they had been treated during the subsequent days, even though the child was 6 years old at the time they were interviewed and much had happened in the intervening period.

Although this is inevitably a sorrowful time for parents, distress is, on occasion, 'aggravated by lack of awareness of the mother's feelings . . . or by the assumption that it was better that she should not give vent to them' (Woodburn, 1973). As the Newcastle study suggests, it appears that staff in maternity units devote 'more energy to making arrangements for the transfer of the child for surgical care than they do to dealing with the shock and bewilderment of the parents', and the point is made that 'as much skill must be applied to the care of the parents as to the child's malformation' (Walker *et al.*, 1971).

Parents' needs at such times are very thoroughly discussed in *Right From the Start*, published by NSMHC (Spain and Wigley, 1975). In brief, parents must be told the truth promptly and the degree of handicap should never be minimized, but at the same time they must always be given hope. Initially, only brief information can be given but as soon as possible after the child has been assessed for treatment, a senior doctor, preferably a pædiatrician or pædiatric surgeon, should discuss the child's condition thoroughly, with both parents present if possible, in order to decide whether or not to operate and to explain fully the consequences of this decision for the child and for the family. Parents will need to have this information repeated to them at intervals since they cannot usually digest all the facts or their implications on first telling, partly because they are distraught but also because the facts in themselves are very complex for someone with no medical background to understand. Many parents find printed information and instructions helpful. This is a good time to suggest to the father the importance of his future role and to encourage him to visit the child in hospital and to attend subsequent out-patient clinics. The whole question of how this service could be improved is discussed in the final section of this chapter.

Many parents will need the help of a social worker or other counsellor at this early stage. Certainly this service must be made available to them, and the social worker should explain who she is, what kind of service she can offer and how she can be contacted so that the mother can refer to her on a future occasion. It is frequently the case that parents have no idea who is their social worker or what is her role, even though many will have encountered her at some stage.

Parents commonly report that in the early weeks they hoped that the child would die, but feel very guilty about this, not realizing that it is a very natural and almost universal feeling. It is important to allow parents to express negative feelings of this kind and to convince them that these are not unnatural, and it is often in this connection that reassurance from another parent is most welcome. As Wing (1966) points out 'such feelings are fully compatible with normal love but the parents may not realize this unless it is clearly explained to them'. If parents can be helped to come to terms with the fact of the handicap in the early weeks and months, if someone is available who can talk to them, frequently if necessary, about their feelings and fears, answer their questions and give them hope, this will go a long way towards preventing unnecessary distress or malfunctioning at a later stage. If parents are not helped to accept the fact of the handicap and of their own negative feelings in the first few months, they may remain ambivalent towards the child, feeling needlessly guilty, and may attempt to compensate for this by being over-solicitous in their management of him, with deleterious effects on the child and on the family well-being.

If the child dies at this early stage, whether or not he is treated surgically, or in the case of a stillbirth, it should not be assumed that this is the end of the problem as far as the parents are concerned, and they should be supported in the same way 'until the period of mourning is over and emotional equilibrium restored' (Walker *et al.*, 1971). In addition, genetic counselling and family-planning advice are just as important for these families as where the child survives, this subject being fully discussed in chapter 2 and later in this section.

The role of the health visitor and other community workers. Within a few days of the birth, parents should be introduced to the health visitor or other domiciliary worker, for example a social worker, or to the community physician who will be responsible for the child's care within the community. The family GP will, of course, wish to be involved and the hospital should encourage him to participate in treatment by ensuring that he has full information on the child's treatment and progress. But unless he takes a particular interest in children, the mother will also require advice from someone who specializes in the care of young children, and the health visitor is the most obvious person to undertake this task.

Although most mothers with handicapped children seem to get little help from health visitors at present, the health visitor can, without question make an invaluable and greatly appreciated contribution, first, because her visits to the home are an accepted part of the care of all children, so her intervention is quite 'nomal'; second, because in a domiciliary visit she is able to give practical advice and counselling often impossible in a busy hospital clinic; and finally because, in her own home, the mother will have more confidence and will be better able to express her problems or discuss her fears. The health visitor can reassure the mother that she will take a general interest in the child's health and will be available for advice about whether the valve is functioning adequately or any other health or management problem. She can also offer immediate practical advice to the mother when the baby returns from hospital on feeding, bathing and handling him, matters which cause much anxiety. As one mother said, 'It's no good sympathy without action' (Fox, 1974) and there are many practical steps which the health visitor or social worker can take in the early weeks which will help to lay the foundation of her relationship with the mother. However it must be recognized that within the present framework of services health visitors in most parts of the country could not offer the detailed information or advice that mothers require, and more will be said in the final section of this chapter about the organizational changes in nursing services which might facilitate the health visitor's involvement in the care of handicapped children.

Family planning and genetic counselling. An issue which must be discussed before the mother leaves the maternity unit is the question of family planning and genetic counselling. Many studies have shown that both of these issues are frequently neglected (Richards and McIntosh, 1973; Spain, 1973; Walker *et al.*, 1971) although parents do act responsibly in respect of genetic counselling if it is offered (Carter and Roberts, 1971). The genetic implications of having a child with spina bifida have been explained in chapter 2 and this sensitive issue is discussed more fully in *Right from the Start* (Spain and Wigley, 1975) from which the following quotation is taken. 'The initiative for seeking these things [family planning and genetic counselling advice] should not be left to the parents, since they may be too preoccupied with the immediate problems to think of the future. The emotional and sexual relationships between parents may be very delicate at this time, with anxiety about the cause, and the worry of possibly having another abnormal child, but the need for mutual comfort is perhaps greater than at any point in their marriage. One's concern must be for the implications this situation has for the future marital integration, as well as for the needs of the moment. More than one approach may be necessary and the pædiatrician, social worker, health visitor and general practitioner should all feel a responsibility in ensuring that the parents do understand any genetic factors and are making use of whatever family planning services are required.'

Of course, family planning advice should never be forced on anyone. However, genetic counselling is essential and this cannot be given sensibly without also ensuring that parents know about contraceptive techniques so that they can delay or prevent a future pregnancy if they so wish. It should not be assumed that if parents fail to ask for advice this means none is wanted. Richards and McIntosh (1973) report that many mothers said they would have accepted family planning if it had been offered and they had known where to go; some were too shy to ask their GP for advice. Fortunately it is possible now to explain to parents that a future pregnancy can be screened and termination offered if the foetus is abnormal (see chapter 2), but that in order to benefit from this service it is most advisable to plan the pregnancy fully. This provides a very positive reason for initiating early discussion of family planning, which can then be seen as a step towards ensuring future healthy offspring rather than simply as a means of preventing conception.

Statutory assistance over housing and other problems. Another matter which must be considered early is the family's housing situation. This problem has been stressed in many studies both in relation to spina bifida (Walker *et al.*, 1971; Woodburn, 1973; Spain, 1973) and to handicap in general (Hewett, 1970; Curran and Swann, 1964). In Curran and Swann's study (1964) of handicapped children in Glasgow it is stated that 'so great was the complicating effect of the bad environmental conditions in which many of the children lived, that it was well-nigh impossible to study the problems inherent in the defect itself, for these were often obscured by superimposed difficulties and side-effects resulting from the conditions in which the family lived'. Quite apart from making certain that there is adequate space for the child and all the equipment that will so rapidly accumulate, and that there are adequate facilities for toileting and washing, it is also essential to ensure 'easy external access and level access to a lavatory inside the house' (Woodburn, 1973). It may not be possible to achieve any necessary rehousing or housing alterations in the early weeks, but it is better to initiate action at this point, anticipating need, rather than waiting till the need becomes urgent.

Other practical statutory assistance which can be offered, such as the attendance allowance, a disposable nappy service, or aids and equipment of various kinds, may not be appropriate or even available for the very young baby, but it is important to let the parents know that these things exist and that they can be provided as the need arises. In some cases there may be an immediate need for financial or other practical help, if the baby is in hospital at some distance from home, necessitating expensive travel or special arrangements to care for other children. Parents might be too depressed to seek help themselves over this, but it is important that the mother visits the baby regularly, and has the opportunity to feed and handle him, and that her other children are not neglected in consequence. The health visitor might be able to mobilize help from neighbours for siblings, and can inquire from the social worker whether hospital endowments or some voluntary agency could help with fares.

Information about child development and about the management of the child. Once the child reaches the age of 3 or 4 months, the parents will require information on child development, advice on how to stimulate the child and what they must do to help him progress. More will be said about this in chapter 6. In this context we must stress that information and advice on child development can save parents a great deal of unnecessary worry and confusion. As one parent said, in relation to an older child, 'How has he got on? You know what I mean, you can't ever be sure . . . you get to such a state you don't hardly know whether they are progressing, or what do they call it, regressing . . . We don't know how a handicapped child of his age should behave' (Fox, 1974).

Parents should not have to rely solely on commonsense on handling their handicapped child, particularly if there is likely to be intellectual impairment. They need to know in advance what to look out for and and also what practical steps they can take to reduce the effects of intellectual and motor abnormalities.

Help for siblings. In the previous chapter the problems of the handicapped child's siblings were discussed. Advice to parents on how to deal with the adverse reactions of their other (non-handicapped) children is also necessary in many cases, and suggestions might be made of ways to minimize these feelings or of compensating them if a certain amount of neglect is unavoidable. In a recent helpful article on this question Parfit (1975a) suggests that the needs of the siblings are for both information and emotional help. The ways in which they can best be helped depends largely on their age in relation to the handicapped child. Where they are older than the handicapped child the need for help is greater, at least in the early stages, than where they are younger. A baby growing up with a handicapped child already in the family will not see the situation as unusual until he begins to overtake the elder in skills, or grows up enough to recognize the reactions of the outside world, but at this point some intervention may be required.

The first essential is for information. Parfit thinks that once a handicap has been diagnosed information must be given to the older siblings as soon as possible (in a way appropriate to their age) about its nature and cause. Younger children should be told about the handicap as soon as they begin to notice differences. Parents may need advice from professionals in doing this. The sibs also need to be helped to know what to tell their friends and teachers. When they are older they need, as much as do the parents (see chapter 2), to talk over any possible genetic implications of the presence of handicap in the family before they themselves get married. Also, suggests Parfit, they must take part in the future plans for the handicapped child since 'many an older sib must dread the thought of being saddled with the responsibility for life of a handicapped adult brother or sister once their parents get too old to carry the burden or die. These fears need to be faced openly . . . and alternative and contingency plans made so that all can plan their lives accordingly.

Inevitably, the presence of the handicapped child will create some difficulties for the siblings and in some cases strong emotional reactions. Again, the way in which siblings are best helped to deal with their feelings will depend on their age. For young children physical reassurance that they are loved and wanted will be more important and, suggests Parfit, 'this is a role the father could make his own, becoming the main support and provider of extra and individual time and attention'. For older children emotional reactions need to be brought into the open where possible through discussions and conversations. As Wing (1966) has pointed out in relation to siblings, 'There is no point in pretending that there is no sadness in the world, but they will learn as well that there is a constructive way to deal with problems.' Presented in such a way the experience will be useful to them in later life, and should not impede their development.

Informal discussions and practical help between parents. Parents can be put in touch with each other on an individual basis from soon after the birth, but later on they may benefit from discussions with others in a group. While the idea of a formal 'discussion group' might well be very off-putting, opportunities can be created where informal discussions can occur. For example, two London boroughs, Lewisham and Greenwich, provide a weekly crèche for spina bifida babies in an infant welfare clinic, and the mothers spend some time chatting together while the children are cared for elsewhere. Sometimes this is just gossip, but the health visitor who runs the crèche can help guide the discussion if a mother introduces deeper issues about her feelings or anxieties.

Issues such as the dangers of an excessively close bond between parent and child or an over-solicitous attitude to him sometimes can also be discussed usefully in group sessions. It is exceedingly difficult for parents to recognize whether the assistance they are giving to the child is essential or whether they are holding back his development by giving too much help. Woodburn (1973) points out, in discussing Schaffer's concept (1964) of the 'too cohesive family', that 'paradoxically such malfunctioning families were likely to get the approval of society since they devoted so much time and effort to the child and they seldom asked for help'. In later years, however, when the child fails to mature emotionally and shows too great a dependency on his family, the parents are often blamed for this. The correct time for professional intervention is in the early months and years of life, and not when the family has fully established its internal relationships. If they have not helped to make parents aware of these dangers at an early stage the professionals must accept some of the responsibility for the resulting problems.

If the group can be encouraged to organize a baby-sitting rota, this can help the parents to overcome any tendency to feel that the child is 'unsafe', if they are not around or that no one else can be trusted with his care. One parent said 'You're frightened to leave her with anyone: neither of us can get out, not together . . . . In five years we've never been outside the door, only to work'. Tizard and Grad (1961) showed that families with a handicapped child at home tended to reduce social contact to a minimum, and this is something that can be avoided if action is taken early on. Reciprocal baby-sitting is something which can easily be arranged on a voluntary basis, but it often requires some professional person to take the initiative in suggesting it or in helping to arrange a rota.

Particularly vulnerable groups. Special attention should be paid to the needs of unmarried mothers or to cases where the marriage may be at risk, for example if the parents are very young or the child was conceived pre-nuptially. Mothers who conceived by accident during the menopause are another group who need extra help. Being older, the physical strain of a handicapped child is more of a problem to them and they are also much more likely to worry about the future than are younger mothers. Also it should not be assumed that the parents of children who are mildly handicapped have no need for counselling or support, since the evidence reviewed in chapter 3 suggests that these families are also vulnerable.

The older pre-school child

Providing the parents with information about the child's condition and about treatment. Perhaps the greatest continuing need of parents is to understand fully the child's medical condition and the reasons for the orthopædic, urinary or other treatment that he receives. Parents commonly feel that the hospital staff does not do enough to help them in this way, as shown in chapter 3. As one mother said, 'they never explain something to you . . . they never take the time to explain' (Fox, 1974). Very often hospital doctors simply do not have much time to spend with any individual patient, nor do they always have a talent for communicating with lay people. Often explanations are given to parents but they cannot comprehend or remember these when they only hear them once and have little opportunity for further questioning. However, as Woodburn (1973) has pointed out medical effort may fail ultimately simply because the family did not understand the implications for them. She uses the example of a urinary diversion which sometimes causes management problems 'greater than those of the incontinence which precedes it. The operation might have a life-saving purpose, but unless the parents could be helped to use the appliance efficiently they were left with apparently even greater practical problems of daily routine than before.' In the Glasgow study (Richards and McIntosh, 1973) only 21 out of 86 mothers felt that they had been given adequate information about the general management of the child. Of the 76 mothers who expressed their views on the child's prognosis, 68 felt that they were expecting the handicap to be 'cured', or at least greatly reduced'. A suitably trained health visitor could obtain additional medical information on the parents' behalf, could elaborate on the explanations given at the hospital, and ensure that the parents do understand the nature of the treatment and why it is necessary. The hospital could use her quite systematically to communicate complex information to the family and to discuss with her the effect of treatment or the child's progress.

Practical help which professionals can provide. Information about how to get practical or financial help must be offered to parents to ensure that they benefit from the attendance allowance, the Family Fund, the mobility allowance a home help service, free disposable nappies or a laundry service, wheelchairs or other equipment, or adaptations to the home. These practical aids can relieve the parents of some of the everyday chores and pressures which can cumulatively produce exhaustion, irritability and depression.

Baby-sitting arrangements of some kind become more important now, together with some day crèche or nursery provision, to give the parents a break from the child's continuous care. Arrangements for some day care in the school holidays is most important if there are older children, so that the mother can devote more time to them and take them on visits. Pre-school experience has many advantages for the development of the child of course, as explained in chapter 6; it can also give the mother an opportunity to compare her child's progress with that of other children of a comparable age. There will be a continuing need for developmental advice and also for advice on common management problems. Counselling of this kind can be given on an individual basis by the health visitor, pædiatrician or social worker, but parent groups can also be beneficial in some cases.

More formal parent discussion groups. Parents can often help each other most at points of particular crisis. It appears that after the birth trauma has been dealt with, the next crisis occurs at about 18 months to 2 years, when the child fails to walk or stand like other children, and then again in the third or fourth year when the choice of school must be made, especially if special schooling is required. The opportunity to discuss their feelings and disappointments with others who have been through the same experience can often be very comforting to parents. However, each family's solution to the problem is likely to be different and these differences must be respected.

At this stage there may be a need for more formal parent groups which can often be provided for the parents of children with different handicaps who share the same pre-school facilities, or attend the same hospital. An example of such a group is given by Wilson (1971) who arranged parent meetings to discuss such things as how to help the child to learn, ways of guarding against overprotection, and society's acceptance of physical handicap. During some sessions speakers were invited to give information about particular topics such as transport or social services. The group was run in conjunction with a recreation programme for the children which facilitated parents' attendance. Where there is no one available to lead a group of this sort, it may be possible to have a parent leader. Groups for mothers with a mentally retarded child have been running successfully in the Southend area, with leadership shared between the community physician and a parent (Crowe, 1975), and provided that guidance is given, this seems quite feasible if the right person can be found.

Community support for the family. Mobilizing support for the family within their own local community is another important activity that could be initiated by the health visitor or other local worker. Families are often apprehensive about the reaction of others to the handicapped child, and are inclined to interpret embarrassment or curiosity as rejection. One mother said 'I think the most important thing for the mother's happiness is to know that people . . . I should think 99 per cent of the general public . . . have sympathy and are kind. That you don't have to hide them away and all that, but that most people want to help you. They're curious but they're not nasty' (Hewett, 1970). Bayley (1973) in his study of families with a mentally retarded member points out that 'the actual help already given by the community was considerable and the potential even greater'. He found that the kind of help most needed by families was with everyday matters such as shopping or keeping an eye on the child from time to time and could best be given by people living close at hand, rather than by statutory services. Social workers could, he suggests, help mobilize this kind of local, neighbourly assistance which is 'complementary to and . . . interwoven with' social services provision. That families do need help even in involving relatives is also indicated in other studies. For example

Burton (1975) points out that among families with a child suffering from cystic fibrosis 'the desire not to hurt relatives by stressing the severity of the disease was widespread . . . this precluded any possibility of mutual assistance in facing up to the illness'. There would of course be direct financial advantages to the Health and Social Services if the local community were encouraged to help. But most important of all would be the knowledge the parents would gain that they were not alone in their struggles, and that the child was lovable and acceptable to those outside the family circle.

Schooling and the post-school years

Incontinence management. A major problem as the spina bifida child grows older is incontinence management. For most boys a penile bag will suffice for the social control of the bladder, but for some boys and nearly all the girls, a urinary diversion will be needed (see chapter 1). Unless the kidneys are at risk it is important that this operation is delayed until both parents have accepted the need for it. People usually find the appliance distasteful and difficult to handle initially, and they can come to terms with this much more readily once they have accepted that there is no alternative. Sometimes the operation has been over-sold to parents and they expect all their troubles to be over once it has been done. It is essential to ensure that parents fully understand what effect the operation will have and are aware in advance of possible problems in managing the appliance. Discussions with other parents and an opportunity to observe them changing the child's appliance would be a great help. The mother should have reached a reasonable level of competence in dealing with the appliance before the child leaves hospital and, whenever possible, the father should also be given some instruction. Once the child is home, domiciliary visits are required to reassure the mother who lacks confidence and to offer information on management. Down Brothers and the other major manufacturers employ a team of nurses who will give advice on the management of appliances including how to avoid odour, how to teach the child to care for his own appliance or related problems. They are willing to visit schools, parent groups or individuals and can be contacted directly (see Appendix G).

Bowel incontinence may well be a greater social problem but very often parents get little help unless it is very severe. Some suggestions on possible management routines are given by Forsythe and Kinley (1970) and also in *Link* magazine (Webster, 1975) and Woodburn (1973) has some useful information as well. It is a question of trial and error with each child to find the right combination of medicines, suppositories or toileting regimes, which will suit him and will also fit in with the family routine. Parents need much reassurance and support over this most distressing problem. Once again, advice from other parents often proves particularly useful but a health visitor who visited regularly could be a great help in suggesting alternative strategies.

This whole area of incontinence is one where it is most essential to involve the father and, if possible, some other adult member of the family or close family friend. Almost invariably at present it is only the mother who knows how to renew the appliance, even though others may know how to empty the bag. This is a great source of stress to the mother (see chapter 3) because it means that she can never be apart from the child for more than a few hours, except when he is at a special school or in hospital. Although in practice this may not be all that different from contact with her other children, the feeling that the child is so completely dependent on her throughout his school life and possibly even later is a great psychological burden. It would make a great difference if at least one other person could be taught to handle the appliance but it may require the intervention of some professional person to bring this about, since the mother may be unwilling to ask anyone else for help. Eventually the child himself must learn how to care for his own appliance. It was suggested in chapter 1 that behaviour modification techniques might be useful in training children with appliances and that parent groups might be formed to teach them the principles of this technique and supervize the child's training. The special school might be the most appropriate place from which to organize this training, so that school and home practice could be co-ordinated to help the child achieve independence as early as possible. Parents of children attending normal school also need this help and these parents might be invited to the training sessions, or possibly a special hospital-based group could be set up for them.

Short-term residential facilities for children. It is important for both the child and his family that he should learn to live independently from them while he is still young and it is also helpful for family harmony if there can be occasional periods of relief from the continual strain of his care. Local residential accommodation should be provided for occasional relief or in times of crisis, but in the absence of this, holiday homes would be a considerable help. Some facilities of this type do exist and information can be obtained from ASBAH headquarters. Nancy Allum's book for parents (1975) also contains some useful addresses. Parents may need some persuasion, initially, to part with their children but are invariably delighted with the outcome and social workers or health visitors should encourage parents to do this.

Liaison with the school. Good liaison between the home and the school is essential during the school years. Regular PTA meetings and individual discussions between the parent and the class teacher would avert much of the misunderstanding and friction which sometimes now occur between parents and staff. Parents would feel reassured if they understood better how the child was faring at school and if his progress were discussed with them from time to time. Information could be given via the school about equipment and services, and parent groups could be organized to discuss particular problems, such as incontinence management.

Advice on helping adolescents. As the child reaches puberty he is likely to become more self-conscious and more subject to moods, and his parents may then be particularly anxious and needful of advice. They will experience pain as they see their child begin to suffer from the limitations that his handicap imposes and they will also have to try to help him become as mature and independent as possible. It is difficult for most parents to accept their child's growing independence during his teens since this conflicts with their natural desire to protect him from painful experiences or possible harm, and this dilemma is multiplied when the child is handicapped so that specially skilled advice may be required at this stage. It is also important that parents are informed about the likelihood of early puberty in girls which occurs sometimes at nine years old, though more commonly at eleven, so that they can discuss the menarche with the girl well in advance.

The organization of services

One of the most striking findings in all the studies of families with a handicapped child is the haphazard nature of provision made for them, and the number of different agencies involved; sometimes services are delivered very well because there happens to be one person – a health visitor, GP, or social worker – who takes an interest and suggests help. Sometimes the parents themselves energetically seek advice and are able to discover the various facilities available. Other parents are not so fortunate and get little assistance of any kind. Although there has recently been a great increase in legislation for the handicapped and much more provision is made now than a few years ago, at least on paper, we do not yet seem to know how best to deliver these services. Consequently, it is perhaps worthwhile considering the organization of services at this point, coupled with suggestions about how they might be made more effective.

Health services

One of the main reasons behind the NHS Reorganization Act of 1973 was the belief that the integration of the hospital, family practitioner and local authority health services under one administrative structure would greatly improve services for those with a chronic condition, such as the handicapped. The reorganized service has not yet had time to demonstrate its capacity for improving the care given to the chronically sick, but it is hoped that the Health Care Planning Teams (HCPT) at district level, and the Joint Consultative Councils, at the area level, will consider the needs of families with a handicapped child and attempt to tailor services to meet their requirements.

The first problem to be considered relates to the policy to be adopted in maternity hospitals when a handicapped child is born. Maternity units already provide special facilities for the care of malformed, immature and delicate infants, and each nurse or doctor in the delivery ward is trained to ensure that all babies who require it receive this special care. What is now needed is an equally well accepted and universal service to cover the needs of the parents during the crisis period immediately following the detection of an abnormality or a perinatal death, and which will guarantee an adequate follow-up when the mother leaves the maternity unit. All maternity staff should be taught how to treat parents when this situation arises and how to initiate the services for families (Spain and Wigley, 1975). The organization of this service need not be identical within every area, but it is essential that some thought be given to who should be responsible (a) for seeing that parents do understand the diagnosis and (b) for ensuring adequate follow-up of the family in the home.

Community–hospital links need to be improved and this is another area which the HCPT should consider. Except in a very few cases, the handicapped child spends most of his time actually in the community and however good hospital services are they can never fully serve his needs. 'The social functioning of the child with spina bifida is ultimately as dependent upon the quality of community pædiatric care as its clinical function is upon that of the hospital specialists' (Walker *et al.*, 1971). A domiciliary visitor of some kind is needed who can discuss the child's progress and interpret hospital instructions. As one mother put it 'Someone who can put it over to you, someone who can call on you in your own home rather than call you to some dreaded old building, with somebody sitting behind a desk, you know' (Fox, 1974). The health visitor seems to be the obvious person for this role, but it is unlikely that a generic health visitor could develop the expertise required since she will so rarely encounter any particular handicap. At present it is likely that she will meet a child with spina bifida not more frequently than once in five or ten years and the same is true of the other major handicapping conditions (Spain, 1975). The syllabus already covered in the general training of health visitors is already very wide-ranging and it would be quite unrealistic to try to give all health visitors a course of training which would allow them to give expert and practical advice for cases that come their way so rarely, and this is presumably why so many mothers find the health visitor of little help.

Some areas have experimented with specialist health visitors of various kinds, sometimes for one specific diagnosis, such as spina bifida or diabetes and sometimes for more general groups such as the handicapped or the elderly. If one or two health visitors within each district were given the opportunity to specialize in this way, they could either take over the care of all such children or act as consultants to the generalist when a handicapped child was born, making joint visits perhaps to the multiply handicapped where necessary. The concept of the specialist health visitor for this group has been advocated in many publications (Richards and McIntosh, 1973; Freeston, 1971; Spain and Wigley, 1975), and families who have experienced this service (which has been operating for a number of years in Lewisham and in the Leeds area) are most enthusiastic.

The duties of the specialist health visitor would include contacting the mother while in the maternity hospital and discussing the child's condition with her (having first established from the treatment hospital the facts of the case); acting in general as the hospital–community link; running a weekly crèche in combination with a mother's club; making contact with the school (special or ordinary) at the appropriate stages to give background information on the child; attending the out-patient clinics with the mother from time to time and liaising with the social worker in the hospital; and using her knowledge of local services or community resources to help the family with any particular problems which arose. She would have to work very closely with the social workers, both at the hospital and in the community, but in practice there seems to be little conflict between their roles in those areas where specialist health visitors are already in existence.

Social services

Many studies have indicated that social workers outside hospitals do not involve themselves very much with handicapped children and their families (Woodburn, 1973; Hewett, 1970; Younghusband *et al.*, 1970). Woodburn states that there was 'little evidence that they [social workers] played a prominent part in the lives of families with spina bifida' and that if they were contacted 'the purpose was usually to request structural alterations to the house'. Parfit (1972) in the course of reviewing services for the young handicapped child states that 'one outstanding impression which needs comment yet once again . . . is the apparent lack of involvement of the social services in provision for the handicapped child and his family'.

When Hewett (1970) was surveying families with a cerebral-palsied child, social work was in the pre-Seebohm reorganization phase. She expressed the hope that the provision of a single social service department would facilitate the delivery of services to the handicapped. However, this does not appear to have occurred and many people are feeling that the move towards the generic concept in social work has been a misguided one. The Seebohm Report did not, in fact, recommend that social workers be generalists, but simply that all social workers should be linked within the same department and that duplication of visitors to the same family should be avoided. Unless there is someone within each area team with the responsibility of overseeing all families with a handicapped child, it seems unlikely that much time will be devoted to this field, because of the constant pressure that departments are under from acute or crisis cases of various kinds.

Woodburn (1973) suggests three functions which the social services departments might fulfil: (i) increasing their own awareness of the needs of families with handicapped children in their area; (ii) providing a useful practical service to parents; and (iii) improving community relationships, by providing the opportunity for dialogues with Parent Associations and by supplying expert help and support to small group discussion among parents. She stresses that intervention on the part of social workers must be confidential and not 'encroach aspects of their personal lives, unless the parents themselves saw this as relevant'.

The main service (outside the hospital) provided by social services departments is in the field of nurseries or playgroups, run either directly by the local authority or by a voluntary body with grant aid, although the proportion of families in need who can be offered this service is still very small. The most common pattern is that a few places are reserved in playgroups or day nurseries especially for handicapped children. However, there is rarely a special programme of education geared to the child's particular needs without which the educational value of the play experience is likely to be relatively low. A good example of the sort of pre-school provision needed by many heavily handicapped spina bifida children is the group set up in Frenchay Hospital, Bristol, spina bifida unit by the social worker there (Ineichen, 1973). Children can attend the playgroup from an early age and a group for mothers is run at the same time, while in the school holidays the premises are used as a club for older spina bifida children.

In addition to pre-school provision families also need help from social services with the day-to-day management of the child, described by Bayley (1973) as 'the daily grind'. What is in fact usually provided is merely a crisis service, rather than a preventive service. It would be naive to imagine that all stress could be eliminated if more preventive work were done but, as Kew (1975) suggests, such a service would help families to 'adjust in a constructive way to potentially damaging experiences. It could develop strengths within the family for coping with its special situation of stress.' Kew goes on to point out that at present 'there is no standard procedure of referral of these families to relevant welfare agencies'. This means that preventive services cannot be offered, and it is essential that arrangements are made between health and social service departments to ensure that handicapped children are referred to the latter, automatically on diagnosis, so that provision can be made.

Facilities should also be provided locally for the temporary residential care of the child; this would give families an occasional break, even if this is only an evening out, and would be a place where the child could go when the mother or a sibling was in hospital. It might be best to provide this in co-operation with the health authorities and one such scheme is described in the final section of this chapter.

Education

The educational needs of the young spina bifida child are dealt with more fully in chapters 7 and 8. However, in the context of service organization it should be noted that, at present, education departments rarely involve themselves in the welfare of handicapped children under two years old and that the provision of nurseries or pre-schooling of any kind for those under the age of five years is still not universal. In *Living with Handicap* (Younghusband *et al.*, 1970), the authors stress the priority that should be given to the needs of the under-fives, declaring that 'There is an urgent need for more pre-school facilities for handicapped children'. In Parfit's (1975b) recent survey of pre-school facilities within the Greater London area, she notes that very little contact between the education and social services departments occurred, where care of children of this age group were concerned. A major problem here is that education departments are often not informed of the presence of a handicapped child until he nears school-age. Again co-operation between the health and education authorities is necessary to overcome this.

Parents' Associations

We have made it clear throughout this chapter that we believe self-help between parents is extremely valuable, both as a therapy and as a source of information. The statutory services should give this principle greater recognition, and encourage the development of parent contacts both informally by putting individuals in touch with each other, and formally by supporting the established voluntary bodies, such as ASBAH.

The voluntary bodies themselves could do more to help parents, as Woodburn (1973) points out. She suggests that parent associations have three main functions: (a) to build up a body of expert advice on management of the child, (b) to offer services for families such as playgroups and holidays and (c) to give parents the opportunity of gaining support and companionship from others in a similar situation. Local groups could do much more to help parents by collecting information about the services available locally, which could be produced as a handout to families, and by the formation of small working parties to discuss particular topics such as the management of bowel incontinence, or how best to explain the handicap to the child himself or his sibling. Information gathered in this way could also be duplicated for the use of others, or used as a basis for further discussion groups.

The need for co-operation

Perhaps the greatest need of all is for greater co-ordination between the three services to avoid the confusion in provision which both parents and professionals face at present, and many people have recognized this need. In *Living with Handicap* (Younghusband *et al.*, 1970) the authors state that '. . . despite instances of good progressive care, the present health education and personal social services do not, within and between them, have sufficient built-in channels of communication and systems of co-ordination'. Kew (1975) in his study of families with handicapped children concludes that 'more co-operation between the existing services is something of a minimum requirement . . . what is really needed is a thoroughly co-ordinated, systematic service designed to meet the needs of the whole family'. The new Joint Consultative Councils and the Health Care Planning Teams could be used as vehicles through which to discuss a planned integration of services. The need for a register of handicapped children with automatic cross-referral between departments has already been mentioned, and discussions on this subject could form the starting point to devising a joint service.

It would probably be wise to provide in each locality one place where the three departments could offer a combined service for the very young handicapped child. This should include a nursery/assessment centre with strong hospital links where the social worker, health visitor and community physician could attend part-time. It could also be a focus for parent groups or other community activities. In this way parents would know that there was one centre from which they could receive advice about all aspects of their child's condition or development. Such a centre could also be a source of advice for the many ordinary playgroups, nurseries and schools which accept handicapped children. There are some examples of schemes of this type already in existence. The Dorothy Gardner Centre in Paddington offers a pre-school service for all local children, whether or not they are handicapped. Nursery provision is included and a pædiatrician specializing in child development is in regular attendance (Tizard, 1975).

In Exeter a centre developed especially for handicapped children under the guidance of the consultant pædiatrician provides a model which could be usefully adopted elsewhere (Brimblecombe, 1974). In this instance the hospital authority provides the premises, and joint staffing is provided by the health, social services and education departments. This unit provides four main services. The first is day care for handicapped or premature infants for two to fours weeks after their discharge as in-patients, where the mother can be given instructions on how to handle the child if this is felt to be necessary. Secondly, nursery facilities are provided for pre-school-age children both for the relief of the mothers and to give them help in learning how to educate their children. Thirdly, short-term residential care is available for children of any age to give parents a break. In this respect the unit to a large extent takes on the role of the extended family. The parents know that if they wish to go out for an evening or to go away for a weekend they can, without formality, arrange for the child to stay in the unit for the appropriate period. This facility is also available for children of school-age especially during holiday times. Fourthly, day care is arranged for school-age children during the holidays, the actual organization being done by volunteers who use primary schools or other suitable premises.

A comprehensive service of this kind can only be provided with the co-operation of all the departments concerned. Difficulties in achieving this will arise because of the different ways in which the three services are financed and administered. However, the examples quoted demonstrate that it is perfectly possible to organize services in this way if the will is there, and parents with a handicapped child have a right to expect that administrative problems will be overcome in the interest of the child and the whole family.

References

Allum, N. (1975), Spina Bifida: *The Treatment and Care of Spina Bifida Children*, Allen and Unwin, London.

Bayley, M., (1973), 'Mental Handicap and Community Care', Routledge and Kegan Paul, London and Boston.

Brimblecombe, F. S. W. (1974), 'Exeter project for handicapped children', *British Medical Journal*, 4, pp. 706–9.

Burton, L. (1975), *The Family Life of Sick Children*, Routledge and Kegan Paul, London and Boston.

Carter, C. O. and Roberts, F. R. (1971), 'Genetic clinic: a follow-up', *Lancet*, i, pp. 281–5.

Crowe, B. (1975), 'Group therapy for parents', *Parent Voice*, 25 (1), pp. 8–9.

Curran, A. P. and Swann, E. (1964), Report to the Carnegie UK Trust.

Forsythe, W. K. and Kinley, J. C. (1970), 'Bowel control of children with spina bifida', *Developmental Medicine and Child Neurology*, 12 (6), pp. 27–31.

Fox, M. (1974), 'They get this training but they don't know how you feel', *Action Research for the Crippled Child*.

Freeston, B. M. (1971), 'An enquiry into the effect of a spina bifida child upon family life', *Developmental Medicine and Child Neurology*, 13, pp. 456–61.

Hewett, S. (1970), *The Family and the Handicapped Child*, Allen and Unwin, London.

Ineichen, R. (1973), 'Towards co-ordinated care of spina bifida children', *Social Work Today*, 4 (11), pp. 321–4.

Kew, S. (1975), *Handicap and Family Crisis*, Pitman, London.

Nordqvist, I. (1972), *Life Together – the Situation of the Handicapped*, Swedish Central Committee for Rehabilitation, Bromma 3, Sweden.

Parfit, J. (1972), *Services for the Young Handicapped Child*, National Children's Bureau.

——, (1975a), 'Siblings of handicapped children', *Special Education*, 2 (1), pp. 19–20.

——, (1975b), 'The integration of handicapped children in Greater London', report of a survey commissioned by the Institute for Research into Mental and Multiple Handicap.

Richards, I. D. G. and McIntosh, H. T. (1973), 'Spina bifida survivors and their parents: a study of problems and services', *Developmental Medicine and Child Neurology*, 15, pp. 292–304.

Schaffer, R. (1964), 'The too-cohesive family, a form of group pathology', *International Journal of Social Psychiatry*, 10, p. 266.

Spain, B. (1973), 'Spina bifida: the need for community support', GLC Intelligence Unit Quarterly Bulletin, 23, pp. 66–71.

——, and Wigley, G. (1975), *Right From the Start*, Association for Mentally Handicapped Children.

Tizard, J. (1975), 'Towards a comprehensive service for young children', *Times Educational Supplement*, 1975.

——, and Grad, J. C., (1961), *The Mentally Handicapped and Their Families*, Maudsley Monograph no. 7, Oxford University Press.

Walker, J. H., Thomas, M. and Russell, I. T. (1971), 'Spina bifida and the parents', *Developmental Medicine and Child Neurology*, 13, pp. 462–76.

Webster, B. (1975), 'Health matters: bowels', *Link*, no. 37, pp. 5 and 7.

Wilson, A. L. (1971), 'Group therapy for parents of handicapped children', *Rehabilitation Literature*, 32 (11), pp. 332–5.

Wing, L. (1966), 'Counselling and the principles of management', in Wing, J. K. (ed.), *Early Childhood Autism*, Pergamon Press, Oxford.

Woodburn, M. (1973), *Social Implications of Spina Bifida – a Study in S.E. Scotland*, Eastern Branch of Scottish Spina Bifida Association, Edinburgh.

Younghusband, E., Davie, R., Birchall, D. and Kellmer Pringle, M. L. (eds.) (1970), *Living with Handicap*, National Bureau for Co-operation in Child Care, London.

3 Abilities, attainments and schooling

5 Intellectual development

It is only comparatively recently that the intellectual development of spina bifida children has been studied in any detail. During the early 1960s it was often believed by pædiatricians, teachers and other professionals (on the basis of very little evidence) that most spina bifida children were of normal intelligence. Even today opinions such as these are often encountered, probably because many spina bifida children are very verbal and so give an initial impression of being 'bright'.

During the last decade, however, a number of research projects have been set up in which the intellectual development of spina bifida children is being looked at in much more detail, partly by means of batteries of standard psychometric and attainment tests and sometimes also through tests or experimental procedures specifically devised to investigate a particular area of functioning. In this country the main large-scale longitudinal studies include Spain's GLC study and the studies of Brian Tew and his colleagues in South Wales. In addition a number of detailed small-scale research studies have been made, for example on visual perception (Miller and Sethi, 1971; Dodds, 1975), short-term memory (Parsons, 1969), and handwriting (Anderson, 1975).

Our main aim in this chapter has been to present, on the basis of research findings, as full a picture as possible of the sorts of strengths and weaknesses in intellectual functioning which characterize spina bifida children, in particular those who also have hydrocephalus. There will of course be exceptions: some spina bifida children may have none or very few of the difficulties described here and may even be of above-average intelligence while others may have much more severe learning problems. However, we shall concentrate upon the majority of children with spina bifida and hydrocephalus, those lying between these extremes, who are likely, both in their intellectual potential and in their attainments to fall into the dull–average or borderline–ESN range. This chapter is primarily concerned with presenting and interpreting research findings rather than with suggesting what can be done to help the children. Those more interested in the latter, whether as parents, teachers, or other professionals may find the chapters which follow (especially chapter 6 on the pre-school years and chapter 8 on teaching spina bifida children) more useful. The chapter begins with a discussion of overall intellectual level and of the relationship between IQ and other variables while the second part of the chapter is about more specific aspects of intellectual development.

Overall intellectual development

Six major points can be made about general intellectual development in spina bifida children: (i) The intelligence of most children tends to be below average. (ii) There are generally marked differences between the intelligence levels of children with and without hydrocephalus; intelligence also varies according to the severity of the hydrocephalus. (iii) Intelligence does not necessarily vary with the severity of the physical handicap unless there is also hydrocephalus. (iv) To some degree there are differences in intelligence related to the nature of the lesion. (v) Differences in intelligence related to the sex of the child have been postulated. (vi) Not all intellectual functions are affected equally, verbal skills tending to be less impaired than performance skills.

(i) *Distribution of intelligence in spina bifida children*

There is now clear evidence from a large number of studies (Badell-Ribera *et al.*, 1966; Burns, 1967; Diller *et al.*, 1969; Spain, 1969, 1970, 1972, 1974; Lorber, 1971; Tew, 1973a, 1973b; Liedholm *et al.*, 1974), that spina bifida children, even when fully treated from birth, do not have a normal distribution of intelligence. Instead their scores are skewed towards the lower end of the IQ range with a peak of scores in the dull and backward range of intelligence. Tew's study (1973a) of fifty-nine 5½-year-old spina bifida children born in South Wales between 1964 and 1966 who had been given comprehensive treatment from birth provides a good example. Children in the control group (matched for age, sex and social class) showed a normal distribution of scores with a mean of 105·9 whereas the spina bifida children had a mean full scale IQ of only 83 (verbal IQ 86 and performance IQ 80). However it must be emphasized that there are individual children and adults with spina bifida, and sometimes hydrocephalus too, of normal or above-average intelligence.

(ii) *The relationship between intelligence and hydrocephalus*
In many studies (e.g. Badell-Ribera *et al.*, 1966; Diller *et al.*, 1969; Laurence and Tew, 1971; Lorber, 1971; Spain, 1974), comparisons have been made between spina bifida children with and without hydrocephalus. The term 'hydrocephalic' may be misleading since, unless otherwise indicated, it might include both children with an initially mild degree of hydrocephalus which has arrested spontaneously, as well as children whose hydrocephalus is severe and progressive. For this reason, it is probably preferable to distinguish between children with and without shunts, since in most cases the presence of a shunt indicates that there was, initially, a significant degree of hydrocephalus. Even so, because some children with shunts may have shown only very mild or doubtful symptoms, neither the shunt/no shunt nor the hydrocephalus/no hydrocephalus categorization can be regarded as a *precise* indication of the severity of hydrocephalus. Whichever contrast is made the findings do, however, indicate quite clearly a strong association between the presence of hydrocephalus and impairment of intellectual functioning.

In Spain's GLC study, for example, children were tested at 6 years of age on the Wechsler Pre-school and Primary Scale of Intelligence (WPPSI) the results for the children with and without shunts being shown in Table 5.1 below.

Table 5.1

		WPPSI		
	N	*Verbal IQ*	*Performance IQ*	*Full Scale IQ*
No Shunt	40	97·5	101·1	99·2
Shunt	86	87·9	80·2	82·9

The results here confirm that the scores of children with shunts are significantly lower than those without, although again it is also important to notice that 35 per cent of the shunted children had verbal and performance IQs of over 85, that is within the normal range of intelligence. For shunted children with Full Scale WPPSI IQs below 80 there was also a significant verbal-performance discrepancy (discussed later in more detail). Similar differences between children with and without shunts were found by Lorber (1971) and Tew and Laurence (1975).

(iii) *The relationship of intelligence to the severity of the physical handicap*

Even if a child is severely physically handicapped he may be of normal or near-normal intelligence if he does not have hydrocephalus, or if, at birth, the hydrocephalus was mild and self-arresting so that a shunt was not required. On the other hand, children with severe physical handicaps coupled with hydrocephalus which required the insertion of a shunt are much more likely to be of dull average intelligence or below. Lorber (1971) has examined these relationships in his 1959–63 series of children (Table 5.2 below). The test used was the Terman-Merrill. Unfortunately details are not given about the age at which the children were tested.

Table 5.2 *Relationship between intelligence, hydrocephalus and severity of physical handicap (From Lorber, 1971)*

Category		*No Hydrocephalus*	*Hydrocephalus No shunt*	*Shunt*	*Total*	*% of Admissions*	*% of Survivors*
1. No handicap		3	1	—	4	1	3
2. Moderate handicap*		9	6	5	20	6	15
3. Severe handicap	IQ 80+	15	15	36	66	20	49
4. Severe handicap	IQ 61–79	2	5	21	28	9	21
5. Extreme handicap	IQ <60	2	1	13	16	5	12
All alive		31	28	75	134	41	100

* The children with 'moderate' handicaps were sometimes incontinent or had a well functioning ileal loop but no chronic infection. They might have motor weakness consistent with walking without calipers. Five of the twenty children in this group had IQs of 75–9, the others higher than this.

These relationships were also investigated in the GLC study and the findings both at 3 years old when the children were tested on hand–eye co-ordination and performance tests of the Griffiths Scale and at 6 years old on the WPPSI (Table 5.3) also showed that the children who were most retarded intellectually were those with a severe physical handicap and a shunt. Once again, however, there were some severely handicapped children with shunts whose performance lay within the normal range.

Table 5.3 *Performance on the WPPSI at 6 years* related to presence of shunt and degree of physical handicap*

	Spina Bifida			
	No Shunt		*Shunt*	
	Phys. Hand.		*Phys. Hand.*	
WPPSI Results	*Min.*	*Mod/Sev.*	*Min.*	*Mod/Sev.*
Mean Verbal Scale Score	97·8	96·6	91·3	86·5
Mean Perf. Scale Score	104.0	92·3	92·6	75·7
Mean Full IQ Score	100·9	94·0	91·2	79·8
Total number	30	10	24	62

* Children too low on ability to be tested on the WPPSI ($N=6$) are excluded, together with three others who could not be tested because of a hearing loss.

(iv) *Intelligence and the type of lesion*

While research evidence suggests that children with meningoceles are likely to fall into the normal range of intelligence and children with myelomeningoceles (by far the largest group) into the low average to backward range (e.g. Laurence and Tew, 1967, 1971; Tew and Laurence, 1972; Tew, 1973a, 1973b) this is not always the case. Some children with meningoceles will be of low ability as part of the normal distribution of intelligence: conversely many children with myelomeningoceles are of average and, in a few cases, above-average ability. Since the terms 'meningocele' and 'myelomeningocele' are often used loosely teachers should not make assumptions about the likelihood of intellectual impairment simply because a child's medical records describe him as having a meningocele or a myelomeningocele.

Children with encephaloceles, the third much smaller group whom teachers may come across, show a very different pattern as regards distribution of IQ scores. By no means all are, as is often assumed, severely intellectually handicapped. Of the 18 encephaloceles in the GLC study half were severely sub-normal, many of these children having marked sensory handicaps. On the other hand, one-third of the group (6 children) had no hydrocephalus and were of normal intelligence.

(v) *Sex differences and intelligence*

It is a well-established finding in the literature on handicap that the incidence of handicapping conditions (for example cerebral palsy, severe subnormality, autism or speech disorders) is higher among boys. Surprisingly, this relationship does not hold for spina bifida or related congenital malformations where more girls are born than boys (the ratio being approximately 1·3 : 1).

Not only do girls seem more likely to develop this condition but among the survivors the girls tend to be more severely handicapped physically, and a higher proportion require valves. In the GLC study over 70 per cent of girls were shunted compared with 50 per cent of boys. Consequently, there were more girls than boys with low IQs.

(vi) *Verbal-performance differences*

The other main feature of intellectual functioning in spina bifida children is that where there is intellectual impairment and particularly in the low-ability children (IQs below 80) all areas of functioning are not equally impaired. Psychologists are often interested in the significance of large 'verbal' and 'performance' discrepancies, the main comparison usually being between scores on the WISC verbal and performance scales, and there is some evidence from the GLC study that spina bifida children, especially those with shunts and with IQs below 80, tend to do significantly better on the verbal than on the performance scale. While this is worth noting, more can be learned by observing spina bifida children functioning on particular WPPSI or WISC subtests and on other standardized tests or experimental tasks designed to explore specific skills.

Different aspects of intellectual development

Introduction

Adults meeting children with spina bifida and hydrocephalus for the first time are often impressed by their apparently superior verbal ability and they may generalize from this to intelligence as a whole. Even those who have known a child over a long period, whether as doctor, teacher or parent, may be deceived by the child's verbal fluency into thinking that he is 'brighter' than he really is. There are of course some spina bifida children of average intelligence or above whose fluency truly reflects general intellectual development, but they are likely to be the exception rather than the rule.

In a book of great insight on the psychological assessment of children with cerebral defects, Taylor (1959) gives a detailed description of 'a child with congenital malformation resulting in hydrocephalus, paraplegia and mental retardation' which is in many ways applicable to children with spina bifida and hydrocephalus. At 15 months (Taylor, 1959, p. 183) John 'is very responsive; he vocalizes a great deal, enjoys company, smiles, and is friendly', but 'his perceptual awareness and comprehension in adaptive tasks rates at approximately the ten- to twelve-month level only, in contrast to the high level of his social skills.'

By four years old his parents are, except for his inability to walk, 'delighted at his progress. Having been warned that the child would develop slowly, they are now triumphant about his responsiveness, his alertness and his pleasant personality. He has talked early, and because of his precocious statements has been found especially entertaining ever since. He has an excellent memory . . . and knows many nursery rhymes. He likes the television, especially the commercials, which he can recite.' However, in a series of tests his performance 'reveals limited comprehension of complex situations. With his reasoning ability hardly on a 3-year level, his form comprehension lower and his verbal facility his main asset only because of his auditory memory, the child's intellectual development at age 4 seems to proceed at a borderline level at best.'

Re-testing at later ages produces the same pattern of findings. Between 6 and 10 years old, for example, Taylor reports (1959, p. 222) that children like John are still 'friendly but slightly tense in the [psychological] examination. They still manage to direct conversation along lines with which they are familiar. They may appear chatty and communicative; they are apt to ask personal questions of the kind often asked by younger children but commonly considered 'nosey' in older ones.' However, 'frequently they do extremely poorly with formboards and on object assembly tests. Usually, they have difficulty with block designs and memory for design tests. Verbal tests which demand reasoning are difficult for them too.' While they can often reproduce almost literally sentences from stories they may be 'unable to explain or repeat in their own words the content of what they recite'.

Summing up, Taylor comments on 'the irregularities in mental functioning' which many of these children display at this and at later ages and which 'add up' to only borderline–normal ratings of intelligence and it is these irregularities which are explored in more detail in the sections which follow.

1. *Verbal ability*

Taylor's comments will have shown that there is much more to verbal ability than simply apparent verbal fluency. In this section the following aspects of verbal ability are considered in turn: (i) auditory perception; (ii) verbal memory; (iii) vocabulary skills; (iv) the development of syntax; (v) the comprehension of language and (vi) hyperverbal behaviour.

(i) *Hearing and auditory perception.* Fortunately, hearing loss is uncommon in spina bifida children, although it may occur. In Woodburn's study for example (1973) only 2 out of 74 children had some degree of hearing defect which had caused moderate anxiety but which was not likely to require special schooling, and in the GLC study two children out of 145, both encephaloceles, were severely deaf, while another with a lumbo-sacral meningocele also required a hearing aid in both ears.

Auditory perception, including the ability to discriminate between and to interpret sounds, seems to develop at least normally in spina bifida children, and possibly at a faster rate than normal. Two aspects of this should be recognized. On the one hand, acuity of hearing and rapid development of the ability to discriminate between sounds is beneficial in that it facilitates language acquisition at an early age, with imitation probably playing a very important part. Thus in Woodburn's study (1973) several parents said that their child had learned to talk at an earlier age than had his sibs. In the GLC study it was noticed that remarkably few children showed articulation defects, when tested, at 3 years.

The other side of the picture is that many parents and teachers have commented to Woodburn and to ourselves that many spina bifida babies as well as pre-school and primary school children are hyper-sensitive to sounds. Cases have been reported where a spina bifida child has become extremely disturbed by the noises of, for example, a hoover, the telephone ringing, loud music on the radio, town bands, school orchestras and puppet voices in a Punch and Judy show. The problem appears to decrease as the children get older but it is not clear whether they actually grow out of this difficulty or simply become better able to tolerate disturbing sounds.

This phenomenon has never been systematically studied: the explanations for it can only be speculative but probably lie in some disturbance of neurological functioning. This could be consequent either on hydrocephalus or on abnormalities arising from the Arnold-Chiari malformation, although the possibility that it is connected with the presence of the shunt cannot yet be completely excluded.

(ii) *Verbal memory.* The ability of young spina bifida children to imitate well and to memorize verbal material, especially rhythmic material such as nursery rhymes, songs, TV commercials and phrases used by adults, suggests that a good verbal memory may be another of their assets. Findings such as those of Purkhiser (1965) who reported that hydrocephalic children were superior to non-hydrocephalics on a digit repetition task led Parsons (1969) to investigate short-term verbal memory in hydrocephalics, in particular where more connective verbal material (rather than random digits) was involved. He concluded that short-term verbal memory in hydrocephalics does not differ significantly from that of non-hydrocephalics and only appears particularly good in relation to their intellectual weaknesses in other areas.

Teachers often comment on the fact that spina bifida children have poor memories in that they seem, for instance in number work, to have forgotten by the next day or even the next hour an 'explanation' recently given to them. The problem here is probably more one of a difficulty in understanding an explanation, or in attention, or of the ability to generalize from one example to another, than an impairment in the ability to remember per se.

Overall the verbal memory of spina bifida or of hydrocephalic children is an area that has not been explored adequately and no definite conclusions can yet be drawn.

(iii) *Vocabulary skills.* One important aspect of language development is the acquisition of vocabulary and here spina bifida children are thought to be relatively unimpaired, although little research has yet been published on this. The children in the GLC study were tested at 3 and 6 years old on the Reynell Developmental Language Scale (Reynell, 1969) which includes a vocabulary subtest. The findings (which have been reported in more detail elsewhere (Spain, 1974)) suggested that the majority of spina bifida children without shunts have normal vocabulary skills at 3 years of age while of the children with shunts, only about one-third have vocabulary skills within the normal range.

Vocabulary was also looked at in Anderson's study. In the English Picture Vocabulary Test (Brimer and Dunn, 1963) in which the child is shown four pictures and asked to point to the one which illustrates a certain word, the mean scores and the range of scores did not differ significantly for the three groups (who were matched for intelligence); however, 75 per cent of the spina bifida children made a score on the EPVT well within the normal range (90+) compared to 55 per cent of the cerebral-palsied children and 51 per cent of the controls. The mean scores of these three groups on the vocabulary and similarities subtests of the WISC were also compared. Again the spina bifida children's vocabulary skills seemed unimpaired (mean 10·1) whereas the control group was well below average (mean 8·5): all three groups, however, were below average on the similarities subtest where reasoning abilities play a greater part.

(iv) *The development of syntax.* One reason for the impression given by most spina bifida children of having normal verbal ability is that they appear to use correct and sometimes quite complex sentence structures. Syntax is very difficult to test, but there is some evidence from the GLC study (Spain, 1974) that their syntax is relatively good. When the children were tested on the Reynell Scale at 3 years old and at 6 years old the findings on the 'structure' (i.e. syntax) subtest of the Expressive Scale suggested that within the whole group use of syntax seemed to be quite normal for the age of the child, even in children with shunts and low performance IQs.

In the GLC study at 6 years old other measures of syntax were used such as sentence length and use of conjunctions which are described in more detail in section (vi). In general they show that spina bifida children are more likely to use complex syntax than normal children matched for ability, although they do not always use it appropriately.

(v) *The comprehension and appropriate use of language.* Those who work with spina bifida children often feel that despite good syntax and quite a wide-ranging vocabulary the children's comprehension of spoken or written language is poor, as is their ability to use language appropriately and with understanding.

This is particularly true of hyperverbal spina bifida children (considered in more detail in section (vi)); is it also true of the more 'typical' spina bifida child?

When the children in the GLC study were 3 years old the Reynell Comprehension Scale was used, which assesses the child's ability to understand what is said to him. On the same test the content subtest of the Expressive Scale (a picture description test) measures the child's capacity for using language in a creative way. The results are shown in Table 5.4 below.

Table 5.4 *Mean scores on the Reynell Scale subtests of 3-year-old spina bifida children*

Groups based on Griffiths Performance Developmental Quotient	*N*	*Reynell Comprehension Mean DQ*	*Reynell Expression Mean DQ*	*Expression Scale subtests (mean raw scores) Structure*	*Vocab.*	*Content*
Children without shunts						
PDQ 80+	27	115·3	109·4	16·8	13·8	9·1
PDQ 50–80	6	80·0	89·0	16·0	11·0	5·0
Children with shunts						
PDQ 80+	29	103·0	97·8	16·6	12·3	6·9
PDQ 50–80	58	82·4	82·4	15·6	10·0	4·0
Mean scores from Reynell norms				16·2	14·0	7·0
Standard error from Reynell norms				15·6–17·1	11·1–17·0	3·2–11·0

This shows that on these two tests it is only the more able children (with or without shunts) who score at or above the average level. The largest group of children, those with a shunt and with a Griffiths Performance DQ below 80, score well below the norm. This contrasts with the subtest measuring use of syntax (structure) where the scores of this latter group come much closer to the norm.

At 6 years old another test of comprehension was used, the Renfrew Bus Story, where children are asked to repeat a story immediately after it has been told to them by the examiner. Their replies are recorded fully and are then analysed to show the total number of words and clauses used, the average sentence length and the number of items of information from the original study which the child remembers and repeats (the Information Score). Table 5.5 below shows that compared with a group of normal children, the spina bifida group used as many words and clauses and only slightly shorter sentences despite the fact that this group had a much higher proportion of children of low ability. However, the information scores of the spina bifida children, particularly those with valves, were poorer than those of the controls. Those giving low information scores were mainly the children rated as 'hyperverbal'.

Table 5.5 *Mean scores on the Renfrew Bus Story Test of 6-year-old spina bifida children*

	Mean scores			
Groups	*Average Sentence length*	*Total no. of words*	*Total no. of clauses*	*Inform. Score*
Spina bifida with valve	8·8	128·0	17·1	20·5
Spina bifida no valve	9·8	130·6	16·5	25·3
Control children	10·1	127·2	17·3	28·1
Renfrew norms	10·7			30·0

(vi) *Hyperverbal behaviour.* Hyperverbal behaviour, often described as 'the cocktail-party syndrome', is an extreme form of this sort of fluent speech coupled with poor understanding. There is a tendency to apply this label indiscriminately to spina bifida children but it must be stressed that not all show it. Tew and Laurence (1972) found evidence of hyperverbal behaviour in 28 per cent of their sample and comment that it was 'a certain indication of below average if not subnormal intelligence'. Although only a proportion of spina bifida children show this syndrome, it has been of considerable interest to researchers.

Long before the term 'cocktail-party syndrome' was coined and also before early surgical treatment of hydrocephalus became common practice, it was recognized by those working in hospitals for severely subnormal children that there was a distinct sub-group of hydrocephalic children who, although grossly retarded, had, surprisingly, acquired some social speech. Their 'conversation', however, tended to be a monologue which was repetitive and limited in its range.

The term 'cocktail-party syndrome' was first applied to hydrocephalic children by Hadenius and his colleagues (1962) and gained wide popularity. They noted in a minority of the children they examined 'a good ability to learn words and talking without knowing what they are talking about'. Matson (1961) made similar observations, and Ingram and Naughton (1962) described children with hydrocephalus associated with cerebral palsy as 'uninhibited', 'chatterboxes' or 'bletherers'.

In later studies hyperverbal behaviour has been looked at in a more systematic way. Fleming (1968) for example used a picture description task, and found that hydrocephalic children had 'difficulty in responding in a consistent and meaningful manner to a specified topic', while many appeared 'to seek distraction from the task' but attempted 'to maintain the flow of language and the conversational relationships'. Swisher and Pinsker (1971) analysed the conversation of a group of children with spina bifida and hydrocephalus and showed that they had a significantly greater output of words and sentences and initiated more conversation than a control group. They also used more bizarre or inappropriate language although this tendency decreased with age.

In a study by Diller and his colleagues (1969) the verbal behaviour of 32 children with spina bifida myelomeningocele was rated by each of four observers, the children being classed as showing normal verbal behaviour or being 'dysverbal' (i.e. hyperverbal). All children rated as dysverbal were hydrocephalics. Dysverbal behaviour tended to occur in socially stressful situations, the children tended to guess rather than say 'I don't know', and behaviour was deviant not only in that the child talked more but also in that he talked irrelevantly. However, this behaviour tended to disappear in adolescence. The dysverbal children were more severely handicapped both neurologically and physically and appeared to spend more time with adults. The authors suggested that neurological damage, motor impairment and parental reactions interacted in producing dysverbal behaviour.

In the GLC study a detailed investigation was made of 6-year-old children rated clinically as 'hyperverbal'. The findings suggest that, overall, about 40 per cent of spina bifida children aged 6 years show this syndrome, though only half that number exhibit it to a marked degree. Typically children rated in this way were female, had shunts, and were poor intellectually, with considerably higher verbal than performance skills. However, those with milder features were often of normal ability. The hyperverbal children tended to be more physically handicapped than the rest and to be rated by teachers as restless, fidgety and inattentive.

Analysis of the children's spontaneous speech showed that the hyperverbal group differed remarkably from a group of normal children matched on the WPPSI for verbal ability. They used quite complex syntax, but often inaccurately, and produced more bizarre utterances, with a tendency to change subject midflow, to give more false starts to sentences and more incomplete sentences. They produced a much higher rate of clichés, or adult-type phrases, although they rarely gave the impression of understanding their meaning.

In Appendix B a recorded extract from the 'conversation' of a child showing this syndrome is given. This is an extreme example but it illustrates that this low-ability child (WISC FS IQ = 55) uses some quite complex sentences, and has an extensive vocabulary. The child declaims rather than converses, tends to drift from one topic to another only loosely related and clearly does not really understand what he is saying. Like Diller *et al.* (1966), Spain concludes that these children exhibit a basic failure in inhibiting irrelevant responses.

2 *Visual Perception*

Introduction. Visual perception has been defined as 'the ability to recognize and use visual stimuli and to interpret these stimuli by relating them to previous experiences' (Goldberg, 1968). Even if a child's receptors – for instance his eyes or ears – are functioning normally, the higher-level processes which determine how the input is organized and incorporated into experience may be working inefficiently and such a child may be said to have perceptual difficulties. Comparatively little research has been carried out into the visuo-perceptual abilities of spina bifida children although in a minority of extreme cases such difficulties are so severe that no one would dispute their existence. One factor which has complicated attempts to assess both visual-perceptual ability and eye–hand co-ordination skills is the high incidence of ocular defects, in particular squint (see chapter 1).

It is not known what effect an early developing squint has on a child's perceptual abilities but some workers believe that it could be important. For example, work carried out by Alberman and Gardiner, (1971), suggested that 'children with squints but no other neurological or mental defects still included an unduly high proportion of poor readers and scored badly on a copying design test, although they performed as well as controls in tests involving intellectual rather than visual ability'. Abercrombie (1963) and Haskell and Hughes (1965) have suggested that difficulties are even greater where the child has an intermittent rather than a constant squint. Problems may persist even when the squint has been corrected; in particular it is thought that children who develop squints within the first year of life (as do most spina bifida children) never achieve binocular vision.

Visuo-perceptual ability: research findings. In most studies of spina bifida children inferences about perception have been based on performances in the Frostig Test, which seeks to measure five operationally defined perceptual skills (Frostig, 1966) these being Subtest I, Eye–Motor Co-ordination; II, Figure–Ground Perception; III, Constancy of Shape; IV, Position in Space; and V, Spatial Relationships. There has been some debate among psychologists about whether this test does measure five specific functions rather than simply one general visual perceptual factor: another problem is that since it is a paper and pencil test children with poor hand control may experience difficulties in actually drawing round the figures (e.g. in the figure–ground discrimination subtest) which may make it harder for them to concentrate on the perceptual aspects of the task. Despite such problems this test is generally felt to be the best available and has been widely used in studies of primary school-aged children with neurological abnormalities.

In the South Wales Study (Tew, 1973a,b) the spina bifida children and their controls were tested on the Frostig Test at $5\frac{1}{2}$ years old. At this age, 'no child with a Wechsler performance quotient under 70 was able to score on any of the subtests' and for this reason twenty-one children had to be excluded. The others, particularly the myelomeningoceles, tended to score very poorly in comparison with the controls, the difference between the mean scores for the two groups ranging 'from 20 months behind on eye–hand co-ordination to a year on the spatial relationships test with an average lag of 17 months' (Tew, 1973a).

In Anderson's study, children with spina bifida and hydrocephalus were tested on subtests I–III of the Frostig Test, and compared with matched groups of non-handicapped and cerebral-palsied 6–9 year olds. No differences were found between the spina bifida children and the controls on the shape constancy subtest but well over half the spina bifida children compared to just over one-third of the non-handicapped group failed to reach Frostig's criterion for normality in the eye–hand co-ordination subtest, and more than two in three scored below the criterion in figure–ground discrimination compared to just under half of the non-handicapped children. A very much higher proportion of the cerebral-palsied group, however, (approximately four in five) had marked difficulties both in the eye–hand co-ordination and figure–ground discrimination subtests and their perceptual problems were clearly more severe than those of the spina bifida children.

A particularly interesting small-scale but detailed study of visual perception in hydrocephalics has recently been made by Jean Dodds (1975). Her study was essentially an attempt to follow up an earlier investigation of visual perception in hydrocephalics carried out by Miller and Sethi (1971). Findings on the Bender-Gestalt Test, the Frostig Test and a series of experimental tasks had led these authors to conclude that visual perception was markedly impaired in hydrocephalic children. In Dodds' study eleven shunted children aged 8–11 years (mean WISC Verbal IQ 88) were compared with a control group closely matched for age, sex and intelligence. The test battery included two tests of figure–ground discrimination (an overlapping figures test and an embedded figures test), a shape constancy test, a test of the children's ability to discriminate between letter-like forms (used by Gibson *et al.*, 1962) and a test in which the child had to pick the 'odd-one-out' in a number of configurations.

The results of the five experiments suggested 'a general trend towards inferior functioning in visual perception in the hydrocephalics', although some aspects of perception caused much more difficulty than others. The task the hydrocephalics found hardest (in fact the only task in Dodd's study where statistically significant differences appeared between the two groups) was the embedded figures task, this aspect of figure–ground discrimination causing much more difficulty than the overlapping figures task. Thus there is now fairly conclusive evidence from several studies (Miller and Sethi, 1971; Tew, 1973a; Anderson, 1975; Dodds, 1975) that the discrimination of figure from background is difficult for many hydrocephalic children. In contrast the hydrocephalic children performed as well as the controls in the shape constancy subtest.

On the other two tasks used in Dodds' study, the discrimination of letter-like forms and the odd-one-out tasks, no significant differences were found between the two groups although there was a trend for the hydrocephalic children to perform more poorly and there was certainly more variation within the spina bifida group. A recent study carried out by Ball (1975) does, however, indicate that hydrocephalic children often have specific difficulty in discriminating between mirror-image symbols.

In an odd-one-out task Dodds noted that the hydrocephalics tended 'to be less effective in rapidly distinguishing which one of a choice of configurations differs in some small detail from the others'. Spain has noticed the same thing in a task where children had to pick out one abstract design from a card containing the test figure plus four similar designs. In order to score the child had to identify the test figure within five seconds. Few children were unable to do the task, but many spina bifida children, particularly those with shunts, could not do it within the time limit.

Since hydrocephalics show, on the WISC Picture Completion Subtest, that they are capable of perceiving which details of a picture were missing, why do they tend to do poorly in an odd-man-out type of task? The answer may lie not so much in impaired perception as in a faulty or inefficient strategy. Work carried out by Anderson (1975) and reported in chapter 9 (p. 246) suggests that hydrocephalic children tend to be very impulsive in choosing which, out of a set of comparison figures, resembles the standard. Dodds also comments that 'scanning ability' may be inferior in the hydrocephalic children. Further work is required before we can conclude whether hydrocephalic children do in fact scan the visual stimuli less efficiently than non-hydrocephalics and, if this is the case, whether and to what extent this is a perceptual problem related to neurological impairment, a problem related to the presence of ocular defects or a matter of an inefficient strategy which the child could be taught to alter.

3 *Visuo-motor and spatial performance skills*

In section 2 we discussed the problems which children with spina bifida and hydrocephalus may have in visuo-perceptual tasks. Often, however, visuo-perceptual and motor skills must be combined, and it is on tasks of this kind that many spina bifida children, especially those with shunts, have marked difficulties from a very early age. The fact that these difficulties *can* be identified at an early age is important since it also means that special help (discussed in detail in chapter 6) can be given early on.

In the GLC study the children were tested at the age of one year on the Griffiths Mental Developmental Test and Spain noted (1970) that the children with valves tended to have lower scores on the hand–eye co-ordination scale than on any other scale (apart from locomotor ability). By the age of 3 years this defect was much more marked, children with shunts showing both poor manipulative ability and inability to appreciate spatial relationships. Table 5.6 shows the distribution of Griffiths Performance Developmental Quotients (PDQs) for children in the different groups related to the presence of a shunt.

Table 5.6 *Variation in performance ability in spina bifida children tested at 3 years old related to presence of shunt and degree of physical handicap*

	Spina Bifida						
Griffiths Perform-mance DQ	*No Shunt Handicap Min.*	*Mod/Sev.*	*Total*	*Shunt Handicap Min.*	*Mod/Sev*	*Total*	*Grand Total*
80+	24	3	27	17	12	29	65
50–79	4	2	6	10	52	62	70
0–49	0	0	0	0	5	5	10
Total	28	5	33	27	69	96	145

Here it can be seen that it is the children with shunts and a moderate or severe physical handicap who tend to do worst on the Griffiths with a large proportion of this group having scores in the 50–79 range. The mean scores for children without shunts were 95·3 on the hand–eye co-ordination scale and 96·5 on the performance scale, whereas corresponding figures for those with shunts were only 79·2 and 79·5. Some items on the Griffiths scale caused particular difficulty. Bead-threading was one; some children were unable to grasp the principle or did so only with difficulty, even when the examiner tried to teach them. At 6 years old 30 per cent of the children with shunts were still having great difficulty in threading beads.

Visuo-motor difficulties are also marked in school-aged children. The poor performance of hydrocephalic children on Subtest I (eye–hand co-ordination) of the Frostig Test has already been noted. Difficulties are also apparent when performance on the WPPSI and WISC subtests which involve visuo-motor skills is examined. In Appendix C we show the performance on the WPPSI or the WISC of spina bifida children in two age-groups. One group are the 6 year olds in Spain's GLC survey, scores for the children with and without shunts and a control group being shown separately. The other scores are for shunted spina bifida children in Anderson's study whose mean subtest scores are compared with those of matched groups of non-handicapped and cerebral-palsied children.

In the GLC study Spain found that children with shunts tended to have higher verbal than performance scores on the WPPSI in contrast to those without shunts and the controls. For the shunted group the subtest on the verbal scale, which gave the most difficulty was arithmetic. Here spatial ability is clearly necessary for success. On the performance scale, items giving the lowest scores were those requiring visuo-spatial skills such as mazes, geometric design and animal house. In the latter children would often begin the task correctly but quickly seemed to forget what they had been asked to do, or became confused over the sequence of activities required for completion of each item. Many children seemed quite incapable of grasping the principle involved on the mazes subtest and were unable to copy any but the simplest designs. When the children were asked to reproduce simple designs with matchsticks, a task requiring a minimum of motor control, children with shunts were markedly poorer than those without, indicating that failure in copying designs were not due simply to poor motor control.

In Anderson's study (1975) the task causing the spina bifida children the greatest difficulty was coding, only four of this group compared to nineteen non-handicapped children making a score of 10 or above. Although the spina bifida children grasped the principle of the task they worked very slowly, frequently losing their place, and the symbols were badly formed. Dodds (1975) makes almost identical observations: 'The low scores . . . were mainly due to the fact that the subjects were laboriously slow in the execution of their task, rather than a large number of mistakes being made . . . The marks drawn by the majority of hydrocephalics, appeared 'shaky' and gave a general appearance of untidiness.'

In both Dodds' and Anderson's studies the block design and object assembly subtests were poorly done. On block design, Dodds (1975) comments that 'the hydrocephalic children more frequently lost points because of slowness in attempting to complete the design rather than because of misplaced blocks. They appeared less confident in using trial and error methods than did the normal children, sometimes seeming unaware that the design they had completed was either grossly incorrect and needed redoing completely, or that part was correct and could be added on to usefully.'

In the object assembly task they 'frequently completed the assembly incorrectly seemingly quite unaware of its incorrectness. Pieces often failed to touch each other or did so only at corners. The control group used trial and error methods much more frequently and successfully than the experimental group did, and seemed to appreciate more readily when pieces were correctly placed. It is likely that spatial visual perception difficulties and visuo–motor co-ordination problems are associated with the low scores in the experimental group.'

All the subtests discussed here make demands upon a number of different skills: block design for example requires analytic and synthetic reasoning ability, visual perceptual ability, visuo–motor co-ordination and close attention, while success in the coding subtest requires in addition good motor control (Lyle and Johnson, 1973) and good short-term memory (Johnson and Lyle, 1973). Further carefully controlled experimentation is needed before the exact nature of the children's difficulties in these subtests can be specified. However the results do indicate very strongly that visuo–motor co-ordination skills and the ability to organize motor actions in space are impaired and this may give rise to difficulties in carrying out many everyday actions such as getting a shirt on the right way round and doing up the buttons or catching a ball, and in school will certainly affect attainments, particularly number work and writing.

4 *Motor (manual) skills*

Many spina bifida children not only have specific visuo–motor difficulties of the kind described in the last section but in addition actual impairment of motor (manual) control. Until comparatively recently it was often assumed that the upper limb function of spina bifida children was normal, but there is now increasing evidence that this is often not so. Evidence on abnormalities in the neurological functioning of the upper limbs provided by Wallace (1973), and the relationship of those abnormalities to the presence of hydrocephalus, and to the Arnold-Chiari malformation, was discussed in chapter 1 (p. 40). Poor hand function has also been noted in many non-clinical situations and in children of all ages. It has been commented on by teachers, psychologists and others working with pre-school children (Rowland, 1973; Spain, 1970) and with school-age children (Sella *et al.*, 1966), as well as by those involved in assessing the aptitudes and abilities of school leavers (Parsons, 1972; Hutchinson, 1975).

In this section the main focus will be on recent research evidence concerning manual ability in spina bifida children. Before looking at the evidence regarding motor control per se, the question of hand preference must be considered.

Hand preference. Teachers frequently comment that spina bifida children are slow to develop clear hand preference and there is now research evidence available to confirm this.

In the GLC study handedness was looked at when the children were 6 years old. The child was asked to write with a pencil, cut with scissors and throw a ball, and the preferred hand was noted. In Anderson's study the handedness of 8- to 10-year-old spina bifida children and their matched controls was investigated in a very similar way. If all the tasks were performed with the same hand the child was scored as right- or left-handed, in all other cases as mixed-handed.

In Table 5.7 below the distribution of handedness of the children in these two studies is shown and compared with data from a study which Belmont and Birch (1963), using very similar tasks, carried out with 'bright normal' children.

Table 5.7 *Handedness in spina bifida and non-handicapped 6–10-year-olds (percentages)*

	GLC Study (6 year old)			*Anderson's Study (7-10 year olds)*		*Belmont and Birch (1963) (5-10 year olds)*		
Handedness	*S.B. with shunts*	*S.B. no shunts*	*Controls*	*S.B. with shunts*	*Controls*	*'Bright normal' children 7yrs*	*8yrs*	*9yrs*
Right	50	75	92	55	80	75	75	82
Left	20	25	6	15	15	4	10	12
Mixed	30	—	2	30	5	21	15	6
Number of children	90	40	49	20	20	28	20	17

The table shows very clearly an abnormally low proportion of pure right-handers in the spina bifida group and an abnormally high proportion of mixed-handers and left-handers even among the older children. In the GLC study, even those children without shunts showed a higher proportion of left-handers than did the controls, but it must be remembered that about half of this group had arrested hydrocephalus.

An extensive literature exists concerning the significance of left or mixed handedness. Annett and Turner (1974) have recently reviewed this and have carried out their own investigation of the relationship between laterality and the growth of intellectual abilities. They point out that two main approaches have been made to the problem. One is to classify general samples of children for laterality and then to look at differences in ability. In the main, findings suggest that there are no differences between right-handers and others with respect to ability. The other approach has been to select children for disabilities and then to compare them with control children for laterality. In studies of this kind an increased incidence of left or mixed handedness has, for example, been found in those of subnormal intelligence, in children with some types of speech defects, and in younger backward readers. However, the increased incidence of left or mixed handedness in groups such as these is not as marked as for children with spina bifida and hydrocephalus.

The reasons for the failure of many spina bifida children to establish hand preference are unclear. Damage to the central nervous system arising from hydrocephalus may play an important part but the exact way in which it does so is not known. We noted earlier (p. 35) that the corpus callosum may not be functioning efficiently in some hydrocephalic children. If, as a result, information from one cerebral hemisphere is not readily available to the other, then specialization of function cannot easily occur within the hemispheres and this might be reflected in the absence of lateralization (i.e. the establishment of preference for using one side of the body).

It is sometimes claimed that ill-defined preference is a sign of general neurological immaturity and this could be the explanation of the mixed handedness of at least some spina bifida children. Alternatively, handedness may be slow to develop simply because young spina bifida children tend to sit late, and then to use one hand as a prop, and overall to get little early practice in manual tasks, and there is some evidence (Lonton, 1976) that as children get older the proportion of mixed-handers declines.

Whatever the reason, the failure to develop preference is likely to retard the development of manual skills and it is important that adults should, after careful observation, decide early on and certainly by the time the child is learning to write which hand he appears to use best and then encourage consistent use of that hand.

Motor control. Very little research has been published specifically on the motor control of spina bifida children perhaps partly because few standardized tests of hand function are available for young children. In the GLC study a series of hand function tests were given to the 6 year olds, including a peg board task, touching thumb and finger tips, putting coins and matches into boxes and drawing vertical lines between horizontal ones (adaptation of the Ozeretzky Test as used by Rutter *et al.*, 1970). On these tests the preferred hand was noted and also the time taken to complete the tasks by each hand separately.

On the timed items, children without shunts scored as well as the controls, while those with valves were significantly poorer, regardless of ability. Many children with shunts found the finger-tip touching task extremely difficult, as did an older group in Anderson's study, and children had trouble in picking up small objects such as matchsticks, or in positioning a peg to get it into the hole in the peg board. Although these were usually children of low ability, skill in this task is probably independent of intellectual ability but it may be related to general neurological maturity. Even shunted children with a clear hand preference were still slower and less skilled than were the controls.

The investigation of hand function problems and, in particular, of writing difficulties was the main focus of research carried out by Anderson (1975). In the first phase of this study 6- to 10-year-old children with spina bifida and hydrocephalus and a closely matched control group were compared on a hand function test standardized for children by Taylor and his colleagues (1973).

The spina bifida children did much more poorly and, although the numbers were fairly small (thirty in each group) and the variation within the spina bifida group considerable, the differences between the two groups reached a high level of statistical significance both for the preferred and non-preferred hand. On most of the subtests only a small proportion of spina bifida children (usually from 5–10 per cent and never more than 14 per cent) scored above the non-handicapped mean, while roughly half the spina bifida children made scores more than two standard deviations below the mean. Overall, more than two in three spina bifida children were markedly slow. The spina bifida children were particularly slow in the picking up small objects test where fine finger movements, efficient release mechanisms and good eye–hand co-ordination are all required. They also had great difficulty in the simulated feeding subtests where beans are scooped up in a spoon. Many held the spoon in an awkward way, and controlled it poorly, while some failed to orient the spoon correctly in order to pick up the beans.

Later in this study the children were given a series of tasks involving use of a pencil. The first was a dotting task (dotting between two circles) for which normative data (Connolly and Stratton, 1968) was available. The main finding (for details see Anderson and Plewis, 1977) was that the spina bifida children performed significantly more slowly than the controls, their dotting speed being comparable to that of normal 6 year olds although their average age was 8·9 years.

Other tests used in the study came much closer to actual handwriting tasks. The simplest was a speed of crossing test first used by Lyle and Johnson (1973), and selected because the perceptual component was minimal and the motor aspect of performance maximized. The child was to fill in as many crosses on a grid of squares as he could in two minutes. As expected, the spina bifida children (mean score = 36·2 per minute) wrote significantly more slowly than the controls (49·3).

Tracing tasks offer a useful means of assessing motor control with a pencil since the child does not have to make any spatial judgments about direction and distance as he does when he copies something and, provided that visual acuity is adequate, poor performance can be attributed mainly to motor dysfunction. In the task devised for this study the children had to trace five sets of unfamiliar symbols, as quickly and as carefully as they could. On all the tasks but one the spina bifida children traced significantly more slowly than the controls and they were also less accurate.

Summing up

The evidence presented in this chapter shows that while those children who have spina bifida but no hydrocephalus, or only a mild degree of hydrocephalus, are likely to show a fairly normal and balanced development of skills, this is not generally true of the great majority of spina bifida children, those with myelomeningocele and a degree of hydrocephalus sufficient to have required early surgery. While some hydrocephalic children are of average or above average intelligence with no specific difficulties, most of this group show marked unevenness of intellectual functioning. Some aspects of verbal ability (the development of syntax and the acquisition of vocabulary skills) seem normal or near normal but other aspects (the comprehension of written or spoken language and the appropriate use of language) are usually less well developed. Certain aspects of perception often appear to be impaired.

On some tasks involving perceptual skills (e.g. picture completion, shape constancy) performance does not differ significantly from that of normal children of comparable overall intellectual ability, while on other perceptual tasks, in particular figure–ground discrimination, there is in many children a marked degree of impairment. Performance on visuo-motor tasks of all kinds is generally poor. Undoubtedly, poor motor control is a major contributory factor although the difficulty is by no means one of executing movements only and there are clear indications that the child's ability to plan and organize his movements in space is impaired.

We are not yet in a position to say how far difficulties of these kinds can be attributed on the one hand to neurological abnormalities (although there can be little doubt that these are involved) and on the other to deprivation of normal experiences resulting both from the children's often severely restricting handicaps and also from social and other factors which prevent them from enjoying the usual range of experiences. What cannot be doubted is that a great deal can be done before the child starts school to minimize many of the difficulties described here, and this is what the following chapter is about.

References

Abercrombie, M. L. M. (1963), in Smith, V. H. (ed.), *Visual Disorders and Cerebral Palsy*, Little Club Clinics in Developmental Medicine, 9, Spastics Society/Heinemann, London.

Alberman, N. B. and Gardiner, P. A. (1971), 'Children with squints. A handicapped group?', *The Practitioner*, 206, pp. 501–6.

Anderson, E. M. (1975), 'Cognitive and motor deficits in children with spina bifida and hydrocephalus with special reference to writing difficulties', unpublished Ph.D. thesis, University of London.

——, and Plewis, I. (1977), 'Impairment of a motor skill in children with spina bifida cystica and hydrocephalus: an exploratory study', *British Journal of Psychology* (in press).

Annett, M. and Turner, A. (1974), 'Laterality and the growth of intellectual abilities', *British Journal of Educational Psychology*, 44 (1), pp. 37–46.

Badell-Ribera, A., Shulman, K. and Paddock, N. (1966), 'The relationship of non-progressive hydrocephalus to intellectual functioning in children with spina bifida cystica', *Paediatrics*, 37, pp. 787–93.

Ball, M. (1975), 'Investigation into the reading abilities and related perceptual abilities of spina bifida children', unpublished report submitted for Masters degree in Child Development, University of London.

Belmont, L. and Birch, H. G. (1963), 'Lateral dominance and right-left awareness in normal children', *Child Development*, 34, pp. 257–70.

Brimer, M. A. and Dunn, L. M. (1963), *Manual for the English Picture Vocabulary Test*, NFER, Windsor, Berks.

Burns, R. (1957), 'The assessment of school placement in children suffering from encephalocele and meningomyelocele in the City of Liverpool', *Developmental Medicine and Child Neurology*, Supplement 13, pp. 23–9.

Connolly, K. and Stratton, P. (1968), 'Developmental changes in associated movements', *Developmental Medicine and Child Neurology* 10, pp. 49–56.

Department of Education and Science (1969), *The Health of the Schoolchild 1966–68*, HMSO, London.

Diller, L., Gordon, W. A., Swinyard, C. and Kastner, S. (1969), *Psychological and Educational Studies with Spina Bifida Children*, Project No. 5-0412, Washington, US Dept. of Health Education and Welfare, US Office of Education.

Dodds, J. (1975), *Hydrocephalic Children and Visual Perception*, unpublished M.Ed. Psychol. Master's dissertation, University of Sussex, 1975.

Fleming, C. P. (1968), 'The verbal behaviour of hydrocephalic children', *Developmental Medicine and Child Neurology*, Supplement 1, pp. 74–82.

Frostig, M. (1966), *Manual for the Marianne Frostig Development Test of Visual Perception*, Consulting Psychologists' Press, Palo Alto, California.

Gibson, E. J., Gibson, J. J., Pick, A. D. and Osser, H. A. (1962), 'Developmental study of the discrimination of letter-like forms', *Journal of Comparative and Physiological Psychology* 55, pp. 897–906.

Goldberg, J. K. (1968), 'Vision, perception and related facts in dyslexia', pp. 90–109 in Keeney, A. H. and Keeney, V. T. (eds.), *Dyslexia: Diagnosis and Treatment of Reading Disorders*, C. V. Mosby, St Louis.

Hadenius, A., Hagberg, B., Hyttnas-Bensch, K. and Sjogren, I. (1962), 'The natural prognosis of infantile hydrocephalus', *Acta Pediatrica* 51, pp. 117–18.

Haskell, S. and Hughes, V. A. (1965), 'Some observations on the performance of squinters and non-squinters on the Wechsler Intelligence Scale for Children', *Perceptual and Motor Skills* 21, pp. 107–12.

Hutchinson, D. (1975), personal communication.

Ingram, T. T. S. and Naughton, J. (1962), 'Pediatric and psychological aspects of cerebral palsy associated with hydrocephalus', *Developmental Medicine and Child Neurology* 4, pp. 287–92.

Johnson, E. G. and Lyle, J. G. (1973), 'Analysis of WISC Coding: 4, Paired associate learning and performance strategies', *Perceptual and Motor Skills*, 37, 695–8.

Kagan, J. (1965), 'Reflection-impulsivity and reading ability in primary grade children', *Child Development*, 36, pp. 609–28.

Laurence, K. M. and Tew, B. J. (1967), 'Follow-up of 65 survivors from 425 cases of spina bifida born in S. Wales between 1956 and 1962', *Developmental Medicine and Child Neurology*, Supplement 13, pp. 1–3.

——, ——, (1971), 'Studies in spina bifida cystica IV', *Archives of Diseases in Childhood*, 47, pp. 128–37.

Laurendeau, M. and Pinard, A. (1970), *The Development of the Concept of Space in the Child*, International University Press Inc., New York.

Liedholm, M., Wessner, G. and Karlberg, P. (1974), 'Mental function in children with myelomeningocele: a preliminary report', *Developmental Medicine and Child Neurology*, Supplement 32, p. 157.

Lonton, A. P., (1976), 'Hand preference in children with myelomeningocele and hydrocephalus', Supplement 37, pp. 143–9.

Lorber, J. (1971), 'Results of treatment of myelomeningocele', *Developmental Medicine and Child Neurology*, 13 (3), pp. 279–303.

Lyle, J. G. and Johnson, E. G. (1973), 'Analysis of WISC Coding: 3, Writing and copying speed and motivation', *Perceptual and Motor Skills*, 36, pp. 211–14.

Matson, D. D. (1961), 'Clinical classification and evaluation of hydrocephalus', in Field, W. S. and Desmond, M. M. (eds.), *Disorders of the Developing Nervous System*, C. C. Thomas, Springfield, Illinois.

Miller, E. and Sethi, L. (1971), 'The effect of hydrocephalus on perception', *Developmental Medicine and Child Neurology*, Supplement 25, pp. 77–81.

Parsons, J. G. (1969), 'Short term verbal memory in hydrocephalic children', *Developmental Medicine and Child Neurology*, Supplement 20, pp. 75–9.

——, (1972), 'Assessment of aptitudes in young people of school leaving age handicapped by hydrocephalus or spina bifida cystica', *Developmental Medicine and Child Neurology*, Supplement 27, pp. 101–8.

Purkhiser, C. A. (1965), 'A comparative investigation of verbal behaviour and psycholinguistic abilities of a group of hydrocephalic children and their matched controls', Ph.D. thesis, Northwestern University, Evanston, Illinois.

Reynell, J. (1969), *Reynell Developmental Language Scale*, NFER, Slough, Bucks.

Rowland, M. (1973), 'Evaluation of playgroup for children with spina bifida', *Social Work Today*, 4 (11), pp. 325–30.

Rutter, M., Graham, P. and Yule, W. (1970), *A Neuropsychiatric Study in Childhood*, Clinics in Developmental Medicine, 35, Spastics Society/Heinemann, London.

Sella, A., Foltz, E. L. and Shurtleff, D. B. (1966), 'A 3 year developmental study of treated and untreated hydrocephalus in children', *Journal of Pediatrics*, 69, p. 887.

Spain, B. (1969), 'Estimating the future school population of spina bifida children within London', Quarterly Bulletin of GLC Research and Intelligence Unit, 7, pp. 18–25.

——, (1970), 'Spina bifida survey', Quarterly Bulletin of GLC Research and Intelligence Unit, 12, pp. 5–12.

——, (1972), 'Verbal and performance ability in pre-school spina bifida children', *Developmental Medicine and Child Neurology*, Supplement 27, p. 155.

——, (1974), 'Verbal and performance ability in pre-school children with spina bifida', *Developmental Medicine and Child Neurology*, 16, pp. 773–80.

Swisher, L. P. and Pinsker, E. J. (1971), 'The language characteristics of hyperverbal hydrocephalic children', *Developmental Medicine and Child Neurology*, 13, pp. 746–55.

Taylor, E. M. (1959), *Psychological Appraisal of Children with Cerebral Defects*, Harvard University Press, Cambridge, Massachusetts.

Taylor, N., Sand, P. L. and Jebsen, R. (1973), 'Evaluation of hand function in children', *Archives of Physical Medicine*, 54, pp. 129–35.

Tew, B. J. (1973a), 'Some psychological consequences of spina bifida and its complications', Proceedings of 31st Bienniel Conference ASE, London.

——, (1973b), 'Spina bifida and hydrocephalus: facts, fallacies and future', *Special Education* 62 (4), pp. 26–31.

——, and Laurence, K. M. (1972), 'The ability and attainments of spina bifida patients born in S. Wales between 1956–62', *Developmental Medicine and Child Neurology*, Supplement 27, pp. 124–131.

Wallace, S. J. (1973), 'The effect of upper limb function on mobility of children with myelomeningocele', *Developmental Medicine and Child Neurology*, Supplement 29, pp. 84–91.

Woodburn, M. (1973), *Social Implications of Spina Bifida – a Study in S.E. Scotland*, Eastern Branch Scottish Spina Bifida Association, Edinburgh.

6 The pre-school years

Introduction

Studies of the normal child's development show that the growth curve for learning does not progress in equal units over time and that the maximum learning per unit of time occurs in the pre-school period. This is partly explained by the fact that the nervous system is not complete at birth but goes on developing during the first few years of life. For example, the cerebellum, that part of the brain which controls fine motor co-ordination (and which is frequently impaired in the spina bifida child), has its fastest growth period post-natally between 0 and 3 years.

However, these (maturational) changes within the body's physiology do not wholly account for the very rapid development of skills in the early years, and the experiences to which the young infant is exposed also play a major part in the rate at which he develops. Psychologists discuss these issues nowadays in terms of 'critical' or 'sensitive' periods for growth (Connolly, 1972) without trying to describe which of these aspects, maturation or experience, is most important. Not only do children develop at a faster rate in the early rather than the later years but environmental influences also exert their maximum impact during these periods of rapid growth.

Many experimental studies have been made by psychologists of the effects upon later development (generally of mammals such as monkeys, dogs and rats) of different kinds of early experiences. Two major approaches have been to study the effects of varying on the one hand the amount of sensory stimulation to which young animals are exposed and on the other the kinds of sensory and social environments in which they are reared. Both point to the conclusion that the right stimulation at the right time is crucial for the optimal development of a skill.

Human infants cannot of course be subjected to experimental deprivation in the way that animals can and the findings from studies on the effects of environment on human development are not so clear cut.

However, recent work by White and others (1970) demonstrates that it is possible to accelerate the rate at which young children acquire certain skills by a careful programme of stimulation, and that similarly children with less stimulation take longer to acquire the same skill. These studies are particularly relevant to the development of the young child with spina bifida, since they are concerned with the development of reaching and grasping in very young infants. Children given extra stimulation in the form of toys and other attractive objects suspended over their cots each day began to reach, grasp and fixate visually at a much earlier age than a control group who did not have these incentives.

Infants who are physically or mentally handicapped need very much the same sensory and social experiences as normal children but because of the limitations imposed on them by their handicaps they are likely to be more dependent upon adult help to ensure that they are exposed to and can benefit from these stimuli. In earlier chapters a detailed account was given of the sorts of physical and intellectual handicaps from which a severely handicapped infant is likely to suffer. How might these reduce his ability to benefit from sensory and other experiences in the early years of life?

Deprivation of experience in the early years

During the first vitally important eighteen months the child's impaired ability to sit up unsupported and to move will mean that, without help, he may spend a much longer period than is normal lying flat on his back in his cot or pram, or in a hospital bed gazing, perhaps, into empty space. Impaired hand control may result in part in a child starting to use his hands later and less successfully than normal infants; he may also appear not to enjoy the usual toys offered to him. A child lying on his back all day, or even in the prone position, cannot easily manipulate objects and when he does so frequently drops them and cannot retrieve them because of his immobility. Most children learn by about one year old that objects have a permanence even when not seen, but before this happens play may be very unrewarding for a spina bifida child and he may even lose interest in toys since they seem to disappear frequently in a most disappointing way. If he has a squint, or other ocular defects, it may be more difficult for him to make sense of visual stimuli. Perceptual problems, and problems of co-ordinating vision and hand movements may also mean that he benefits less or more slowly from experiences than a normal child.

It is essential, therefore, that the child is helped to achieve a sitting posture at the correct age, not only by early exercises to strengthen the relevant muscles, but also by using a special chair or sitting apparatus if necessary, so that by six or seven months of age he can have the experience of sitting in an upright position. This enables him to see more of his surroundings and to play with objects using both hands freely. Many spina bifida children cannot sit unsupported even by the age of two years. In the GLC study half of the children could not sit safely on an ordinary kitchen chair at this age, and most of these needed to use one hand as a prop if sitting unsupported on the floor, consequently manipulating objects with only one hand. If such children reach forward to pick up a toy they may be unable to pull themselves upright again without adult help. These children had little opportunity to use both hands together and to develop normal manipulative skills. Most parents do buy some type of special chair for their child but it is not always the most satisfactory one in terms of giving maximum support and a large area for play at the appropriate height. Advice to parents about this must be given during the first six months and a list of books which suggest appropriate chairs, toys and other aids is given in Appendix G. For the very young child it is not difficult to improvise a suitable chair. A block of firm foam rubber with a curve cut out of it makes an excellent and very portable chair which supports the child on three sides and can be enlarged (by cutting back the foam) as he grows. A low table makes a better play surface than the floor if the child cannot pull himself upright and this can be made by sawing the legs off a coffee table, or from a large tray with the legs screwed or stuck underneath.

Most children in the GLC study (over 90 per cent) could, by the age of two, get about the floor in some fashion, either self-propelled or by means of a low-wheeled buggy or 'chariot' which they had learnt to manipulate. However, only a third could stand without support and an even smaller proportion could walk in any useful sense. Nearly 40 per cent of the children could not stand at all at this age, even with adult help or with calipers, and 50 per cent could not climb down from an ordinary chair unassisted. Most normal children stand around the age of a year and walk and climb well before the age of two, so the experience of the majority of handicapped children is already quite restricted even during the first two years of life.

By three years most children were still unable to stand without adult support, in or out of calipers. Only one third could walk any appreciable distance out of doors and over 40 per cent could not walk at all or only a few steps. Over 75 per cent of the children had, in effect, to be carried everywhere once outside the living-room or kitchen. Even at six years old only 47 per cent of the children could get about the house in some way without restriction, and 20 per cent were virtually confined to one or two rooms. This means not only that the child's chances of exploring his environment are very restricted: it also reduces his chances of achieving personal independence.

Hunt (1973) gives a vivid description of restrictions of this kind: 'the main deprivation of the paraplegic child was due to immobility. He usually moved by dragging himself along by his arms [and] spent much of the day confined to a trolley at floor level or to a chair. Outdoor activities were infrequent and companionship limited. Opportunities for investigation and experimentation were restricted to trolley level or chair range, and the child's occupation depended largely on what was provided by his mother . . . In many . . . lack of trunk control meant that one hand or elbow was needed for a prop, leaving only one hand free for play.'

The distance that the child could actually walk was also examined in the GLC study (Table 6.1) this factor being important not only because it will affect his ability to explore his own environment in and near to home, and to share in the social experiences of his peers, but also for later school placement.

Table 6.1 *Distance child can walk at four years. GLC Spina Bifida Survey*

	N	%
Completely mobile	36	25
Could walk to shops or school	20	14
Around home including stairs	39	27
Around house a little	21	15
2 or 3 steps only	14	9
Not at all	15	10

Here we see that less than 40 per cent were completely mobile or could walk a short distance outdoors, while 29 per cent had no useful walking even at the age of four.

The data presented so far shows how the motor impairment itself may deprive the spina bifida child of sensory-motor or social stimulation in the pre-school period. An examination of other activities in relation to the degree of locomotor handicap reveals further how the handicapped child's whole experience in the early years may be affected by the consequences of his physical condition. Even in eating, an activity not obviously related to the locomotor handicap, the two year old with spina bifida shows developmental delay, since 15 per cent of children could not or did not feed themselves with a spoon and a further 22 per cent required considerable help with feeding. At the age of three years (when most normal children have mastered this skill) the child's ability to use a spoon and fork was examined in relation to the degree of motor impairment and the results are shown in Table 6.2.

Table 6.2 *Percentage of 3 year olds able to use a spoon and fork, GLC Spina Bifida Survey*

Degree of locomotor handicaps	*Unable to use any implement*	*Uses spoon only*	*Uses spoon and fork with reasonable skill*	*Total %*	*Total N*
Mod/severe	2·7	43	55	100·0	68
Mild or none	0	14	86	100·0	48

Whether the child eats at table with the family or in a special chair on his own was also related to handicap; only 4 per cent of those who were mildly handicapped did not eat at the table with the rest of the family compared with 35 per cent of the more severely handicapped. Another area investigated in this survey was the sleeping arrangements made for the child. Here it was found that none of the less handicapped children slept in their parents' bed at 3 years and only 15 per cent slept in their parents' room, whereas over 30 per cent of the more handicapped children slept in their parents' room and some even in the same bed.

A number of other questions which mothers were asked about their 3 year olds also brought out the differences between the mildly and the moderately/severely handicapped children. A much higher proportion of mildly than of severely handicapped children were reported as being adventurous; conversely a higher proportion of severely handicapped children were either fearful or simply did not attempt to do new things (Table 6.3).

Overall, during the pre-school years when the child's most intensive learning experiences take place, spina bifida children are liable, because of their physical handicaps, to be deprived of many normal experiences.

Table 6.3 *Percentage of 3 year olds said to be adventurous, GLC Spina Bifida Survey*

Degree of locomotor handicap	*Adventurous*	*Does not do new things*	*Fearful*	*Total %*	*N*
Mod/severe	56	22	22	100·0	68
Mild/none	88	8	4	100·0	48

In many cases they are also likely to be hampered by the intellectual problems which were discussed in the previous chapter, and emotional and behavioural problems, particularly distractability (discussed in chapters 8 and 9), may also prevent them from benefitting fully from the experiences which are presented to them. Fortunately, parents and professionals working with spina bifida children can do an enormous amount to prevent such deprivation of experiences from occurring and in the next section we describe, first, what can be done in the home to facilitate the pre-school child's development and, second, what use can be made of facilities outside the home, in particular through pre-school 'education' in all its forms.

Helping pre-school spina bifida children in the home: the role of the parents

The role of the parents in the training and treatment of pre-school children handicapped in a variety of ways is now being increasingly recognized and is likely to be even more fully developed in the future (e.g. Patterson and Gullion, 1968; Johnson and Katz, 1973; Seifert, 1973; Cunningham, 1975). Parents of blind and deaf children are usually given considerable guidance about how to help their children in the early years, but this has not been the case for physically handicapped children. We probably now know enough about the sorts of problems which spina bifida children are likely to have – some of them obvious, others like perceptual deficits and poor eye–hand co-ordination, less so – to be able to be much more specific about the ways in which parents can help the child to minimize these problems. Because the basis for many important skills is laid in the first eighteen months of life, parents should, very early on, be given practical help and guidance about how they can encourage the development of the child. Active and informed involvement in the child's management is also likely to make it easier for the parents to accept the child's handicaps, and this in turn will benefit his social development. Even where there is a primary organic problem such as hydrocephalus or cerebral palsy it must not be assumed that intellectual retardation is inevitable or that it cannot be improved by early intervention, particularly in those areas where we know that the child's physiological endowment is weakest.

It is therefore essential that parents receive developmental advice and information about the management of the child during the early years. Most parents have only a hazy notion of the sequence of development in normal children, especially if it is their first child. The activities appropriate for each stage of development are usually dictated by the child himself: he insists on sitting, walking and feeding himself at a particular age and usually manages to ensure that his parents co-operate with him in his efforts to achieve independence. Because of his physical limitations a handicapped child cannot 'teach' his parents what his developmental needs are in the same way as a normal child does, therefore his parents must receive instructions if they are to help him achieve the appropriate behaviours in sequence and, as far as possible, at the same age as other children.

Because parents of a handicapped child are quite naturally fearful that the child will come to harm, they often tend to restrict his exploratory or motor development. They need a great deal of information and encouragement if they are to allow him to attempt new activities which might be slightly dangerous, such as learning how to fall safely or to climb furniture or stairs. Also the activities of a handicapped child are likely to be much more parent-controlled than is true of a normal child, and he does not have the opportunity to do 'forbidden' things, which are often a very important part of intellectual and emotional development.

It is often difficult for parents to take their handicapped child outside the house because of the problem of travelling, of accessibility or of facilities for changing him. Unless they have a car, families often cannot visit relatives or friends or places of interest to children such as parks, zoos or museums as often as they would like. These children and their families need special help if the child is to gain a normal experience of the outside world.

A handicapped child whose physical needs make him very dependent on his parents is often treated as being younger than he actually is (see also chapter 9). Such children are often emotionally immature in consequence and this may have repercussions upon intellectual development. Parents very often hesitate to make demands on the child or to insist that he become more independent or mature because they do not wish to distress or frustrate him. In consequence, some handicapped children are not stretched at home; they may not learn that real intellectual effort is often required in order to achieve something and that this effort can be very rewarding.

Help and advice for parents in the pre-school period is, therefore, most important. As was pointed out in chapter 4, they must be assisted in increasing their self-confidence in their own competence and fathers as well as mothers need to be involved. Parents of quite normal children usually experience misgivings from time to time about their own capabilities. Parents of handicapped children very often feel inadequate to cope with the task of bringing them up or at a loss to know how best to help them. They should be given some background information and techniques and taught how to observe and assess their child's progress. (Schedules are now being developed specifically for this purpose and examples are to be found in Appendix E.)

A visit to the home is invaluable to anyone working with parents. This will allow the 'expert' to see what the child is doing at home, how he spends his day and what limitations or resources exist within the home. The way the parent interacts with the child and the way the child behaves at home may well be quite different from the impression given during hospital or clinic attendances. On home territory the parents are usually more relaxed and better able to present their viewpoint. Advice given in the home can be more practical and specific and therefore more informative and useful, and parents can be helped to see how they can use ordinary household objects and furniture to help their child develop the relevant skills, or where minor adaptations could give the child more freedom or independence.

Those with experience in working with parents (e.g. Patterson and Gullion, 1973; Cunningham, 1975) have found that parents need practical and not just verbal teaching in developing training programmes for their child. Discussions or talks explaining the principles of child development are important, as is printed information which the parents can take home to read or discuss at their leisure, but of much greater value are actual demonstrations to the parents of those child-management or observational techniques which they need to develop. Video-tapes can be very useful but there is no substitute for practical demonstrations, particularly those involving the child himself in his own home.

Play activities in the home

Play for handicapped children: general principles

Jill Norris in her introduction to the excellent booklet on toys and play activities for handicapped children produced by the Toy Libraries Association (from which many of the ideas in this section are taken) points out that 'play experiences needed by handicapped children are largely the same as those of normal children only in slow motion and with different accents; so what will help them most is not so much a "special" toy but the right amount of the right toy at the right time presented in the right way'. The play experiences needed by handicapped children may differ slightly from those of normal children in a number of ways.

Firstly, the handicapped child often needs to be provided with carefully planned stimulation earlier than parents might feel was necessary with normal children. Secondly, he will probably need more repetitive play experiences than normal children to reinforce the skills that play teaches. Thirdly, he may need to be presented with more provoking (attention-catching) situations, to stimulate his reactions. Fourthly, since handicapped children often lack the initiative to sustain play on their own he may need more encouragement, praise and support in his play activities. More detailed examples will be given in the paragraphs which follow.

Activities and play for spina bifida infants

(a) *Encouraging visual awareness.* Babies have to learn first to fixate their gaze on an object and then to follow the object with their eyes, horizontally at first and then vertically. Initially, until he can sit or hold objects, himself the baby will depend on adults to enrich the space around him with different sights and sounds which will encourage him to focus, to follow with his eyes and in general to become more aware of his environment. Research has shown that even tiny babies register more when they are sitting up, so that the baby should be propped up in his pram or in a baby-chair in the room where his mother is working from as early as possible. The development of fixation and following skills will be encouraged if: (i) his behaviour is rewarded by the mother (by smiling, cuddling, cooing, etc.); (ii) the child is exposed to the right stimuli. These will of course include his mother's face and the feeding bottle but also objects suspended above his cot or pram or tied to it so that he does not lose them. Since he may have visual or perceptual problems, objects with a big visual impact in shiny materials and bold primary colours can be selected. Jill Norris suggests that parents can begin by turning the baby's head to the electric light, the window and the mirror or by suspending in front of him a simple red ball within his range, for random knocking or kicking. Objects should not only be suspended across the cot but on either side as well and the child encouraged to reach for objects on the left side with his right hand and vice versa. Following skills can be encouraged by getting the baby to follow with his eyes a moving torch or bubbles or an object suspended from a string, or by hanging a mobile or other hanging objects within sight and hearing. The position from which the child lies and watches them can be changed, and he can be picked up and shown the objects from different angles. Musical and moving toys can also be used.

(b) *Encouraging body and tactile awareness.* Infants become aware of their own body and separate identity by playing with their toes, fingers and so on. Later it is helpful to sit the baby in front of a mirror and to point to and name the different parts of his face and body. He should also be encouraged to 'explore' his mother's face, clothes and parts of the body. A study of myelomeningocele children aged 5 to 7 years (Barnitt, 1975) suggested deficiencies in 'body image', that is, in the child's awareness of the relationship of the different parts of his body to each other. Training over a relatively short period resulted in large improvements and there is no reason why the development of a correct body-image should not be encouraged early on in life. The child's attention should also be drawn to his lower limbs (for example bells could be tied to his ankles) as otherwise, owing to lack of sensation, he may hardly be aware of their existence.

It is also important to encourage the awareness of tactile sensations, especially as there is evidence (e.g. Miller and Sethi, 1971) that in some spina bifida children tactile sensation is poor. It is possible that early tactile stimulation may help to improve the hand function. While there is as yet no experimental evidence of this for spina bifida children, work with young cerebral-palsied children (Barrett and Jones, 1967) suggests the benefits upon hand function which can be gained by encouraging tactile awareness.

There are many ways of doing this and the materials needed are present in every home. Jill Norris gives a wide range of ideas in her booklet on toys for handicapped children. She points out that 'as soon as he can use his hands the child will need objects and toys to grasp, squeeze, wave about, roll, open and shut, and drop – as well as things to suck, lick, bite, chew and generally explore with his mouth. So at this stage add to his range of tactile experiences as much as possible by letting him handle different shapes, sizes, textures (smooth, soft, hard and rough) and weights. These can be hung from a coat-hanger above his cot or pram . . . within handling range or even from a net above his cot . . . He will also enjoy at this stage squeezing a sponge at bathtime. All this is just as important as stimulating him by sight and sound.' Seifert (1973) points out that mealtimes can also provide much tactile stimulation and that long before a spoon can be used the baby is able to finger feed, this giving him sensations of different textures and shapes. Later on water-play will give the child a whole new range of tactile experience and movement.

(c) *Encouraging eye–hand co-ordination.* Research evidence reported in the last chapter suggested that eye–hand co-ordination is poor in many spina bifida children. There is reason to believe that this is due in part to lack of normal experiences and not simply to neurological damage, so that this is an area in which early encouragement is particularly important. As noted earlier, the ability to grasp or reach for an object can be developed or retarded according to the child's experience. Generally, normal infants will briefly grasp an object placed in the hand in the latter part of the third month. If by the fourth month the baby has made no attempt to grasp anything, his fingers and hands can be curled firmly around toys of different sizes, and he can be encouraged to keep hold of them. The toys should not be too small, and square or cylindrical objects may be best. Following this, the baby will begin to open his hands in anticipation of getting an object and later to reach for objects and these actions should always be encouraged by the object itself and by praise. He will be discouraged if the object is too heavy and best results will be obtained if it is fairly large, but easy to grasp and lightweight.

From about the seventh month the baby should, from a well-supported sitting position at a large hard play surface at the appropriate height (see p. 147), be encouraged to reach for objects with one hand at a time, to pick up an object from a surface and to transfer it from hand to hand. By the age of nine or ten months, finer finger movements will be developing. Use of the pincer grasp can be encouraged by offering bite-sized pieces of food and giving them to the baby only when he uses this grasp. An infant also needs practice in poking and pushing, and in using his fingers separately, starting at this stage with the index finger. Many children keep their fingers clenched in the early days and fine finger movements cannot develop until the child has learnt to release his grasp. Spina bifida children sometimes have difficulty in doing this and it is a skill which needs to be practised and rewarded. It can be encouraged for example, by getting the child to drop an object into a container which makes a noise.

We have described in some detail some of the skills which spina bifida children can be helped to develop during the vital first 12 months of life. If parents know the sequence in which certain skills can be expected and how they can be encouraged then they can do a great deal to get the infant off to an excellent start.

Play activities for older spina bifida pre-school children and infants
From the age of about 18 months to 7 years a spina bifida child will, like any other child, need a very wide range of play experiences and below a brief description is given of some activities which should be particularly encouraged in the light of what is known about these children's strengths and weaknesses. Again, many of these ideas are taken from Jill Norris's booklet on toys and play for handicapped children.

(i) *Play to develop visual skills and the perception of form.* Skill in distinguishing shapes, sizes, patterns and colours is a first step in learning to read. Many spina bifida children will need to spend much longer at the stages where they play with three-dimensional objects before they go on to purely two-dimensional sorting games such as lotto. So in the early stages the child should be encouraged to manipulate and explore solid shapes made for example of wood or plastic, and form-boards will be useful too. At a slightly later stage he will be able to progress to matching shapes cut from wood or card with pictures. He can also be encouraged to identify shapes in the environment, for instance finding all the square shapes or objects he can see in the kitchen. Once he can cope with purely visual sorting he will start to benefit from pairing games like snap or picture dominoes, colour-grading games being the easiest ones to start with.

(ii) *Play to develop tactile skills.* Many games can be invented at home to increase the child's tactile sensitivity. Games can be played involving the tactile discrimination of different woodblock shapes, familiar objects can be hidden under a cloth or buried in a bowl of sand and identified by touch. If the child fails to identify them properly, then he is allowed to look at the object and relate what he feels to what he sees before the objects are again hidden. It is in this way that he builds up a tactile-visual image. Another game is to ask the child to pick out a particular texture from different materials, or loose materials such as gravel, sand, beans and sawdust can be identified. It is better to make games like these fairly short, perhaps five or ten minutes only, and to play them often rather than to risk the child becoming bored and inattentive. Not only will they encourage better co-ordination and a greater awareness of the hands but also perceptual and language skills.

(iii) *Play to develop eye–hand co-ordination skills and manual dexterity.* Eye–hand co-ordination in making both large and small movements should be developed. Throwing and catching games are important since they train a child to judge distance, adapt his muscles, keep his eye on the ball and keep his balance, but should begin in a very simple way, for instance with a large soft cushion which is easy to catch, progressing down through small soft objects to large balls and then to small balls. The child may need to be supported in case he falls sideways. Eye–hand co-ordination in large movements is also encouraged by getting the child to clap his hands to music, or bang musical instruments and again he should be encouraged to use both hands together. Since dressing and undressing often cause difficulties, dressing-up clothes are useful and the child's awareness of his own body is encouraged if he can look at himself wearing them in a mirror. Other bilateral activities suggested by Jill Norris include playing with extra large but not too heavy bricks, and cooking, weighing and sieving. Water and sand play will also encourage the use of both hands together and each one separately.

In some of these activities adaptations will be needed so that they can be done from a sitting position or from a position where the child is standing propped up, and the child must always be well supported.

The child also needs to be encouraged in activities which require finer finger control provided that too much is not asked of him. Constructional toys such as hammer toys, simple stacking and fitting toys, simple jigsaws with large pieces and posting boxes may all be useful. Other activities to encourage include bead threading and peg boards (initially big pegs and very large beads will be needed), and modelling.

Play-doh, brick-building, glove puppets, tearing paper, cutting and pasting, all help eye–hand co-ordination skills and for older children finger-painting, colouring pictures (with an emphasis, if the child has developed the necessary control, on keeping inside the lines rather than only free imaginative painting), joining up dot pictures, and tracing may be useful.

(iv) *Play to develop spatial and number skills.* Many spina bifida children experience great difficulty at school with number work (see chapter 8). Norris points out that before the child is able to grasp the abstract concepts of number and measurement he will need a lot of practical experience with measuring, e.g. with sand and water (different polythene bottles, jugs, cups and sieves in the bath) and if possible with simple cooking, as well as experience in handling three dimensional shapes and bricks. It may also benefit him to play with weighing and balance scales if these are strongly made, and it will help him to grasp the concepts involved if these are always stated verbally, for example 'this is the heavier one'.

Many spina bifida children, probably partly because of specific perceptual difficulties and also because of restricted mobility, have a very poor understanding of space and direction. Children over two years old will respond to prepositions such as under, beside, behind, and games can be played using these directions in which the child is asked to find familiar objects hidden in the room. Rail tracks or a large dolls' house can also help to give ideas of forward, backward, up, down, next to and so on. Directional difficulties are often seen when the child tries to dress himself and dressing-up games should be encouraged.

(v) *Other types of play.* There is sometimes a danger that those who work with handicapped children will forget that the essential thing about play is that it is enjoyable. A great deal of the play of young normal children is dominated by the sheer joy of activity for its own sake, and this must have some biological function. Play also allows the child to release tensions of various kinds, to be creative perhaps in a noisy or messy way or simply to relax.

All children need the chance to express themselves in 'messy' play; spina bifida children need a lot of encouragement before they will express themselves freely with painting, drawing, clay or finger painting, and, of course, with sand or water. Children can also often work through their fears by means of play; with many spina bifida children games connected with hospitals, and nurses' and doctors' kits are very popular. As with other children, dressing-up, dolls' prams and of course the opportunity to use real household equipment will all help the children to develop socially. What is much more difficult to provide a severely handicapped child with is the kind of play, involving gross motor skills, which engages so much of a normal child's time, but even heavily handicapped children can experience some of the exhilaration created by movement by means of swings, slides or chariots, and many good ideas for this sort of exciting play can be seen in adventure playgrounds for handicapped children. Suggestions are available from the Handicapped Adventure Playground Association as well as in Arvid Bengtsson's book (1972).

(vi) *Helping children who are hyperverbal and distractable.* The problem of distractability is commonly reported in spina bifida children and is dealt with in more detail in chapters 8 and 9. However, since findings from the GLC survey showed that this problem was noticed even as early as at 3 years old by both parents and professionals, it seemed important to us to discuss the problem in relationship to play. Parents who have been alerted to this problem can do a great deal to improve the child's concentration and also to inhibit irrelevant speech from quite an early age.

The problem of distractability might be considerably reduced if parents and other adults always encouraged the child to *listen* and to *attend* from an early age. Telling or reading stories to young children is a good way of doing this; the child needs to be encouraged to listen without making too many interruptions, and asked about the story from time to time to make sure that he has understood. Making a child re-tell the story is another way of checking that he has understood, while adult comments on what he says will help him to distinguish relevant from unimportant detail.

In other activities, such as drawing, painting or building, the child should be encouraged to keep his attention on the task and to persist in what he is doing. A child will not enjoy an activity or want to do it again unless he has some success (e.g. completion of a puzzle). He must therefore be encouraged to do all he can by himself but may be helped to finish tasks when necessary. A story should, like these other activities, be kept short so that he can succeed in listening to it all. Failure will lead to boredom, flagging concentration and a loss of interest in that activity next time. The length of the activity or story can be gradually increased as the child's concentration improves.

While it is quite natural for a child to talk about what he is doing and this speech may actually facilitate his performance, parents and other adults should, as far as possible, ignore chatter about things not related to the activity engaged in. This must be done gently; encouragement and praise should be given when he is doing well and lapses should be ignored. Although questions must be answered if they are important for the child's understanding, an adult can respond to questions or remarks which do not seem important by a remark such as 'Ssh, never mind about that, let's get on with what we're doing.' If the child has difficulty in comprehending an instruction, it is best to re-phrase it or elaborate on it until he does understand. Similarly, if he cannot answer a question immediately, the adult should continue to provide the child with additional information until he can arrive at a solution by himself.

It would be best if this advice could be conveyed to the whole family and not just the parents, so that within the family circle a consistent approach is adopted. It is all too easy for other relatives or visitors to laugh at the child's idiosyncracies of speech and so reinforce the behaviour it is hoped to eliminate.

Summing up: general points about play

(1) An enormous amount of learning takes place through play in the pre-school years. Parents buy toys anyway but they need to be aware of what kinds of play and what kinds of toys will be most helpful in developing which skills, so that money is not wasted on useless or frustrating objects. They also need information about the areas of development in which spina bifida children are likely to have difficulties and so need lots of practice and encouragement.

(2) A child must be well motivated in order to benefit from play, that is, it must be fun for him, and it must hold his attention. Below, a number of points are listed which will help to ensure that play is both fun and beneficial for a spina bifida child.

(i) The child should be positioned securely so that he is not anxious about falling over and is able to use both hands freely.

(ii) The activities involved need to be well within his capacity so that he has the satisfaction of completing a task. The toy or activity should, in other words, be in some way rewarding. It is also important that the child is 'stretched' sometimes: on these occasions social rewards may help to hold his interest.

(iii) The objects or subjects must be meaningful to him.
(iv) Distractions should be removed before the toys are got out and, particularly if perceptual difficulties are suspected, the toys presented on a plain background.
(v) The toys themselves should be visually clear, for example books or puzzles selected in which the outlines of the pictures are well defined.
(vi) He also needs to be allowed to learn from his own mistakes and to do things in his own way.
(vii) Any one activity or toy should be experienced for a short time only but, on many occasions.
(viii) Play activities should be encouraged when the child is at his best not when he is fatigued or hungry.
(3) Parents can help their children to learn to play most effectively through trying to increase their own ability to observe accurately what the child is doing. In some areas parent groups have been set up with this as one of their functions. By observing and recording the child's reactions to different toys and activities, the interest shown in them, the length of time he is able to concentrate on them, the time of day when he seems to co-operate best, and perhaps any major difficulties he experiences, the parents will, first, learn more themselves about how best to help their child to play, and, second, will have information which may be very helpful to the pædiatrician, psychologist, teacher, therapist or other professionals who are also working with the child.

Intervention/assessment programmes for use by parents

In this section we felt it would be useful to discuss briefly two actual programmes or schedules specifically designed for use by parents in the home. There are, of course, many other programmes available, for example the sorts of activities described by Seifert (1973) but those outlined below have been included because they illustrate a programme designed specifically for spina bifida children, as well as one which could be used by parents of children handicapped in a variety of ways.

The first is a programme designed to foster eye–hand co-ordination during the first twelve months of life in young children with spina bifida (Rosenbaum, Barnitt and Brand, 1975). The principles used in designing this programme were that: (i) there should be a developmental orientation, that is 'an approach based on clear understanding of the principles and patterns of normal child development; an assessment of the present developmental achievements of a handicapped child; and a programme designed to build upon current abilities in a developmentally appropriate sequence and rate' (Rosenbaum and Rosenbloom, 1973); (ii) there should be flexibility, i.e. it should take individual variations into account; (iii) the equipment needed should be readily available; and (iv) the programme must be simple and easy for parents to carry out in the home.

Part of this programme is shown in detail in Appendix D but basically it was designed to improve eye–hand co-ordination through a series of activities carried out by the parents with the child over the first twelve months of life. During the first three months specific training was given in visual fixation, visual following and grasping an object placed in the hands. Over the second three months grasping and playing with objects, reaching for and grasping objects and mouthing were trained. The next skills (months 7–9) to be trained were a unidextrous approach, the transfer of objects from hand to hand, the simultaneous retention of two objects, and the understanding of object permanence, while in months 10–12 the skills concentrated on were the use of a pincer grip, the use of the index finger, and training in the release of objects.

The programme was used in a research study based at Queen Elizabeth Hospital, Hackney (Rosenbaum *et al.*, 1975). Although the findings, in terms of accelerated learning gains, were inconclusive owing to the small size of the sample and difficulties in interpreting the results, there was a clear suggestion that these children did improve compared to others similarly handicapped who were not given help of this kind. What the study did demonstrate quite clearly was that it is feasible to give developmental advice to parents and that they understand and welcome help of this kind.

Another schedule for use by parents which we thought particularly useful is the one designed by Jeffree and McConkey (1976), of the Hester Adrian Research Centre. This consists of a series of charts for parents to complete, the aims of the charts being (i) to enable parents to record their child's present level of development in the major 'areas' of development, (ii) to direct the parents' observation of their child and draw their attention to aspects of development which they may have overlooked and (iii) to give parents an indication of the 'stages' children pass through in the development of basic skills. This will be of help when formulating appropriate teaching objectives for their child. Examples from the schedule are shown in Appendix E.

The pre-school spina bifida child outside the home

The previous section was concerned only with the young spina bifida child's experiences within the home, usually in a one-to-one situation with an adult. In this section we turn to peer contacts outside the home in playgroups, nursery schools and other organized groups, the general term pre-school education being used to refer to all these types of early experiences. Three main aspects of pre-school education are examined, firstly the extent to which spina bifida children are, in different parts of the country, getting pre-school education at all and the main problems involved when they are not, secondly the advantages and disadvantages, particularly as viewed by the parents, and finally the different ways in which pre-school education has been organized for spina bifida and other handicapped children.

Number of spina bifida children having pre-school education

In the GLC study mothers were first asked about nursery education when the child was three years old and again the following year. At three years old (see Table 6.4) there was no difference in the proportion of children with and without a locomotor handicap who were attending pre-school groups. However, about half the children in each of these categories were not attending at all. These mothers were asked if they would like their children to attend, or to attend more frequently if attendance was minimal (half day a week). Over 80 per cent of mothers wanted more nursery education, irrespective of the degree of handicap. At four years old the proportion of children receiving pre-school education had increased considerably (Table 6.4) and in addition a small number of children were weekly or full-time boarders at a residential school for spina bifida children.

Data on pre-school education for spina bifida children from a number of other studies shows that the amount of provision available varies considerably from one part of the country to the other. Freeston's figures (1971) for four year olds are similar to Spain's three year olds. Of the 38 four year olds with spina bifida in the Sheffield area whose parents she interviewed, 65 per cent were not attending anywhere although five of these had been promised vacancies in the near future. This indicated that about half the four year olds in her study were likely to have some pre-school experience. 75 per cent of the mothers whose children had not yet been placed or had been offered places in the near future would have liked their children to have had some pre-school education.

Table 6.4 *Percentage of spina bifida children attending pre-school groups at 3 and 4 years. GLC Spina Bifida Survey*

	At 3 years		*At 4 years*	
	No or mild handicap	*Mod. or severe handicap*	*No or mild handicap*	*Mod. or severe handicap*
Not at all	55	58	40	40
Half day a week	8	4	3	0
Part time	20	14	17	10
Full time	17	24	40	48
Boards full or part time	0	0	0	2
Total %	100·0	100·0	100·0	100·0
Total N	75	57	62	73

Useful information about nursery education is provided by Woodburn (1973) in her south-east Scotland study, details being shown in Table 6.5.

Table 6.5 *Pre-school education experience of myelomeningocele children (From Woodburn 1973)*

	Age Group			
	3 and 4 year olds		*5, 6 and 7 year olds*	
Nursery Experience	*N*	*%*	*N*	*%*
Never attended	5*	29·3	5	21·6
Attended in past	1	5·9	14	61·0
Currently attending	11	64·8	4†	17·4
Total children	17	100·0	23	100·0

* Three were on the waiting list.

† Two about to transfer to normal school. Two to have an extra year in a nursery class.

This table shows that some sort of nursery education was available for 70 per cent of the 3–4 year olds (and would probably be available for a further 18 per cent when vacancies arose) and had been available for 78 per cent of the children now 5–7. Just over one-third of the children attended for a full day every day of the week, another third half a day every day and all but one of the others for two or three days a week. Over two-thirds of the children attended nurseries or groups run by the local authority.

In contrast, among the fifteen myelomeningocele children aged 8–11 years old at the time of the study, only 31 per cent had had any pre-school education and all but one of these lived inside the city boundaries, while none of the children over the age of 11 years had had such experience at all. Overall, Woodburn found that there was 'relatively little difficulty for those now of nursery school age in gaining entry, although there might still be some difficulties for those living in the country'. Where a child had not attended a nursery this was most often because there was no nursery within reach, frequently the case for children living outside the city boundaries.

In some parts of the country facilities are available for most handicapped children who want them. Thus a study carried out in the Hester Adrian Research Centre, Manchester (Mittler, 1976) showed that of the 150 mentally handicapped children known to the LEA, 82 per cent of the 4 year olds and 64 per cent of the 3 year olds were having some pre-school education. However, it must also be recognized that provision is extremely patchy. Further, the mere fact that a child is receiving some sort of nursery education says nothing in itself about the quality of what is being provided, nor about its appropriateness in his particular case. Arrangements are often made by the mother without any guidance which means the child may not be attending the sort of group which can help him most. Also, as we point out later in this section, staff in nursery centres generally lack advice as to how handicapped children can be integrated into a group and are often not given the resources which would enable them to cope.

Advantages and disadvantages of pre-school education

Over recent years the importance of pre-school education for all children, but in particular handicapped children, has been stressed. In *Living with Handicap* (Younghusband *et al.*, 1970) 'the urgent need for more pre-school facilities for handicapped children', was noted: the DHSS in their report *The Management of the Child with Spina Bifida* (1973) strongly recommend nursery education; and the Committee of Enquiry into Special Education (Warnock Committee) is collecting detailed evidence on this question.

Advantages
Most parents of spina bifida children find pre-school education valuable: thus 88 per cent of the mothers of myelomeningocele children in Woodburn's study (1973) whose children had had nursery education felt that it had been beneficial while of the other 5 mothers 3 had felt equivocal and only 2 that there were no advantages. The sorts of benefits which have been reported by parents, teachers, social workers and others and which are discussed in the following sections include advantages both to the children and to their mothers.

Advantages to children

(i) *Gains in social development.* In Woodburn's study 39 per cent of the mothers remarked on the child's gains in social development, for example that being in a pre-school group had 'brought him on' and 'taught him to play with others'.

There is a very great danger that without nursery education spina bifida children may become isolated from their peers. Rowland (1973) states that of eleven spina bifida children attending a special hospital playgroup in Bristol, seven, before attending, had had no playmaes at all. In the GLC study, mothers were asked about how frequently the child played with his sibs or peers at three years old. Of the 57 children with no handicap or only a mild handicap 80 per cent did so, compared to only 58 per cent of the moderately/severely handicapped children and for 16 per cent of the latter group (compared to only 5 per cent of the former) peer group contacts had been confined to experience in a playgroup. This finding indicates that severity of handicap does affect opportunities for social play and that playgroup experience is very important.

The quality of play at 3 years was also looked at, the mothers of those children who did have play opportunities being asked whether they felt that their children had difficulties when playing with other children. Their replies suggested that although 21 per cent of the severely handicapped children had some problems in playing with others compared to only 6 per cent of those who were less handicapped, the percentage who had marked problems was about the same (2 per cent) for both groups.

Clearly then, spina bifida children do stand to gain a great deal socially through suitable nursery placement. Elizabeth Grantham (1971) the Medical Adviser to the Peterborough and District Branch of the

Pre-school Playgroups Association notes that on first joining a normal playgroup a handicapped child tends 'just to sit and watch the other children – this alone is often a novel experience. He then begins to copy other children's activities and gradually he joins in with group activities – singing, games, action stories and so on – later in creative imaginative play with a small group. By these means he begins to develop a relationship with other children.' However it cannot be assumed that a very handicapped child will be able to do this automatically and he may need considerable help in learning to interact socially with other children.

(ii) *Emotional gains.* In her very detailed study of twelve spina bifida children attending a special hospital playgroup in Bristol, Rowland (1973) found that most of the children were very dependent on their mothers partly because they had to rely on them for physical care. All those mothers whose children had become less dependent over the past year attributed this to the playgroup and Woodburn (1973) and Grantham (1971) were also told by many mothers that their children had become less clinging and dependent. However, the children in Rowland's study (1973) who had marked behaviour problems of other kinds did not improve, and this suggests that where there are very specific problems then very specific help will be needed and placement in a playgroup will not in itself bring about improvements.

(iii) *Gains in motor development.* Both in the Bristol playgroup (Rowland, 1973) and in Woodburn's study (1973) several mothers commented on the physical gains, especially in mobility, made by the child, attributing this to the stimulation given by other children. Grantham (1971) has described the part played by imitation of other children. She watched 'an athetoid child, just able to walk with support, swing all over a climbing frame and a spina bifida child throw down her crutches, struggle up the steps of a slide, go whizzing down and shuffle on her bottom back to the steps again. These children watched the non-handicapped children for a long time before they attempted to copy but when they found they could do it too their whole horizon widened.' Many spina bifida children have had no experience of rough-and-tumble games at home and pre-school groups may be useful in this respect; it may be even more useful for parents to learn that they can take part safely in such activities.

Sophie Levitt, a physiotherapist, has recently reported a series of long-term observations made in a handicapped children's adventure playground (1975). She emphasizes that what such a playgroup offers is 'an enrichment of movements already established'. While few of the children she observed developed a new range of movements they did get opportunities to use movements which were unlikely to occur in other circumstances. She also noticed, however, that the adults helping in the playgroup often did not wait for the children to make their own efforts at motor activities but were over-eager to help them. One reason for this was that the adults lacked knowledge of the motor abilities present in each child: for example many children who could start the motor skill of getting up from the ground on their own, or even complete this, were not given the chance to do so but were immediately picked up by an adult. The result was that many children waited for adults to help them rather than attempting a movement on their own. This suggests that adults in playgroups should allow children the maximum opportunity for independence, intervening only when the child is in danger.

(iv) *Children better prepared for entry to school.* There can be little doubt, from the descriptions above, that spina bifida children who had nursery education will, intellectually, physically and, most important of all, socially, be better prepared for entry to school. Laurence (1973) notes that spina bifida children who had had playgroup experience 'were usually able to make a smooth transition to normal schools' and this has been a typical finding. Mothers of the children in the GLC study were asked when the child was six years old if they had noticed any improvements since he started school: for those without pre-school experience improvements were noted, whereas for those who had had such experience the improvement had been noted earlier on when the child first started in a pre-school group and was then seen as a continuous process.

(v) *Increase in the child's overall development.* The great majority of children attending the pre-school groups described by these writers undoubtedly enjoyed their experiences there. Mothers frequently mentioned that the child loved going, was unhappy if he had to stay at home and talked a lot about his activities at the nursery. The main aim of the playgroup teacher in the Frenchay hospital nursery was 'to increase the field of play for the children through the development of mobility, building up of visual discrimination, improvement of manual dexterity, development of self-reliance and encouragement of speech'. The social worker who assessed the gains of the twelve spina bifida children attending noted that, after a year, they were able to play more creatively and took a greater interest in the things around them.

(vi) *Need for evaluation and research.* While these and the other observations reported in this section are perfectly valid there is also a need for much more precise evaluations of the benefits gained by handicapped children from playgroup experiences. So far there has been comparatively little research of this kind; Levitt's study (1975) is one example of the kind of contribution which research can make, another being the study of cerebral-palsied children carried out by Barrett and her colleagues (1967) in California. Here the effects of group experience in a small confined space was studied, an area of the nursery 6 feet by 5 feet being partitioned off for twelve individuals and called 'the little playhouse'. The ten young cerebral-palsied children who participated over a 4½-month period 'enjoyed the experience and improved in social awareness and peer interaction, and in social, verbal and motor ability'. Only research could answer the important question of whether spina bifida children might also benefit from a similar situation.

Advantages to the mothers of pre-school education

(i) *Source of support.* The need of mothers for understanding and support has already been discussed in chapter 4. The child's attendance at a nursery or playgroup offers many mothers an additional source of support and practical help and may also lessen her possible isolation through the contacts she makes there with other parents (perhaps both of handicapped and non-handicapped children) and with the staff at the nursery.

(ii) *Relieves mother: gives her some time off.* Many spina bifida children make enormous demands on their mothers' time. In a survey of families in the Sheffield area Freeston (1971) compared the attention needs of spina bifida children with those who were normal or who had cerebral palsy. Her findings showed that a much larger proportion of spina bifida children either could not be left at all or could only be left for about half an hour than was true of either normal or cerebral-palsied children and that none of the spina bifida 4 year olds, compared to nearly half the normal and one-third of the cerebral-palsied children could be left for more than an hour.

This means that many mothers of young spina bifida children have virtually no time off from the handicapped child in which to relax, to get on with other household chores, or to give some uninterrupted attention to their other children. Woodburn (1973) found that in a large number of cases the child's attendance at a playgroup did mean that the mother got some relief from daily management and felt that as a result she coped better with the handicapped child and had more time to spend with his sibs. It is also good for mothers to realize that their children can be cared for competently by others.

(iii) *Gives mother better understanding of the child.* In evaluating the benefits derived by mothers and children attending the Frenchay unit, Rowland (1973) comments on the fact that the mothers of handicapped children may have expectancies which are either too high or too low because of a failure to understand the nature of the child's difficulties. Some of the mothers at the Frenchay unit felt that their contacts with the nursery staff had helped to give them a much better understanding of the nature of the child's problems (and hence an increase in their self-confidence in bringing him up) than they had gained from professionals such as GPs or Health Visitors. By observing a child with his peers a mother is forced to make comparisons and if the child is retarded it is much better that she learns this through her own observations than that she is simply told by an 'expert'.

Disadvantages of pre-school education

On the whole, mothers of spina bifida children find that the advantages of pre-school education greatly outweigh the disadvantages. In Woodburn's study (1973) one quarter of the mothers of myelomeningocele children thought that there were no disadvantages. Two main problems were mentioned by the others, one being the effort involved in getting to the nursery and the other the practical problems presented by the journey itself. Changes in the child's behaviour may occasionally worry mothers; the problem is not one of the child settling in badly but rather that mothers sometimes mention that the child has become 'naughty' since attending. Since many spina bifida children are too passive this is generally a change to be welcomed, although a mixed blessing to the mother.

The nature of pre-school provision

So far the relative merits of different ways of making pre-school provision for spina bifida children have not been discussed. In the next chapter detailed consideration is given to the complex question of school placement and at this stage only a short account will be given of the different possibilities as regards pre-school placement.

Groups specifically for handicapped children

In some hospitals playgroups or nursery classes have been set up for children with specific handicaps, whilst in others the children have a variety of handicaps. Local authorities and voluntary organizations may also make special nursery provision of different kinds, for example 'opportunity' playgroups specifically for handicapped children, and an increasing number of special schools have special classes for handicapped children of pre-school age. An example of a very specialized facility is the playgroup for spina bifida children set up at Frenchay Hospital, Bristol. Rowland (1973) reports that most of the mothers of the children attending preferred a playgroup for spina bifida children rather than an ordinary playgroup since there was a trained nursery teacher in charge, and the children would get more individual attention there, whereas they would not, they thought, keep up in an ordinary group and might be trampled on and Rowland herself (1973) felt that placement in an ordinary playgroup would not have been suitable for these children.

Ordinary pre-school facilities

In contrast, the great majority of the children in the south-east Scotland survey (Woodburn, 1973) were attending ordinary pre-school facilities and their mothers were, on the whole, well satisfied with this placement. Many other examples could be given of ordinary playgroups and nursery schools which have had great success in integrating individual children or small groups of children with severe mental and physical handicaps. Parfit (1975) quotes Dr Ronald Faulkner, one of those responsible for the recent interest of the Pre-school Playgroups Association in accepting handicapped children, as pointing out that in 1974 half of the pre-school playgroups in England were each taking 1–4 handicapped children.

Grantham (1971) a medical adviser to a local playgroup association also feels that attendance in ordinary playgroups is very important and that 'the aim should be to get them [handicapped children] to think of themselves as part of the community, doing what all other children do, not to regard themselves as special or odd'. However, she makes a crucial point when she says that ordinary playgroups will need extra help and support if they are to cater for handicapped children, and suggests that no more than about 10 per cent of any group should consist of 'problem' cases (not all disabled children being, of course, problem cases, and not all problem cases being disabled children). The help given to groups should include provision of a welfare assistant or extra helper and also full backing from experts in dealing with any problems which may arise. In some cases this expertise might be provided by the staff of a local special school.

Unfortunately, as is pointed out by the Pre-School Playgroups Association, many groups accept handicapped children at the request of pædiatricians, assessment centre staff, social workers and others and then receive no further advice, and the PPA frequently stress that playgroup leaders feel a need for far more support and advice for handicapped children in their groups than they generally receive. This came out particularly clearly in Parfit's survey (1975) of the integration of handicapped children in ordinary pre-school facilities and in ordinary schools in London. She points out that expert help and information for those working with integrated children is 'remarkable more for its absence than its availability', gaps in back-up services being stressed particularly by the social services department staff. In one borough, for example, excellent back-up services were available to the staff of the local special school for physically handicapped children, whereas there was a total absence of such services for the staff of those day nurseries and private playgroups in the same area which were taking handicapped children.

There are two main ways in which this situation can be improved. One is that those working in pre-school facilities of different kinds should be given further training in the care of the handicapped child. This is at present being planned by the NNEB in a higher diploma course and carried out on an in-service basis in a few Colleges of Further Education as well as by voluntary societies, but such opportunities are still grossly insufficient. The other way of improving the quality of care available to handicapped children in ordinary pre-school facilities is to make better use of those 'experts' who could provide back-up services and this is discussed in the section which follows.

Liaison between the 'experts' and ordinary playgroup staff

In a number of areas a good deal of attention is being paid to ways in which close links can be established between, on the one hand, specialized facilities for handicapped children and, on the other, ordinary 'community' playgroups and other forms of pre-school provision. The Pre-school Playgroups Association gives examples of hospitals in Poole, Peterborough and Oxford which do this and although there must be others they appear to be exceptions and generally, reports the PPA, it is unusual for pædiatric staff to visit groups, to arrange advisory help, or to request progress reports. It is suggested that the reasons for this are lack of time, the belief that the local authority does all that is necessary and diffidence combined with ignorance of the tremendous variation in quality of playgroups.

Raikes (1973) has described how close liaison was developed between remedial and community (i.e. ordinary) playgroups in Poole, where there is a comprehensive diagnostic and therapeutic unit for pre-school children. The team staffing this unit is hospital-based but works with families at home as well as in hospital, where there is also a treatment unit and a remedial playgroup.

This small hospital playgroup has two main functions: to help children with developmental problems, and to help the physiotherapists and OTs to liaise with the local community pre-school playgroup organizers. Close links have been developed with co-operative playgroup leaders enabling the hospital staff to pass on practical details about management problems to the playgroups and to receive in return feedback from the play-leaders about the child's progress. None of the children suitable for community playgroups has been refused a place and all are well integrated and accepted by the other children. Increasing numbers of playgroup organizers now visit the assessment unit, and plans were being made for equally close links to be developed with teachers of reception classes or special units in infant schools.

There are of course problems even when expert help is available. Standards vary greatly and there are a number of playgroups where organizers are not sufficiently trained. A less frequently encountered problem is the feeling in some groups and in some LEAs that children with any type of developmental abnormality should be isolated in 'special' groups which, Raikes believes, may only increase the problem for the child and his family.

Clearly, the onus should be on the education authority, the health district or area and the social services departments to liaise in providing early help for handicapped children. The Health Care Planning Teams at health district level and the Joint Consultative Committees at area level might well be the appropriate bodies to discuss this type of liaison. What really matters is not who takes the initiative but that some initiative on this matter is taken.

It will be necessary for the three authorities involved, Health, Social Services and Education, to discuss, first, how to improve the methods for the early detection of handicap, and second, how children thought to be at risk or clearly handicapped should be registered, and how the information about them gained by each of the authorities should be pooled. Third, the question of cross-referral and confidentiality will need to be raised. In practice, it is rarely unnecessary to take any action without the parents' consent, since they are usually only too anxious to receive help and advice, provided that this is offered sympathetically. If there were liaison of this kind, a register with combined referrals from health and social services could be provided to the LEA (with parental consent) as soon as the diagnosis was made. This would enable the LEA to offer a service to parents as soon as they were ready to receive it, either on a domiciliary basis or through pre-schooling. This is current practice in most areas for the deaf or blind child and there is no logical reason why it cannot be extended to all handicapped children. Appropriate pre-school education should always be provided as near the child's home as possible, and, as stated earlier, the aim should be to give the child some experience of mixing with normal children of the same age.

Finally, what is essential and what is frequently lacking at the moment is that the three authorities should work closely together in deciding exactly how a combined service to families with a young handicapped child should be delivered, the aim being that such a service would include the best that each has to offer. What is also needed is a central pool of information (which can be used both by professionals and by parents) on the services which are available in a particular area.

References

Barnitt, R. (1975), 'Body-image disorders in children with spina bifida and hydrocephalus', dissertation submitted for B.Sc. (Psychology), University of London.

Barrett, M. L. and Jones, M. H. (1967), 'The sensory story. A multisensory training procedure for toddlers', *Developmental Medicine and Child Neurology*, 9, pp. 448–56.

——, Hunt, V. L. and Jones, M. L. (1967), 'Behavioural growth of cerebral-palsied children from group experience in a confined space', *Developmental Medicine and Child Neurology*, 9 (1), pp. 50–8.

Bengtsson, A. (1972), *Adventure Playgrounds*, Crosby Lockwood, St Albans, Herts.

Connolly, K. (1972), 'Learning and the concept of critical periods in infancy', *Developmental Medicine and Child Neurology*, 14 (6), pp. 705–14.

Cunningham, C. C. (1975), 'Parents as therapists and educators', in Kiernan, C. C. and Woodford, P. (eds.), *Behaviour Modification with the Severely Retarded*, Excerpta Medica/North Holland, Amsterdam/Elsevier.

DHSS (1973), *Management of the Child with Spina Bifida.*

Freeston, B. M. (1971), 'An enquiry into the effect of a spina bifida child on family life', *Developmental Medicine and Child Neurology*, 13, pp. 456–61.

Grantham, E. (1971), 'Handicapped children in pre-school playgroups', *British Medical Journal*, 4, pp. 346–8.

Hunt, G. M. (1973), 'Implications of the treatment of myelomeningocele for the child and his family', *Lancet* ii, pp. 1308–10.

Jeffree, D. M. and McConkey, R. (1976), *Parental Involvement Project Development Charts*, Hodder and Stoughton, London.

Johnson, C. A. and Katz, R. G. (1973), 'Using parents as change agents for their children, a review', *Journal of Child Psychology and Psychiatry*, 14, pp. 181–200.

Laurence, E. (1973), 'School placement of spina bifida children', in Palmer, J. (ed.), *Special Education and the Community Services*, Ron Jones, Publ., Ferndale.

Levitt, S. (1975), 'A study of gross motor skills of cerebral-palsied children in an adventure playground for handicapped children', *Child: Care, Health and Development*, 1, pp. 29–43.

Miller, E. and Sethi, L. (1971), 'Tactile matching in children with hydrocephalus', *Neuropaediat*, 3, pp. 191–4.

Mittler, P. (1976), 'The early education of severely subnormal children', in *Proceedings of International Conference on Special Education '75: the New Frontiers*. Publication of the Joint Council for Education of Handicapped Children.

Norris, J. (undated), *Choosing Toys and Activities for Handicapped Children*, Toy Libraries Association.

Parfit, J. (1975), 'The integration of handicapped children in Greater London', report of a survey commissioned by the Institute for Research into Mental and Multiple Handicap, London.

Patterson, G. and Gullion, M. (1968), *Living with Children: New Models for Parents and Teachers*, Research Press, Champaign, Illinois.

Raikes, A. (1973), 'Liaison between remedial and community playgroups', paper given at Spastics Society study group on promoting better movement in children with motor handicap at Nottingham University, September 1973.

Rosenbaum, P., Barnitt, R. and Brand, H. L. (1975), 'A developmental intervention programme designed to overcome the effects of impaired movement in spina bifida infants', ch. 13 in Holt, K. S. (ed.), *Movement and Child Development,* Clinics in Developmental Medicine, 55, Spastics International Medical Publications/Heinemann, London.

——, and Rosenbloom, L. (1973), 'An intervention programme to aid the development of children with motor disability', paper given at the Spastics Society study group on promoting better movement in children with motor handicap, University of Nottingham, September 1973.

Rowland, M. (1973), 'Evaluation of playgroup for children with spina bifida', *Social Work Today,* 4 (11), pp. 325–30.

Seifert, A. (1973), 'Sensory-motor stimulation for the young handicapped child', *Occupational Therapy,* 37, pp. 559–71.

White, B. (1970), 'Experience and the development of motor mechanisms in infancy', in Connolly, K. (ed.), *Mechanisms of Motor Skill Development,* Academic Press, London.

Woodburn, M. (1973), *Social Implications of Spina Bifida – a Study in S.E. Scotland,* Eastern Branch Scottish Spina Bifida Association, Edinburgh.

7 Choosing a school

> Any class of young persons marked by an infirmity . . . depend more than ordinary persons do for their happiness and for their support, upon the ties of kindred, of friendship and of neighbourhood. All these, therefore, ought to be nourished and strengthened during childhood and youth – for it is then, and then only, that they take such deep root as to become strong and life lasting . . . Beware how you needlessly sever any of these ties . . . lest you make a homeless man, a wanderer and a stranger.

The speaker was Samuel Howe, the date 1866, the occasion laying a cornerstone of the New York Institution for the Blind. Now, over 100 years later, a very similar problem presents itself for a completely different group of young persons who at that time rarely survived birth, children with spina bifida. How can their need to put down roots in childhood and youth in their own neighbourhoods be reconciled with the equally clear needs of many of them for very special kinds of help at school?

In this country the choice open to most physically handicapped children is still, in many areas, a strikingly polarized one. On the one hand is the 'special' school for the physically handicapped, offering an environment which is entirely geared towards meeting the specialized needs of a particular group of handicapped pupils. On the other is the 'ordinary' school, based essentially on the assumption of physical, social and emotional and intellectual 'normality', even if the range of what is accepted as 'normal' in any or all of these dimensions is becoming increasingly wider.

This situation is changing slowly. Increasing numbers of physically handicapped children are being accepted in ordinary schools and a number of local authorities are making available more special provision within ordinary schools, although wide variations exist between one area and another in the extent to which this is being done and also in the form that this special provision takes. Another encouraging sign is the recognition that the initial placement is not the final one and that frequent reviews of the appropriateness of a particular placement are necessary.

Within the special schools the situation has also been changing over the last fifteen years. The proportion of children with conditions such as polio, or diseases of the bones or joints which produced physical but not intellectual impairment has been markedly declining while there has been an increase in the survival rate of more multiply handicapped children, in particular those with spina bifida. This has meant that in most PH schools about two-thirds of the pupils, at least in the primary departments, are likely to have either spina bifida (usually with hydrocephalus) or cerebral palsy, the other major physically handicapping condition in childhood. The special schools are thus coping increasingly with children who may have both physical and intellectual handicaps.

Since the issue of school placement for physically handicapped pupils is such an important, complex and, at present, controversial one, it is looked at in some detail in this chapter. We begin by discussing the attitudes of those concerned, secondly consider the extent to which the special needs of spina bifida children can be met by different kinds of schools, thirdly we turn to the way in which placement decisions are arrived at and finally look at what is actually happening to spina bifida children as regards school placement.

Attitudes to different types of schooling

Recent years have seen, on the one hand, a greater pressure from disabled people themselves, as well as from parents of handicapped children, for ordinary school placement, coupled with pressure for improvements in the facilities offered to disabled children by ordinary schools and, on the other, clearly expressed anxieties on the part of professionals working closely with disabled children about the adverse medical or social or educational effects which might result from inappropriate placement.

(a) *The attitudes of disabled people*

Very little evidence is available about what disabled children themselves feel about school placement. In a study of disabled children in ordinary primary schools (Anderson, 1973) the great majority of children were reported by their parents as being happy at school; however, had parents with children of the same age in special schools been asked the same question an equally affirmative answer would probably have been given. The views of disabled teenagers in different kinds of schools have never been systematically explored on a large scale but there is some evidence that many teenagers in special schools would like more opportunities to mix with their peers but feel, at the same time, some natural apprehension about ordinary school placement.

Dorner (1976), for example, in his interviews with spina bifida teenagers found that while most of those at special schools were strongly in favour of greater integration, and would have liked to go to ordinary schools, they felt at the same time that they would not have been able to manage. However, four moderately or severely handicapped teenagers had attended ordinary schools because of their parents' insistence and 'all felt it had been the right decision'. The Head of one special school (Hall, 1975, personal communication), which has for several years been placing an increasingly large number of disabled pupils in the local comprehensive school reports that initially the pupils were very anxious about the move but after about six weeks in the comprehensive school were happily settled there, and 'found every excuse' why they should not return to the special school even for physiotherapy as had been arranged.

Other sources of information on this question come from disabled students in further education and from organizations set up by disabled adults such as the Association of Disabled Professionals or the Union of the Physically Impaired Against Segregation. These bodies are unanimous in their conviction that the proper place to educate all children – including all handicapped children – is in ordinary schools, and in pressing strongly for more special provision to be made for such children in ordinary rather than special schools. Although the point is sometimes made that these are the views of exceptionally competent and articulate disabled people who are better able than many to cope emotionally and intellectually with an ordinary school environment, there is no evidence that their views differ from those of other disabled adults.

(b) *Parent attitudes*

An earlier study of disabled children (Anderson, 1973) offered strong evidence that large numbers of parents prefer ordinary to special school placement, although only a comparatively small proportion of those interviewed were parents of spina bifida children. Dr. Boothman, (1975) herself handicapped by spina bifida, states that most parents of spina bifida children would prefer the child to attend an ordinary school and there is considerable evidence that this is the case. In Glasgow, for example, Richards and McIntosh (1973) interviewed seventy-six mothers of spina bifida children. Most of these mothers 'felt strongly that their children should attend normal schools and that incontinence should not exclude them from doing so.'

Useful information about parent attitudes also comes from Woodburn's study of spina bifida children in south-east Scotland (1973) where the parents of children of 4 years old or older were asked what they saw as the benefits and disadvantages of ordinary schools, special day schools and special residential schools. The advantages most frequently commented on by the parents of myelomeningocele children were the normal standard of education (58 per cent) the unsheltered environment enabling children to face the realities of life (30·5 per cent); mixing with local friends (22 per cent) and educating other people in their ideas about handicap (18 per cent). One quarter of the parents thought ordinary school placement had no advantages; these were the parents of children whose physical or educational handicaps were of such a degree that ordinary education was just not seen as feasible.

The main disadvantages of ordinary schools reported by parents included the difficulties in incontinence management (43 per cent) and sometimes (but not always) management of a urinary diversion. 39 per cent saw some educational disadvantages, the main ones mentioned being the child's inability, because of physical limitations, to participate fully in class activities; the fact that teachers were not specially trained; and the fact that they could not, because of the class size, give the child the extra individual help he might need. Other disadvantages mentioned quite frequently were problems with other children (28 per cent) including being teased, knocked over and overprotected; old, inconvenient buildings (23·6 per cent) and transport problems (20 per cent).

Of the parents with views on day special schools about one-fifth saw no advantages. Those who did see advantages most frequently mentioned educational advantages, and advantages in incontinence management. Some parents commented that the staff were better equipped for the general management of handicapped children, some thought it was socially advantageous for the child to mix with others like himself and a small number mentioned the suitability of the building, and the availability of transport and physiotherapy.

The disadvantage about day special schooling most frequently mentioned was that special schools were inferior educationally; there were more parents who felt this than who saw educational advantages.

Reasons given were that these schools were too much geared to handicap, that teacher expectations were low, and that the general atmosphere was over-protective and unchallenging. Social disadvantages were commented on too, some parents feeling that special school placement made the child more conscious of his handicap and some finding that it isolated him from neighbourhood peers.

Few parents had had to consider residential schools as a real possibility and of the eight parents with experience of this, none thought it the ideal answer, although three mentioned that such placement could afford some relief to the parents and five that it offered the child companionship and an independence training and social programme well suited to his needs. However, as Woodburn (1973) comments, the need for residential schooling is comparatively small.

The views expressed by the parents in Woodburn's study are very similar indeed to those of the parents of the disabled children attending ordinary schools in Anderson's study (1973). This suggests that the mothers of spina bifida children perceive alternative forms of schooling in much the same way as do mothers of children with other handicaps, although they do see special schools as having an unchallenged advantage in incontinence management.

Parental attitudes will of course be influenced by what is actually available and the range of alternatives differs greatly from one area to another. In parts of the country where local authorities have made a determined effort to make special provision for handicapped children in ordinary schools, this type of placement is generally preferred to special school placement. However, in areas where the only choice is between a day special school or an ordinary school with no extra help, parents who initially express a wish for ordinary school placement may modify their views as the child gets older.

There is some evidence of this from the GLC survey which was carried out in an area exceptionally well served with special schools and where, in consequence, as Parfit (1975) found, little special provision has been made for disabled children in ordinary schools. When the child was 3 years old over half of all the GLC parents of spina bifida children expressed a wish for ordinary day school placement and even in the case of those whose children had moderate or severe physical handicaps, nearly one-third did not want special school placement.

By the age of 6, however, the picture was somewhat different. All children were now at school, 40 per cent being in ordinary schools, 52 per cent in day PH schools and the others wholly residential or weekly boarders. Few parents had major complaints, although parents of special school children sometimes expressed anxiety about academic standards. In some cases ordinary school placement had only been agreed following a struggle between the parents and the LEA. On the whole, however, parents accepted the philosophy of the LEA and it was only a few vocal, persistent and articulate parents who had succeeded in placing a moderately handicapped child in an ordinary school.

It is important to understand the reasons for parental views on school placement, and not to label them as 'unrealistic', or 'irrational'. For most parents of handicapped children, the school placement decision is a 'crisis' point in the child's history. Roskies's (1972) interviews with the mothers of thalidomide children showed that next to the interviews on the birth-period, the most anxiety-provoking topic for mothers was discussion of their future plans and expectancies, in particular as regards schooling. Interestingly, the mothers who felt the most stress were those whose children were 'marginal' in terms of acceptance in the normal community.

Ordinary school placement is usually perceived as likely to facilitate society's acceptance of the child, or, at worst, the child's ability to cope with society's ambivalence. This came out clearly in a previous study (Anderson, 1973) where, in one mother's words: 'The younger they live with normal people the quicker they'll adapt. They're always going to get comments, and the younger they accept it the better.' Special school placement, on the other hand, is often seen as socially 'stigmatizing'. In this mothers are, to a large degree, only being realistic, since society does view children attending special schools or at least certain categories of special schools as being not only different but also, if one is being honest, inferior. Since greater stigma attaches, in our society, to mental than to physical handicap, mothers are particularly anxious that their children should not go to schools where they may be identified with 'mentally handicapped' or 'retarded' children. Interestingly, the same stigma does not (at least yet) appear to attach to special classes within ordinary schools and mothers are generally much more accepting of special provision within an ordinary school than in a separate institution.

Another major fact influencing attitudes about school placement is the mother's perception of education as providing one means by which a child can compensate for his disability, and more often than not it is the ordinary school which is seen as offering the greater chances of compensation. Once more, it is the association of the special schools with mental handicap which makes many parents doubtful about placement there.

The assumption that the other children in the special school *will* be of poorer ability or, put in another way, the tendency for parents of physically handicapped children to over-estimate their child's intellectual ability is an extremely common one. Tew (1973), for example, found that the parents of spina bifida children most likely to over-estimate their children's abilities were those with children whose IQs were between 60 and 80, that is, children 'who may show evidence of apparent normality in some aspects of behaviour although overall their functional level is well below average for their age'. When he compared parents' estimates of the child's mental age (converted to an IQ score) with their WISC Full Scale IQs he found for children in the 60–80 IQ range that in every case the parents had estimated the child to be in the normal range of intelligence. He comments on the fact that 'while parents often come to terms with their child's physical handicaps in a realistic manner over a period of time . . . the evidence of mental handicap in addition to the physical disability is not similarly acknowledged'. The tendency to over-estimate ability is not confined to parents of children with spina bifida but has been reported in many other studies of physically handicapped children (e.g. Boles, 1959; Jensen and Kogan, 1962; Barclay and Vaught, 1964; Keith and Markie, 1969; Roskies, 1972).

Sometimes there may be specific reasons for this. In Tew's study it was the parents of children whose expressive language was good compared with their other achievements who were particularly likely to over-estimate ability, as doctors, teachers and others may also do. However, more general factors affecting a mother's perception of her child's ability may also be operating. The child's developmental progress probably differed from that of other children and the mother may see him as slow to develop rather than as limited in ability, particularly if he has had to spend long periods in hospital. After her initial shock and pessimism at the child's birth, every positive achievement is likely to be given great emphasis, so that the standards she uses to evaluate intelligence are not necessarily those applied to normal children unless a mother is encouraged and helped to do this.

(c) *Attitudes of professionals*

The most up-to-date and useful discussion of official policy regarding the placement of handicapped children is found in the DES booklet

(1974) *Integrating Handicapped Children* and it has, of course, long been Departmental policy that 'no child should be sent to a special school who can be satisfactorily educated in an ordinary school'. When it comes to actual placement decisions, however, a great deal hangs on the phrase 'satisfactorily educated' and the attitudes of professionals often vary enormously. Some have a strong belief in the value of 'integrated' education and will press for special provision to be made to enable a child to attend an ordinary school, while others tend to see special schools as having more to offer. Attitudes will also be influenced by the sort of provision actually available.

Not infrequently, parents and professionals (for example a medical officer or psychologist) conflict over the appropriateness of a particular placement recommendation, especially when special provision is recommended because a child is intellectually retarded. Conflict could be reduced if professionals explained more carefully to parents the function of the tests and either immediately afterwards or in a follow-up session discussed with them the findings and their implications.

In fact it should never be necessary for a professional to have to tell an unsuspecting mother that her three or four year old is retarded: instead the mother should, from early on, have been asked what she thinks, and encouraged to make comparisons with other children the same age so that it is *she* who can point out to the professional those ways in which her child's progress differs from that of his peers. If the child has attended some form of pre-school provision where there are also non-handicapped children (see chapter 6) it will be much easier for her to do this.

Roskies (1972) suggests that many professionals have a rather clear (although often subconscious) concept of what a 'good' mother is, regarding her as someone who is able to adjust to the existing social system. Thus if she lives in an area where provision is in the form of special schools, a 'good' mother will see the advantages of this system whereas if the area is not well-endowed in this respect she is more likely to be considered 'good' if she accepts ordinary school placement without showing too much anxiety. Hewett, in her study of cerebral-palsied children (1970) expresses very clearly the contradictory nature of the role which the 'good' mother must play: 'The parents and later the child himself, must walk a tight-rope between acceptance of the fact that he is different from other children and insistence that he should be like them in as many ways as possible. If they emphasize his differences continuously, make allowances for his disability and learn a habit of helping and shielding, they may be labelled as over-protective; if they minimize his handicap . . . and speak with optimism of his mental attainment or physical prospects they may be judged to have failed to accept the situation'. It is small wonder that mothers are sometimes unable to play such a complex and contradictory role, and are too readily labelled (often in connection with school-placement decisions) as 'over-protective' or 'difficult' and 'over-demanding' and there is a need to educate professionals in more understanding attitudes.

The other group of professionals whose views should, but at least until recently have not usually influenced placement decisions (except insofar as they have the right to refuse to accept a child), are head and class teachers. Comparatively little research has been done on their views about where handicapped children should be placed although Anderson's study (1973) suggested that after first-hand experience of a disabled child in their class the great majority of teachers favoured ordinary school placement.

This is much less likely to be true of teachers with no first-hand experience of handicap especially those who are already under a great deal of stress, for example, teachers in city schools. They cannot be expected to welcome the idea of accepting handicapped children into their classes unless they can be assured of regular back-up services. Even then they may feel apprehensive, and research suggests (Haring *et al.*, 1958; Thomas, 1975) that favourable attitudes will not be produced simply by giving teachers information about the handicapped but that it must be coupled with direct experience with them. Knowledge without experience, suggests Thomas (who is head of a special education department in a College of Education), is only likely to increase teacher anxiety.

This finding has important implications when ordinary school placement seems appropriate for a child with spina bifida. It suggests that the head and class teacher of the receiving school are most likely to accept such a child happily if they have had, in addition to information about him, some actual prior experience with him. They can, for example, invite both mother and child to visit the school before the final decision is made and can also visit the child in his home setting. In addition, it is very valuable for the teacher or teachers concerned to be given the chance to spend one or two mornings or afternoons with the child in his pre-school group setting, whether this is a playgroup or nursery school, both as observers and if possible as participants. Teachers' attitudes are also likely to be more favourable if it is made clear that the child will initially attend an ordinary school for a trial period.

Meeting the special needs of spina bifida children in different types of school settings

The existing range of school settings in which a spina bifida child might conceivably be placed can be summarized as follows, beginning with the most specialized:

A (i) Boarding special school for spina bifida children.
(ii) Boarding special school for physically handicapped children.
(iii) Boarding or day special school for ESN(M) or ESN(S) children.
(iv) Day special school for PH children.

B (i) Special class/unit for PH children in ordinary school.
(ii) Special 'remedial' class in ordinary school.
(iii) Ordinary class in ordinary school with physical adaptations, ancillary care staff and special teaching facilities (e.g. 'resource' room).
(iv) Ordinary class in ordinary school with physical adaptations and ancillary care staff only.

C (i) Ordinary class with special individual arrangements (e.g. ancillary help).
(ii) Ordinary class with no special arrangements.

Grouped together under *A* are the special schools. These vary in the extent to which they provide for children with similar or widely differing handicaps, in their size and in the extent to which they have formal and informal contacts with ordinary schools. Contrasting with them are the type *C* settings, placement in an ordinary class in an ordinary school sometimes with and sometimes without special individual arrangements, and somewhere in between come the *B* settings. These represent, or could represent very much a half-way house, resembling *C* in that the child attends an ordinary school and *A* in that arrangements have been made in that school for a *group* of children with special needs. At present spina bifida children are placed most often in either the *A* or *C* type of setting, especially *A* (iv), day PH school, and *C* (ii), ordinary class. One reason for this is that comparatively few local authorities make provision of the *B* type, i.e. for *groups* of handicapped children within ordinary schools.

(a) *Educational needs*

In chapter 5 it was pointed out that while children with spina bifida but no hydrocephalus will probably be of normal intelligence, those with hydrocephalus are much more likely to have some degree of intellectual retardation, and to fall into the IQ range 70–90 (although there will of course be exceptions). These children will generally differ from other slow learners in that their intellectual development tends to be uneven with verbal skills generally being superior to perceptual and visuo-motor skills. The effect of these specific learning difficulties upon the children's attainments and the ways in which teachers can help are discussed in detail in chapter 8: the point we wish to emphasize here is that many spina bifida children are likely to need extra teaching help either on an individual basis or in a small group.

Special schools and special classes for PH children in ordinary schools are organized so as to be able to provide such help. The classes are usually small and although not all the teachers have special qualifications many have considerable experience with handicapped children. Little evidence is available about the relative merits of special classes, and special schools but research (Cope and Anderson, 1977) suggests that in terms of attainment closely matched groups of spina bifida children in special schools and in special classes were doing equally well.

Special help is much less likely to be available for a spina bifida child in an ordinary class. If his learning difficulties are not severe the class-teacher may well be able to cope on her own, especially at the infant stage when work is less formal. As the child grows older, however, or if the initial assessment indicates that he is likely to have marked learning difficulties then the ordinary class is unlikely to provide a suitable environment unless arrangements have been made to provide the class teacher with adequate back-up services from within or outside the school. She will need not only the fullest possible advance information about the child before he enters the class, but also must know whom exactly she can consult for expert help if the need arises. The back-up services which are available are discussed in chapter 8. These may be sufficient, although in contrast to countries such as Sweden, Denmark and the USA where there has been a much greater emphasis on integration (Anderson, 1976) little effort has been made in this country to organize special teaching help for physically handicapped children in ordinary schools.

Frequent and long absences from school are quite common in spina bifida children and intensive compensatory education may be needed if the child is not to fall further and further behind. Woodburn (1973) notes that orthopaedic operations in particular cause disruption to schooling, not simply because of the period in hospital but because of the long period of immobility in plaster at home. Sometimes LEAs plan compensatory education in advance and provide a home teacher in close contact with the class-teacher, and sometimes they provide special transport to school, but often this does not happen and long periods of school may be missed. Wherever the child is at school the question both of the necessity and of the timing of surgery should be fully discussed by all those professionals concerned and account should be taken of the child's educational as well as of his medical interests.

(b) *Medical and physical needs*

We start with incontinence as this was, for mothers, such a major problem. Needs are of two main kinds. First the toilets must be physically suitable. There must be facilities to enable a person to change the child there, they must be accessible to a child in a wheelchair and, most important, the child must have privacy. Secondly, there will usually be a need for either total or partial toileting assistance, including assistance in the management of the appliance if the child has one, and training in independence. 'Accidents' in class can occur and the child should always know that there is an adult at hand (and who this is) with the responsibility for seeing that he gets the help he requires. The class-teacher should also know about his problem even if she is not the person who will actually help him and when a child changes class this information must be passed on to the new teacher.

Special schools are geared to meet these needs, and usually ordinary schools also when provision for groups of handicapped children have been made. In ordinary schools where children have been placed individually or in twos or threes the problem may be greater, although it can be coped with successfully (Laurence, 1973; Welbourn, 1975). The appointment of welfare assistants to help such children was discussed in an earlier study (Anderson, 1973) and increasing numbers of local authorities appear to be making such arrangements. In a Scottish Education Department Report (1975) on secondary education for PH children in Scotland one of the major recommendations (para. 40) is that 'where children but for toileting problems, would be appropriately placed in an ordinary school, consideration should be given to the employment of welfare assistants or auxiliaries to provide the necessary help to enable the children to attend ordinary schools. This is especially important in the case of spina bifida children'.

Even then, as Welbourn (1975) points out, difficulties can arise. In her study she found that 'The younger children with incontinence attended school in nappies. The welfare assistants went off duty during the school dinner hour so in most cases these children had to return home at midday to be changed. The school was scarcely aware of any problem. Urinary appliances, particularly penile bags, often caused embarrassment by leaking. The older children learned to manage their appliances themselves just before or soon after promotion to junior school. We were fortunate in having few major bowel problems, but one 8-year-old child was still in special day school solely on account of bowel incontinence.'

Impaired mobility is the second major physical problem likely to affect school placement decisions. This raises questions firstly of access and movement around the different parts of a school and secondly of the provision of the appropriate treatment. Special schools are usually purpose-built; daily physiotherapy is available on the premises and often swimming too; the opportunity exists for close liaison between teachers and therapists and emphasis is usually laid on making the children as mobile as possible. In addition the physical and recreational activities at the school are especially geared to the needs of disabled children.

For children in ordinary schools, difficulties may arise in connection with transport and access; with the provision of physiotherapy; and in the field of physical activities generally. Some of the problems are met more easily than others. Most LEAs are willing to provide special transport, usually by taxi, for disabled children attending ordinary schools, and in the Scottish Education Department Report (1975) this was another major recommendation.

Physical adaptations needed to school buildings may include, in addition to special toilet facilities, the provision of at least one level entrance or, if necessary, a ramp with suitable handrails, while ramps may also be needed within the building. In secondary schools, in particular, a lift may be needed. When new buildings are being designed it should be possible to provide ramps, handrails and special toilet facilities at no great additional cost but lifts will be costly. It may be necessary to choose one or two schools in an area in which to make extensive adaptations and a few LEAs are beginning to do this. While the capital costs of such adaptations may seem high, the long-term savings should be much greater, but, unfortunately, proper cost-analyses are rarely carried out. Problems sometimes arise because adaptations have been made at the primary but not the secondary level with the result that disabled children leaving primary school have had to transfer to special schools, and it is very important that when provision is being planned it encompasses the whole school age range.

The extent to which a spina bifida child needs physiotherapy may be a major factor determining whether or not he can attend an ordinary school. In special schools (and for some special classes) physiotherapy is provided on the premises, daily if required. For an individual child in an ordinary school it is much more difficult to provide intensive physiotherapy, although it is often possible for the child to attend a local hospital for physiotherapy once a week: if this is done the treatment sessions should if possible be arranged outside school hours or during activities in which the child cannot participate fully.

It is preferable, though, for arrangements to be made within the school, and this will involve the use of peripatetic therapists. Other countries provide interesting ideas about how this could be done. In Calgary, Alberta (a city of about half a million), four hospital-based 'mobile teams', each comprising a physiotherapist, occupational therapist and speech therapist, provide a service to handicapped children who have been placed in ordinary schools, while the Ingham School District, Michigan, provides similar peripatetic services, their therapists being employed by the special education division of the LEA. In this country some use is made of peripatetic physiotherapists. Scotland, for example, has mobile physiotherapy units, and in south Gloucestershire Welbourn (1975) describes how 'peripatetic physiotherapists employed by the county council visited each [spina bifida] child weekly, at home, during the pre-school years, and subsequently at school, supervizing his daily activity programme, and in suitable cases instructed the welfare assistant how to continue'. However, in the main such services are not well developed.

Impaired mobility will also mean that many spina bifida children will need careful supervision and general help outside the classroom. In ordinary schools, this may involve the appointment of a welfare assistant to assist the child in getting around the school, in participating as fully as possible in PE, music and movement and games, in dressing, at mealtimes, and so on. The welfare assistant may also have general supervisory duties and, depending on a child's particular needs, special duties such as keeping an eye on his fluid intake and his diet.

In an increasing number of LEAs, handicapped children attending ordinary schools are being provided with welfare assistants on the medical officer's recommendation. The system generally seems to work, but could be improved if short training-courses for assistants were set up, since untrained assistants often fail to encourage the child to be as active and independent as he might because of anxiety lest he hurt himself.

(c) *Social and emotional needs*

Placement decisions must take into account a particular child's social and emotional needs and also the social climate of the school in which placement is a possibility. A severely handicapped child in an ordinary school will have to accept the fact that there will be some activities in which he will not be able to participate, and may face a special kind of stress if he is the only disabled child in the school: on the other hand, if he is the only child in his immediate neighbourhood who attends a special school, this may also make him feel 'different'.

For a child attending an ordinary school, two periods are likely to be particularly stressful. The first is, of course, when he starts school. As Kershaw (1973) points out, the restricted social experiences of many handicapped children may mean they are socially immature on entering school and unready for a group environment. A child 'may have been impeded in joining with his peers in play, his parents may have taken him about in their normal activities less than they would if he had had no disability, or he may have been over-indulged at home'. However, increasing numbers of handicapped children are now receiving integrated pre-school education and may experience little stress on starting in infant school.

The other potentially stressful period comes when the child has to change schools. The move from infant to junior school does not usually cause problems if the child moves up with his peers and if there is good liaison between his old and new class teacher. The move to a secondary school is potentially much more stressful and a period of emotional, social and sometimes educational regression may occur.

In the Scottish Education Department Report (1975) it is emphasized that it is much more difficult to achieve a suitable social climate in a secondary school than a suitable physical environment. In order to achieve this 'the attitudes of head teacher and staff and pupils are all-important. Sympathy is not enough. An informed attitude on the part of all concerned – handicapped and non-handicapped – has to be sought. There is a danger of over-protection in some aspects and insufficient attention in others. The head teacher and his staff must be willing to make certain organizational adjustments to ensure a full and satisfying role for the handicapped child in the life of the school as a first consideration. The staff and pupils of the school must have an understanding of the nature of the handicap, and it is vital that a member of the guidance staff of the school be given a specific duty for helping the handicapped pupil, acting as a link between home, school and the specialist services. To be successful, integration involves a great deal of effort, foresight and understanding on the part of all concerned at school and at home.'

The school placement decision

The initial placement decision

The process leading to a decision about the initial placement of a handicapped child (sometimes described as 'ascertainment'), involves three stages: discovery (finding out which children have disabilities which may call for special help), diagnosis (determining the nature and causes of the disabilities), and assessment (determination of the effect of the disabilities on the child's functioning, and consideration of the nature of any special educational requirement).

Until very recently the decision about the sort of education the child required was a medical one. Dissatisfaction with this state of affairs has been growing and in 1975 the DES issued a draft circular on the assessment question (DES, 1975) which recommends to LEAs what should be welcome and far-reaching changes in the assessment process. In this circular it is recognized that four kinds of people have particularly crucial contributions to make, the parents, psychologists, teachers and doctors, although it is recognized that information from others such as the GP, health visitor or social worker may also be useful. Parents, it is stated, 'should be brought into the picture early on and kept in the picture; their advice should be asked and their legal rights explained to them. In these ways their morale as parents will be raised instead of lowered, and their child will benefit as a result'.

The roles of the school doctor, the educational psychologist and teachers are much more clearly defined than hitherto, reports from all of these being required where appropriate. (A teacher's report will not of course be available for the initial assessment but it is required when placements are being reviewed.) It is recognized in this circular that teachers of handicapped children (in ordinary and special schools) have often had little information about them and the three forms which are to be filled in by the school doctor, educational psychologist and head teacher are intended to be passed to teachers and specifically designed to give the latter information which will be helpful and constructive.

If local authorities follow the recommendation in this circular the problems which, in the past, have been frequently raised by parents should be considerably eased. However, at present a commonly recurring problem is that many parents feel that they receive inadequate help and support in finding the right placement for the child. In Sheffield, for example, Freeston (1971) found that although all the thirty-eight four-year-old spina bifida children in her study were known to the LEA (since they were attending at the Sheffield Children's Hospital where they were reviewed annually, and a copy of the letter from the pædiatrician to the GP had been sent to the Medical Officer of Health) 40 per cent of the mothers had had no contact with the LEA. Not even a routine letter had been sent to confirm that the authority was aware of the child's condition and would be giving consideration to his special educational needs.

In the GLC study the situation seemed to be little better. At 3 years old 5 children were already in school, 26 had been assessed for schooling and appointments had been made for a further 11. However, 83 children (39 with moderate or severe handicaps and 44 with mild or minimal handicaps) had not and their mothers had no idea what the procedure for assessment for schooling would be. They were worried because they felt that they should be putting the child's name down for a particular school, but did not know which one. This was in contrast to the procedure for their non-handicapped children which was very simple and understood by everyone. Parents were also very nervous of approaching special schools to ask to look around or talk to staff even when they were encouraged to do so by the interviewer.

The conflict which may arise between parents and the professionals doing the assessment as to what the most appropriate placement is has already been referred to; a further problem is that even when parents and professionals agree there may be difficulty in finding a school willing to accept the child. In both cases part of the problem is often that the placement decision is presented both to the parents and to the school as a *fait accompli.* The mother is told what sort of placement is considered suitable, often after little consultation, and the head or the class-teacher is 'informed' that a spina bifida child will be arriving next term. Although in some areas consultation procedures are excellent all too often this is not the case.

The new assessment procedure should help greatly but other points are worth considering. It should be made clear that when some sort of initial decision about placement is arrived at this should be regarded as a suggestion only. If an ordinary school has been suggested, both the doctor and the educational psychologist should visit it to discuss the placement with the head and class-teacher concerned. Next the mother and child should visit the school to discuss the placement with the head and class-teacher. Only after this has been done, and after the staff have actually met the child should a final decision about placement be taken. The class-teacher may then want to see the child in his pre-school setting. It is also helpful if the placement is initially for a trial period, if the mother can assure the teacher of close support and if the doctor makes it clear to schools that he is willing to provide information, advice and general support.

Reviews of placement, transfer between schools and flexibility of arrangements

In the new DES circular on assessment (DES, 1975) it is emphasized that no placement should be assumed to be final and that the progress of handicapped children, wherever they are placed, should be the subject of regular systematic review. 'This should take place annually and should preferably not involve formal procedures which might unsettle the child and his parents.' A similar recommendation is made in the Scottish Education Department report (1975).

The time at which a child moves from primary to secondary education is a particularly important time for proper assessment. The child's views should be taken into account at this stage, he should be given full information about the different possibilities and if a move to a different kind of school is being seriously considered he should be properly prepared. If he is in an ordinary school the staff there in conjunction with the ascertainment team should anticipate the difficulties which might be encountered at the secondary level. Among the questions which need to be asked are questions about access, about how the child will get around the school, about the availability of personal assistance and remedial teaching if needed and about the attitudes of the secondary school staff and pupils. Liaison is needed between his primary and secondary school; information about the child must be passed on to the secondary school and the new head can also be invited to send the person who will be responsible for the child (e.g. a form teacher or 'house' master) to meet the child in his old school the term before the move takes place. The child and his parents should also be encouraged to visit the secondary school in advance, perhaps with a neighbour who is already there or a friend who will be going up with him.

It is very helpful if arrangements can be made as flexible as possible. One aspect of a flexible approach is the building up of closer liaison between ordinary and special schools. It was noted in the Scottish Education Report (1975) that small special schools find it difficult to provide a reasonable range of secondary education subjects for the pupils. For this reason, these schools 'must look outwards towards ordinary schools. We were impressed by several instances of pupils in special schools going out for certain subjects to the secondary school. Where the disability of the child does not permit this, specialist subject teachers from ordinary schools should come to the special schools. To facilitate this each special school should have a formal association with an ordinary secondary school.'

School placement of spina bifida children: selected research reports

To end this chapter survey findings are discussed which show what is actually happening to spina bifida children in different areas.

In the GLC study overall, 39 per cent of children were attending ordinary schools at the age of 6 years. However, of those children still living within the ILEA area at school entry, only 30 per cent were in ordinary schools, compared with 40 per cent of those in the outer London boroughs and 58 per cent of those living outside the GLC area. The type of school placement is shown in Table 7.1 below.

This shows that only 30 per cent of the children living in London were in ordinary schools in contrast to 58 per cent who had been placed in day schools for the physically handicapped. A much higher proportion of the girls (60 per cent) than of the boys (30 per cent) were in some form of special education, this being in line with national findings (*Health of the Schoolchild*, 1966–68). As noted earlier spina bifida children now comprise an increasingly large proportion of children in day PH schools (Table 7.2).

Table 7.1 *School placement at 6 years old of children in the GLC Spina Bifida Survey*

	*Ordinary**	*Day PH†*	*ESN/ SSN*	*Residen-tial‡*	*Total*
Males	29	28	2	2	61
Females	33	46	6	9	94
Total	62	74	8	11	155
Percentage	40·0	46·4	5·1	7·0	
% ILEA only	29·4	53·6	2·4	14·6	41
% Outer London Boroughs	40·0	52·0	4·4	3·3	90
% Outside GLC	58·0	21·0	12·5	8·5	24

* Includes two children in special units.
† Includes four weekly boarders
‡ Includes three illegitimate children, four very severely subnormal, and one in care for non-accidental injury.

Table 7.2 *Percentage of cerebral palsied and spina bifida children in ILEA day PH schools in 1973, as % of all day PH pupils (From Spain, 1973)*

	Age-groups			
	Below 5	*5–11*	*12+*	*Total*
Spina bifida	30	21	10	19
Cerebral palsy	30	45	50	45
Other	40	34	40	36
Total	100	100	100	100

Of the 58 children seen in ordinary schools, 28 had no apparent handicap. However, even where the child was quite badly handicapped very little information had been given to the teachers about the nature of the problem, other than what they were able to glean from the parents themselves. Over 50 per cent of teachers said that they wanted more information about the child's medical condition. When asked if the school should have been helped in some way to absorb the child, 25 per cent said yes, including all teachers of children with obvious handicaps.

All teachers of children who were incontinent and also had locomotor handicaps felt that they needed more information or assistance or both. 11 of the 26 children who were incontinent were not helped by anyone on the school staff and either a sibling or the parent took the whole responsibility. In at least 6 cases it was felt that this placed an unnecessary burden on the mother. Despite the lack of help to schools all these children had been absorbed successfully, in the sense that the child, teacher and parent were satisfied with the placement, even though there were sometimes outstanding problems. With but one exception, all the teachers were in favour of integration and this teacher had to manage, without any assistance, a doubly incontinent child.

It is well known that placement policy as well as the availability of special provision varies greatly from one part of the country to another and a few examples are quoted of the situation in other areas including Cambridgeshire, South Wales, Glasgow and south-east Scotland.

In Cambridgeshire, Hunt (1973) looked at the social and family problems of a series of 77 children with spina bifida myelomeningocele. 32 of these were of school age and the main types of placement are shown below in relation to intelligence.

Table 7.3 *Schooling and intelligence of 32 children aged over 5 years, surgically treated for myelomeningocele (From Hunt, 1973)*

	Type of Schooling			
IQ	*County primary school*	*Special PH day school*	*Other schools**	*Total*
Normal (80–126)	11	8	0	19
ESN (50–80)	2	4	3	9
SSN (<50)	0	0	4	4
% of total	40·6	37·5	21·9	100·0

* Other – included two boarding PH schools, two mental subnormality hospital schools, two ESN/SSN day schools and one nursery school.

Most of the children in this study were moderately or severely handicapped: 24 of the 32 spent most of their school life in wheelchairs and only 8 could walk independently with or without aids. Only 3 were both continent and able to use the school toilet independently. Despite this, most were happily placed, although a few were unpopular either because of incontinence or behaviour difficulties.

South Wales provides an example of an area where there are few day special schools. The result is that a high proportion of spina bifida children in the earlier Tew and Laurence study (1972) were attending ordinary schools. Sex differences, however, were marked, with very few spina bifida boys but almost half of the girls in special residential schools. Of the children born between 1964 and 1966, 49 per cent were, at 7 years old, attending special schools, just over three-quarters of these being children with shunts (Tew and Laurence, 1975).

While the lack of special day schools in South Wales was of course one reason for the somewhat higher proportion of children there in ordinary schools as compared to London, this could not however have been true of Glasgow which is well equipped with special schools. Nevertheless, Findlay (1969) noted that of 133 school-age children in the city with spina bifida cystica, 64 per cent were in ordinary schools and 32 per cent in special schools (the reverse of the ILEA figures), while 4 per cent received home tuition.

Woodburn's study (1973) of spina bifida in south-east Scotland gives a detailed breakdown of school placement (Table 7.4). One disturbing feature here was that nearly 16 per cent of the myelomeningoceles had not been placed by the age of 5, and the most serious criticism of schooling was usually that placement had been unnecessarily delayed.

Table 7.4 *Primary schooling at age 5 for children with spina bifida myelomeningocele (From Woodburn, 1973)*

	Type of Schooling						
	Ordinary School	*Special Day School*	*Special Resid. School*	*Still in Nursery*	*Home teacher or other*	*No schooling 5th yr.*	*Total*
N	17	13	2	5*	8	8	53*
%	33·3	25·5	3·9	9·8	15·7	15·7	103·9*

* Includes two for whom arrangements had been made to admit to normal school during year and who are also coded under that heading.

Although many problems relating to school placement do still exist and although what happens to a child depends too much upon where he happens to live, the situation is improving. Increasing numbers of spina bifida children now have the chance of pre-school education; there is a greater awareness that assessment for education should be a team-based decision and that educational psychologists, teachers, social workers and above all parents should be fully consulted in addition to medical staff; the need for more frequent reviews of the suitability of a particular placement is being recognized; many special schools are trying to build up contacts with ordinary schools; and local authorities are doing more to make ordinary schools suitable for handicapped pupils.

Two final points can be made. First, there is no doubt that many of the advantages of special schools which were discussed in this chapter *could* be provided within the ordinary school system. The different ways in which this could be done (and is actually being done in some other countries) have been described elsewhere (Anderson, 1973, 1976) and the current trend in this direction in this country is to be welcomed. Second, however, well-established systems of special provision tend to change only slowly. Many spina bifida children do need specialized teaching help and other special arrangements, and at present such help is, with few exceptions, only available in special schools. It is important therefore that existing special schools should do all that they can to arrange joint activities with neighbouring ordinary schools, especially at the secondary level when, as we discuss in chapter 9, social isolation can become an acute problem for many teenagers with spina bifida.

References

Anderson, E. M. (1973), *The Disabled Schoolchild: A Study of Integration in Primary Schools*, Methuen, London.

——, (1976), 'Special schools or special schooling for the handicapped child?', *Journal of Child Psychology and Psychiatry* 17, pp. 151–5.

Barclay, A. and Vaught, G. (1964), 'Maternal estimates of future achievement in cerebral-palsied children', *American Journal of Mental Deficiency*, 69, pp. 62–5.

Boles, G. (1959), 'Personality factors in mothers of cerebral-palsied children', *Genetic Psychology Monographs*, 59, pp. 159–218.

Boothman, R., (1975), 'Some observations on the management of the child with a Spina Bifida'. *British Medical Journal*, No. 5950, 1, pp. 145–6.

Cope, C. and Anderson, E. M., (1977), *Special Units in Ordinary Schools. An Exploratory Study of Special Provision for Disabled Children*, Institute of Education, London.

DES (1969), *Health of the Schoolchild*, 1966–68, HMSO, London.

——, (1974), *Integrating Handicapped Children*, DES Educ. Information.

——, (1975), 'The discovery of handicapped pupils and the assessment of their needs', Circular 2/75, DES.

Dorner, S. (1976), 'Adolescents with spina bifida – how they see their situation', *Archives of Diseases in Childhood*, 51, pp. 439–44.

Findlay, J. A. (1969), 'An appraisal of the management of spina bifida cystica', *Developmental Medicine and Child Neurology*, Supplement 20, pp. 86–90.

Freeston, B. M. (1971), 'An enquiry into the effect of a spina bifida child on family life', *Developmental Medicine and Child Neurology*, 13, pp. 456–61.

Hall, M. J. (1975), personal communication.

Haring, N. G., Stern, G. G. and Cruickshank, W. M. (1958), *Attitudes of Educators Towards Exceptional Children*, Syracuse University Press, New York.

Hewett, S. (1970), *The Family and the Handicapped Child*, Allen and Unwin, London.

Hunt, G. M. (1973), 'Implications of the treatment of myelomeningocele for the child and his family', *Lancet* ii, pp. 1308–10.

Jensen, G. D. and Kogan, K. L. (1962), 'Parental estimates of the future achievement of children with cerebral palsy', *Journal of Mental Deficiency Research*, 6 (1), pp. 56–64.

Keith, R. A. and Markie, G. S. (1969), 'Parental and professional assessment of functioning in cerebral palsy', *Developmental Medicine and Child Neurology*, 11 (6), pp. 735–42.

Kershaw, J. D. (1973), 'Handicapped children in the ordinary school', ch. 1 in Varma, V. (ed.), *Stresses in Children*, University of London Press.

Laurence, E. (1973), 'School placement of spina bifida children', in Palmer, J. (ed.), *Special Education and the Community Services*, Ron Jones Publ., Ferndale.

Parfit, J. (1975), 'The integration of handicapped children in Greater London', report of a survey commissioned by the Institute for Research into Mental and Multiple Handicap.

Richards, I. D. G. and McIntosh, H. T. (1973), 'Spina bifida survivors and their parents, a study of problems and services', *Developmental Medicine and Child Neurology*, 15, pp. 293–304.

Roskies, E. (1972), *Abnormality and normality. The Mothering of Thalidomide Children*, Cornell University Press, New York.

Scott, M., Roberts, M. C. C. and Tew, B. (1975), 'Psychosexual problems in adolescent spina bifida patients with special reference to the effect of urinary diversion on patient attitudes', paper given at the annual meeting of the Society for Research into Spina Bifida and Hydrocephalus, Glasgow, 25–28 June 1975.

Scottish Education Department Report (1975), *The Secondary Education of Physically Handicapped Children in Scotland*, HMSO, Edinburgh.

Tew, B. J. (1973), 'Some psychological consequences of spina bifida and its complications', Proceedings of the 31st Bienniel Conference of the Association for Special Education, London.

——, and Laurence, K. M. (1975), 'The effects of hydrocephalus on intelligence, visual perception and school attainment, *Developmental Medicine and Child Neurology*, Supplement 35, pp. 129–34.

Thomas, D. N. (1975), 'The teacher and the handicapped child', ch. 14 in Loring, J. and Burn, G. (eds.), *The Integration of Handicapped Children in Society*, Routledge and Kegan Paul, London.

Welbourn, H. (1975), 'Spina bifida children attending ordinary schools', *British Medical Journal*, 1, pp. 142–5.

Woodburn, M. (1973), *Social Implications of Spina Bifida – a study in S.E. Scotland*, Eastern Branch Scottish Spina Bifida Association, Edinburgh.

8 Teaching children with spina bifida

In this chapter, which focuses on spina bifida children in the classroom, we have tried to alert parents, teachers and other professionals to the sorts of learning difficulties which research evidence suggests that some spina bifida children may have and to offer some positive suggestions about the ways in which teachers can help them. Many of the difficulties described here are clearly related to the effects of hydrocephalus on intellectual functioning (see chapter 5). However, evidence from other studies (e.g. Pless and Pinkerton, 1975, pp. 101–3; Burton, 1975, pp. 169–71) suggests that children of normal intelligence with chronic handicaps not involving neurological impairment may be considerably retarded in their school attainments.

Since all aspects of classroom performance could not be covered in one chapter we have concentrated on a few areas of particular importance to the child's development. These are first the three Rs, reading, writing and number work, and finally an area which frequently causes anxieties to teachers in ordinary schools with physically handicapped children in their classes, games and PE. The concluding section of the chapter is about the ways in which teachers can help children with learning difficulties to develop their skills in school.

Reading

Introduction

Comparatively little research has been done on the reading abilities of spina bifida children and the data which is available is often hard to interpret and sometimes at first sight, even conflicting. One reason for this is that there are a number of variables which are likely to have a major affect on reading attainments in spina bifida children which researchers do not always take into account. These include the child's overall IQ, whether or not he has hydrocephalus, the sort of school he attends and the method of teaching used. Another problem is that in most studies the children have been quite young when reading was looked at so that their attainments are anyway still minimal. A further problem is that since reading difficulties affect quite a large proportion of non-handicapped children, with considerable variations from one part of the country to another (Davie *et al.*, 1972), it is really necessary to use a control group to be able to interpret what is happening. Often, however, control groups are either not used at all or are, in some respects, inadequate.

On the whole the research findings suggest that spina bifida children tend to be poor readers: however so much depends upon whether or not the child has hydrocephalus and also upon the degree of hydrocephalus that the question 'are spina bifida children poor readers?' is not a very meaningful one, a much more useful question being 'which spina bifida children are likely to have reading difficulties or to be "at risk" in this respect?' It is with this question in mind that research findings are discussed in the following section.

Research on reading

One of the first studies of reading to be reported comes from New York (Diller *et al.*, 1969). In this study a group of children with spina bifida and hydrocephalus aged 5–15 years were compared to a group with spina bifida only and a group with congenital limb amputations: results indicated that, on average, the hydrocephalic children were retarded by about eighteen months in reading, whilst the other groups had no major problems.

In this country Tew and Laurence (1972) carried out a study in South Wales (using the Neale Analysis of Reading Ability, 1966) which gave broadly similar findings. However, since the 58 children in the study had been born between 1956 and 1962 and had received later treatment than is usual today, the findings for them are not necessarily typical. The general picture resembled the New York findings in that a large proportion of the myelomeningoceles (37·5 per cent) were retarded in reading by between one and four years. What was surprising was that an even higher proportion (47 per cent) of meningoceles were retarded to the same extent, a finding which the authors were unable to explain. Unfortunately no control group was used in this study.

Of more interest are the findings from a study in South Wales (Tew and Laurence, 1975) in which data has been collected on 56 spina bifida children born between 1964 and 1966 and a control group who were matched for sex, place in family, locality and father's social class but not for intelligence. At 7 years old the children were tested on the Vernon Reading Test and the Schonell Spelling Test. The children without shunts tended to do slightly worse on these tests than the controls whereas those with shunts were very much poorer, more than 60 per cent of the shunt-treated group being unable to read a simple three-letter word by the age of 7. Details for reading are shown in Table 8.1 below: the results for spelling (not shown here) followed a very similar pattern.

Table 8.1 *Reading attainments at 7 years old of spina bifida and control group children (from Tew and Laurence, 1975)*

		Spina Bifida		
		No Shunts		
	Controls (*N*=56)	*No signs of hydro.* (*N*=20)	*Arrested hydro.* (*N*=8)	*Shunts* (*N*=28)
Reading age (yrs/mths) of scorers	6·11	6·5	6·4	5·7
Number of non-scorers	3	4	2	18
Mean WPPSI IQ	105·9	89·9	83·8	70·0*

* Mean is for 31 children.

Reading attainment was looked at in the GLC survey when the children reached the age of about 6 years. As the children were so young, standardized tests were not used: instead, the class-teacher was asked to place the child into one of three categories: (a) those who could not read at all, (b) those who could read flash cards or were on a first 'look and say' reader, and (c) those who were using more advanced readers.

Although teachers' assessments of reading ability do not give as accurate a picture as standardized test results the findings are interesting, particularly as it was possible to break down the findings for those with and without valves and those in special and in ordinary schools (Table 8.2).

with and without valves and those in day PH and in ordinary schools most like the controls in terms of IQ and school placement (i.e. no valve in ordinary school) have made quite a good start with reading, although they are a little behind the controls. Secondly, the children with the

Table 8.2 *Reading attainments in 6-year-old spina bifida children in the GLC survey*

		*Spina bifida children**			
		In ordinary schools		*In day PH schools*	
Status as reader	*Controls** %	*No valve* %	*Valve* %	*No valve* %	*Valve* %
Non-reader	0·0	10·0	22·2	28·5	37·5
Words only	31·8	20·0	22·2	43·0	48·0
Reader	68·2	70·0	55·6	28·5	14·5
Total %	100·0	100·0	100·0	100·0	100·0
No. in each group	22	20	18	7	48
Mean FS WPPSI IQ	109·3	102·2	94·1	95·9	79·6

* Data was only available for a sample of children.

greatest problem in learning to read are those in day PH schools with valves and a mean WPPSI IQ of about 80: 38 per cent were not reading at all and only 15 per cent were using readers.

Results for slightly older children (6½–9 year olds, mean age 7·8 years) are available from Anderson's study where the children were tested on the Neale Analysis of Reading Ability. In this study the spina bifida children (all of whom had valves) were closely matched for intelligence as well as for age and sex with groups of non-handicapped and of cerebral-palsied children. All but three of the spina bifida and three of the cerebral-palsied children were in special schools. The reverse was true for the controls; the majority were in ordinary schools but five had been placed in ESN schools.

In computing the scores non-readers were treated as if they had scored at the floor level of the test, i.e. at 6·0 years. There were in fact 6 non-readers in the spina bifida group, 5 in the cerebral-palsied group and 9 in the non-handicapped group. On average the spina bifida children (mean WISC IQ 88·3) were reading at a level within a month of their chronological age while the cerebral-palsied children and the non-handicapped children were, on average, 7 months and 12 months behind respectively. In terms of percentages the proportion of children in each group reading at or above their chronological age was 41 per cent for the spina bifida children, 28 per cent for the cerebral-palsied group and only 14 per cent for the non-handicapped children (mean WISC FS IQ 92·7). The poor spina bifida and cerebral-palsied readers tended to be children at the lower end of the IQ range, whereas almost half of the non-readers in the control group had IQs of 90+.

A similar pattern of results (overall, poorer performance in the control group than in the two handicapped groups) was obtained for reading comprehension although there was a marked tendency for the spina bifida children to have reading accuracy scores which were higher than their reading comprehension scores, whereas the reverse was true for the cerebral-palsied children, with the non-handicapped group somewhere in between. This suggests that the spina bifida children's grasp of the mechanics of reading was better than their comprehension of what they read. This difference was replicated by Ball (1975), although overall the hydrocephalic children in her study were much poorer readers than those in Anderson's study.

Research providing interesting data on reading attainments has recently been carried out by Cope (1977). In her study children attending special units for the physically handicapped in ordinary schools were compared with children in special schools matched individually for intelligence, age and the nature and severity of the handicap. The study included 15 juniors in each kind of placement who had spina bifida and valves (mean WISC FS IQs being 78·8 in the unit children and 80·0 in the special school children). The unit children were, on average, retarded by 19 months in reading and the special school children by 24 months. In the units 50 per cent of the spina bifida children were retarded by over 18 months and in the special schools 75 per cent. Four of the unit children and none of those in the special schools were reading at a level above their chronological age.

There has not been enough research on reading in spina bifida children for any very firm conclusions to be drawn but the studies reviewed here indicate that it is unwise to generalize. It is more useful to distinguish between two groups of spina bifida children. First, there is quite a large group, including most children without valves and the more able children with valves, who are unlikely to have any serious difficulty in learning to read. The little evidence available so far suggests that where reading is concerned these children do at least as well if not better in ordinary than in special schools.

Secondly there is an equally large group of children who are much more likely to be slow in learning to read and who are at risk of falling increasingly behind their peers. Most of these children will have hydrocephalus controlled by a valve and WISC Full Scale IQs below about 80, and they tend to be the same children in whom marked differences in verbal and 'performance' ability are found.

In chapter 5 the comparatively good verbal ability of spina bifida children was noted. Since, in reading, a child 'decodes' a set of symbols into a language with which he is familiar, the more verbally fluent he is, the more likely he is to be successful. He will be better able to guess at a word from fewer sound cues and his familiarity with syntax will be helpful. Since vocabulary and syntax tend to be well developed in spina bifida children we might expect them to learn to read fairly easily. Other factors discussed earlier, however, will make it more difficult for the child to become a fluent reader. Ocular defects, particularly squinting, may cause problems. More importantly, good visual discrimination ability is important when a child is learning to read, and spina bifida children with severe perceptual difficulties may make very slow progress, especially if their perceptual problems have not been diagnosed, and if they have had inadequate pre-reading training in making visual discriminations. Ball (1975) for example, found that hydrocephalic children frequently had specific problems of discriminating between mirror-image letters at a much later age than would normally be expected and she suggests that these problems are 'a primary factor in these children's reading retardation'. However, children can be taught to discriminate between reversible letters if specific teaching programmes are used (e.g. Henrickson and Muehl, 1962; Jones *et al.*, 1966).

An important aspect of reading is that children have to learn to attend selectively to the relevant visual cues. Those with difficulties in distinguishing 'figure' from 'ground' may find it hard to keep the relevant cues in mind and may be easily distracted by background cues on the page. Since many spina bifida children have some degree of figure–ground discrimination difficulty, it is important to keep the teaching materials as simple as possible.

Reading is often taught by a combination of the look-and-say and phonic approaches with, as the children progress, a change from an emphasis on the former to an emphasis on the latter. Children with visual discrimination difficulties may not be able to benefit at the usual age from the look-and-say approach, and a mainly phonic approach from the start may be more appropriate for them and may capitalize on their relatively good auditory skills.

Overall, however, there is no reason why most spina bifida children should not become adequate readers. What is more of a danger is that reading comprehension will not keep pace with reading fluency. Teachers and parents need to be aware of this and should always try to make sure that the child has a good understanding of what he is reading or of what is read to him.

In this context the findings in a recent experiment carried out by Riding and Shore (1974) are interesting. The purpose of the experiment was to find out how the comprehension of a story or piece of prose which was read aloud might be increased in children of below-average intelligence. The authors hypothesized that comprehension might be improved (i) if verbally presented material was supplemented by pictorial aids and (ii) if the presentation rate was slowed down. In their experiment they took 100 ESN children (age-range 9–16 years, mean age 14 years, mean IQ 68) and compared these two methods. One group of children was presented with pictures of some of the objects described in the passage at the moment when the object was mentioned. Another group had the passage read to them at a slower rate than usual, a third group had the pictures *and* the slow presentation and the fourth group normal presentation and no pictures. The authors found that both the inclusion of visual material and decreasing the presentation rate produced improvements in understanding, the greatest improvement being in the group who had both the pictures and the slower rate of presentation.

Number work

In the case of number work, research evidence is more conclusive. The studies carried out by Diller and his colleagues in New York (1969), by Tew and Laurence (1972, 1975) in South Wales as well as Cope's study (1977) of children with spina bifida and valves in special schools and special units in ordinary schools concur in suggesting that number work difficulties are particularly marked for children with spina bifida and hydrocephalus.

In the New York study these children were on average 2½ years behind children with spina bifida and no hydrocephalus while in the earlier South Wales study 78 per cent of the myelomeningoceles and 65 per cent of the meningoceles were retarded by more than a year in arithmetic on the Vernon Graded Arithmetic-Mathematics Test (Vernon, 1971). Findings in the South Wales study for children aged 7 years (Tew and Laurence, 1975) who were tested on the NFER 'Mathematics Attainment Test A' showed that even children with spina bifida only and no hydrocephalus had somewhat lower arithmetic quotients than the controls (mean of 94·9 compared to 105·5). The children with the greatest difficulties were those with spina bifida and shunts, 13 of the 28 children failing to score at all on the scale and the mean score for the others being only 79·9. Tew and Laurence also noted that 'about one third of the spina bifida cases were wholly incapable of simple counting at the age of seven'.

These findings are consistently confirmed by discussions with teachers who almost always report arithmetic problems as being much greater than reading problems. They are also confirmed by findings for spina bifida children on the arithmetic subtest of the WPPSI and the WISC. As reported in chapter 5 the children in our own research studies who had valves and mean IQs between about 60 and 90 tended to do extremely poorly on this subtest, while those without valves, or with valves but IQs in the 90s or above were only slightly poorer than the non-handicapped children.

It is a well established fact that brain-damaged children in general do tend to have poor achievements in number work. In an earlier study of physically handicapped children in ordinary schools (Anderson, 1973) in which teacher ratings of arithmetic ability were used, 78·1 per cent of the physically handicapped children with neurological abnormalities (either cerebral-palsied children or those with spina bifida and hydrocephalus) were rated by teachers as being of well below average ability in number work compared to only 29·5 per cent of the PH children without neurological abnormalities and 30·8 per cent of the control group children.

Taken together, the findings from different studies suggest that approximately 3 in 4 children with spina bifida and hydrocephalus are likely to have considerable difficulty in number work and that in this they very much resemble cerebral-palsied children of a similar overall intelligence level.

Haskell (1972) has discussed in some detail the factors which may lead to poor arithmetic performance in neurologically abnormal children and most of these are applicable to children with spina bifida and hydrocephalus. Some are factors which operate mainly in the pre-school period, some once the child has started school, and some at both these times.

Firstly, as discussed in detail in chapter 6, there is a danger that unless preventive action is taken spina bifida children may have impoverished pre-school experiences, especially sensory-motor experiences, arising from restricted mobility, impaired hand control and frequent hospitalization. As a result the child may not be ready to start number work at the usual age.

Secondly, a number of problems specifically associated with spina bifida and hydrocephalus may have an adverse effect upon number work. Ocular defects, particularly squint, may lead to reduced efficiency in simple tasks involving movements of the eyes. Perceptual, visuomotor and motor problems may work together to make it difficult for the child to carry out the sort of operations required in the early stages of number work. Most operations, for example constructing a model with rods, require that the child has reasonable visual discrimination skills (which enable him to distinguish differences in the length of the rods) as well as reasonable hand–eye co-ordination and motor control (so that he can set out the rods in a certain way), and these are often the very skills which are poorly developed in many spina bifida children. At a slightly later stage, as number work becomes more formal and written work increases, a child with poor spatial ability may find it difficult to set out sums properly and to arrange the figures in the appropriate columns.

Thirdly, in addition to these rather specific problems, there are behavioural and motivational factors which have to be taken into account. Distractability is a common problem in hydrocephalic children as in most brain-damaged children, and failure to concentrate will particularly affect arithmetic attainment since 'one of the major determinants of success in working sums is the degree to which the pupil can keep his mind persistently on the task in hand' (Schonell and Schonell, 1957).

Finally, frequent absences from school will affect progress in number work perhaps more than in the acquisition of other skills, since each step necessitates understanding of the previous steps. However, although some spina bifida children do have frequent absences, especially in the early years, Tew and Laurence (1975) found the attendance rate of the spina bifida children in their study very similar to that of the controls.

What can teachers do to help spina bifida children with number work problems? Below we list a number of suggestions made by a teacher of spina bifida children with experience in this area (Stollard, personal communication, 1975).

She begins by pointing out that 'pre-school experience is the key to successful concept formation in all children and this is a major area where spina bifida children are impoverished'. Because the physical handicap impedes a child's mobility and limits the extent to which he can gain personal knowledge of space and distance 'the ground work for the appreciation of distance and spatial orientation may be lacking in his early pre-school years'. The child's experience with 'messy' play through which the pre-school child can develop concepts of volume and weight etc. may also be lacking. It is necessary to give the child additional experience at school with sand, water, building bricks and of 'handling objects of varying shapes, weights, texture and smell'.

Since spatial, ocular and manipulative problems are likely to be common it is necessary to establish first what the child is able to do readily and a check-list of simple perceptual-motor tasks should be devised, including such things as 'can cut with scissors', 'can stick gummed shapes', 'can use glue', so that absent skills can be taught. In teaching discrimination and spatial skills, it is useful to start with solid objects which can be taken apart and put together again, before progressing to simple jig-saws. Experience in looking for differences and similarities between objects will help him later with matching and sorting operations in pre-number work and with symbol discrimination.

Since many spina bifida children have difficulty in comprehending the principles behind number operations it is necessary for the teacher to start an exercise using very concrete examples gradually increasing the number of different situations where the principle can be applied in order to help the child to generalize or transfer. It is best to use a wide range of common objects such as shells, beads, sticks, etc. in order to stress the relevance of number operations. The application of tables can be taught with simple practical examples such as four records playing for three minutes each or the number of wheels on seven cars. The young child may be asked to carry out practical exercises at home, for example, counting square objects in the kitchen, so that number work is not seen simply as an abstract activity confined to the classroom.

Because spina bifida children are very distractable, especially when asked to do tasks like number work which they find difficult, special attention must be given to the question of motivation. The child can be asked to do a task for a specified length of time, with a previously agreed reward if he succeeds, and the time can gradually be lengthened. Distractions should be reduced to a minimum and the use of a tape-recorder or the Synchrofax 'talking page' with headphones may also help the child to attend to instructions and may improve motivation, whilst freeing the teacher to work with other children. Individual work programmes are essential to ensure that the child is never asked to do things far beyond his level and so that he is frequently rewarded by his success. If the child must be absent for long periods at home or in hospital, work can be prepared from the child's own programme to be continued there.

Although many spina bifida children are verbally fluent they do not always understand what is said and similarly while reading with mechanical skill they may not comprehend well. Therefore it is particularly important to ensure that the child does understand spoken and written instructions. Before he is allowed to proceed on his own, it is helpful if the teacher first demonstrates the task followed by an explanation of each process, after which the child must demonstrate an example with a verbal commentary, since verbalization will help the child to define the sequence of activities required. Written instructions should be kept to a minimum.

Once a skill has been mastered the child needs as many opportunities as possible to generalize the concept so that he can internalize the process and abstract the principle involved. The technical vocabulary used should always be defined clearly and strictly adhered to in order to minimize confusion in transfer. It is also helpful to make use of pictorial representation of principles which can be applied in different situations.

The children may also have difficulty in learning how to write number symbols, and it is sometimes helpful to give a child wooden stencils or cardboard cut-outs to trace, or to use numbers cut out of sandpaper or other textured materials for the child to trace with his finger, thus getting kinæsthetic experience. Numbers drawn as a series of small arrowheads indicating the direction the pencil should follow sometimes help to give the child the idea of a set pattern of movement for a particular symbol. When the stage is reached at which operational symbols are introduced spina bifida children who have perceptual problems may find it difficult to make the necessary discriminations (e.g. between + and ×) and these signs should be used at first in conjunction with their written names.

In general, these children are likely to have difficulty setting out materials because of spatial problems and writing may be laborious for them (see next section). At first the teacher may have to write out or set down most of the work the child has done. She can also help the child by showing him how the action he has carried out can be represented pictorially in the form, for example, of a graph or chart, thus minimizing actual writing demands, and this will also give the child visual recall cues about actions he has performed before. Later the child must be helped to record his work himself. Published material in the form of general texts, workbooks or workcards is unlikely to be useful as it stands, since there tends to be too much information on any one page, and too much reliance on written instructions, nor is the work usually broken down into sufficiently small steps. However it can provide helpful ideas and diagrams which can then be adapted to suit the needs of individual children.

Finally, it may be necessary to curtail the syllabus for the less able children, concentrating on those concepts which are necessary for day-to-day tasks, such as how to multiply and divide, money, time, weight, etc. However, spina bifida children should never be allowed to feel that they 'can't do numbers'. If they are given constant reward and encouragement, if tasks are broken down into small steps, if distractions are minimized and the child is not asked to do things far beyond his level or for too long a period, these children can be taught the basic number concepts. They will, however, probably need to be taught each step in the process, since they are generally not capable of discovering relationships for themselves without help. At the same time, each child must continually be asked for a little more effort, so that he becomes used to looking for relationships between operations and attempts to discover for himself the next step to follow. The chapter by Gulliford (1969) on mathematics in his book *Backwardness and Educational Failure* gives a detailed discussion on the ways in which children acquire mathematical concepts and how a slower learner may be helped, as does Galperin's article (1957) in Simon's book *Psychology in the Soviet Union*.

Writing

Today, the teaching of handwriting is generally neglected in primary schools. This neglect is reflected by the absence of research both on the development of writing skills in non-handicapped children, and on handwriting problems in children with handicaps of different kinds. This has certainly been true where spina bifida children are concerned despite the increasing evidence from classroom observations that these children often have more difficulty in learning to write than in learning to read. Most teachers would probably agree that spina bifida children often find writing assignments laborious, that the quantity of written work produced is small and the quality of the handwriting poor. Handwriting problems will of course affect almost everything that a child does in school and can be an immense source of frustration and misery to the child, and it is important that a child is given appropriate help in this area as early on as possible.

Research findings

Writing was not looked at in detail in the GLC survey but information was collected on three points: first, on the child's ability to write his name (full name, first name only, or neither), second, on how many letters he could write, and third, on whether he could write freehand, or needed to copy or did neither. As Table 8.3 shows, the spina bifida children without valves who were in ordinary schools were doing almost as well as the control group children, although a rather smaller proportion could write freehand. The group in ordinary schools with valves resembled the group in day PH schools without valves although a higher proportion of the ordinary school children knew at least ten of their letters. The most striking finding was the very small proportion of those children in special schools who had valves and were more intellectually handicapped (mean WPPSI IQ 80) who could do these things.

Table 8.3 *Percentage of children in the GLC study able to carry out certain writing tasks at 6 years*

	Controls	*Spina bifida children*			
		Ordinary school		*Day PH school*	
		No valve	*Valve*	*No valve*	*Valve*
	(*N*=22)	(*N*=26)	(*N*=23)	(*N*=10)	(*N*=58)
Writes full name	55·1	46·2	30·4	30·0	12·1
Writes 10 or more letters	73·4	69·2	60·9	40·0	15·5
Writes free hand	50·0	38·5	30·4	30·0	3·4
WPPSI IQ Mean FS	109·3	102·2	94·1	95·9	79·6

Much more detailed information on writing skills was provided by Anderson's study (1975) where twenty 8–10 year olds with spina bifida and hydrocephalus were compared with non-handicapped children individually matched for intelligence, age and sex.

The children were asked first to carry out some simple tasks involving the ability to write (from dictation and then by copying) single letters, digits and then reversible words (e.g. tub, saw). Almost identical tasks had been used in a study of normal 7½–8½ year olds carried out by Chapman and his colleagues (Chapman *et al.*, 1970; Chapman and Wedell, 1972). The letters and digits were each scored as correct or incorrect and the nature of the error (omissions, substitutions, rotations and poorly formed letters or digits) was recorded. No major differences between the groups were found and overall the spina bifida children seemed to 'know' their letters and digits slightly better than the controls. Rotation errors were of particular interest: altogether three of the twenty spina bifida children had clear reversal problems compared to four of the controls. However, whereas the non-handicapped reversers were all children under 8 years of age, two of the three spina bifida reversers were 9 years old, and they were all children of lower overall ability. Their reversals were mainly of letters or numbers involving correct orientation of the diagonal (z,s,3,7), whereas the non-handicapped children more often had problems with d,b,p and 9.

Although the spina bifida children were capable of producing the correct letter or digit the quality of the penmanship tended to be poorer than for the controls and to examine this in more detail more complex tasks (in which speed was also an element) were introduced, and a more rigorous scoring system devised.

All children were given the 'copying a sentence subtest' from the Daniels and Diack Standard Reading Test Battery (1960). They were asked to copy in their best writing and while doing so were unobtrusively timed. As expected, the non-handicapped children copied the sentence significantly faster than the spina bifida children, the average time taken being 38 seconds compared to 56 seconds.

The quality of the writing was looked at in several ways. First, two independent adults were given pairs of sentences, one written by a spina bifida child and one by his matched control, and asked to choose the one with the 'better' handwriting. Neither rater knew which child was which. There was high inter-rater agreement and in two out of every three pairs the non-handicapped child was selected as the better writer. Below two examples are reproduced in which the non-handicapped child's writing was rated as superior by both raters. The time taken to write the sentence is shown in brackets and below each pair of sentences are shown the age of the child as well as his reading age on the Neale Test. These examples show clearly the overall faster and superior writing of the non-handicapped children. In those cases where the spina bifida child was rated as superior the differences in the quality of writing was much less marked.

Figure 8.1 *Example 1*

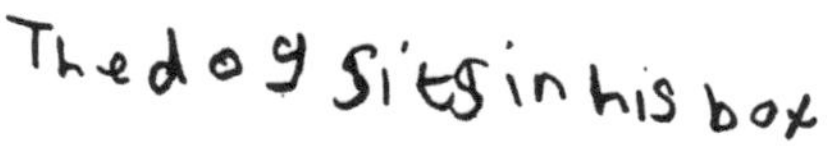

(54 secs)

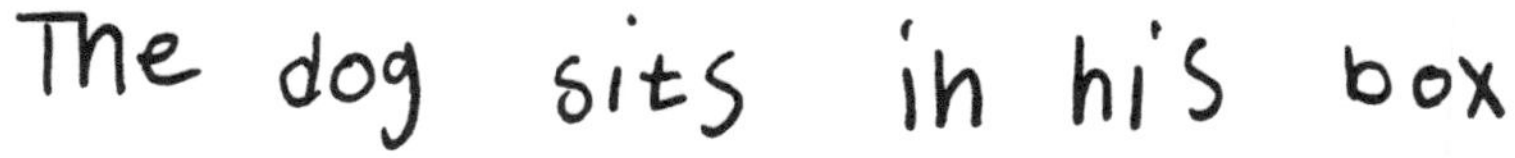

(30 secs)

Spina Bifida Girl (above): 10·2 years; Reading age 8·2 years.
Non-handicapped Girl (below): 9·8 years; Reading age 8·4 years.

Example 2

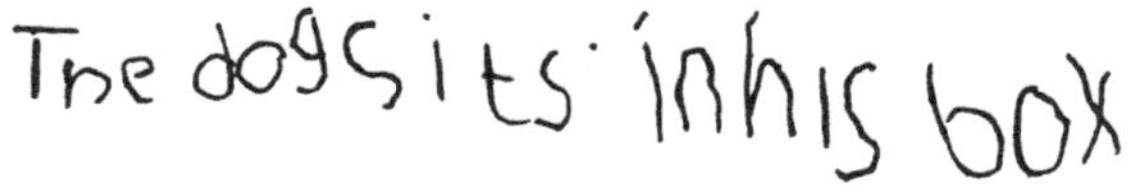

(85 secs)

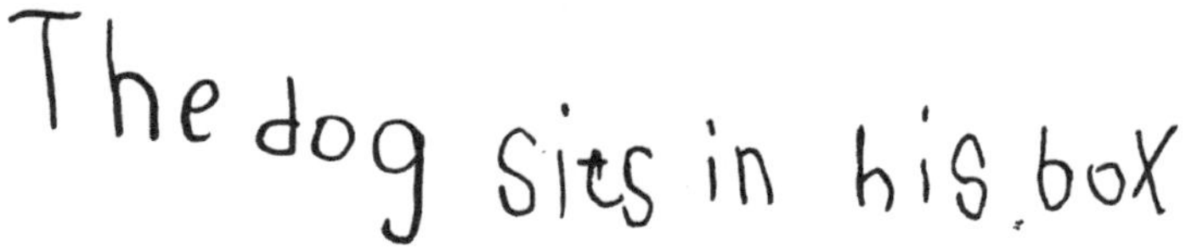

(45 secs)

Spina Bifida Boy (above): 7·9 years; Reading age 8·5 years.
Non-handicapped Boy (below): 7·11 years; Reading age 6·8 years.

Next the raters scored each sentence out of 30. The correlations between the raters' scores were quite high (0·72 for the spina bifida group and 0·70 for the non-handicapped group) and in both cases the mean score of the non-handicapped children was significantly higher than that of the spina bifida children.

An objective scoring method was also devised especially for the study, points being awarded for two main aspects of handwriting, the 'spatial qualities' of the writing and the 'letter formation qualities'. The spatial qualities score took into account the alignment of the words on the page, the spacing of the words and the spacing of the letters within the words, while the letter formation qualities total score included the formation of individual letters, uniformity of letter size, uniformity of the slant and the quality of the stroke. High correlations were found between the 'subjective' scores assigned by the raters and the scores arrived at when the 'objective' scoring method was used, the objective method having the advantage that different aspects of writing could be analysed separately.

After all the children had shown that they could copy a simple sentence they were asked to copy 6 different sentences. This time the child was asked to write not only as well but also as quickly as possible. Once again, large and very consistent differences between the groups were found in the speed of writing: this is best expressed by saying that the spina bifida children required the same time to write two sentences as the controls did to write three whether or not they knew they were being timed. In both groups there was a tendency for the girls to write faster than the boys, and the older children faster than the younger ones.

Significant differences were also found between the two groups in the quality of the writing, the distribution of the total writing scores being shown in Table 8.4 below.

Table 8.4 *Distribution of sentence copying scores in matched groups of spina bifida and non-handicapped children*

	0–39		40–59		60–79		80+	
Groups	N	%	N	%	N	%	N	%
S.B. (N=20)	3	15	4	20	9	45	4	20
N.H. (N=20)	1	5	2	10	5	25	12	60

When the different components of the total score were analysed separately, much greater differences were found between the groups for the 'spatial' qualities component of the score than for the 'letter formation' component. The spina bifida children were much poorer in spacing the words and also in spacing the letters and aligning the words correctly.

Much more information was obtained from this study than it has been possible to discuss here but two final points can be made. The first is that at least two out of three even of the more able children with spina bifida and hydrocephalus (mean WISC IQ 88) had marked handwriting problems when compared to normal children *of the same age and intelligence level.* Secondly, it would be wrong to conclude from these findings that all children with spina bifida and hydrocephalus are poor writers. Within both groups of children, but particularly in the spina bifida group, there was a great deal of within-group variation. A final example is given below in which the handwriting of two spina bifida boys with a similar mean WISC IQ is compared.

Figure 8.2 *Copying a sentence: within-group variation.*

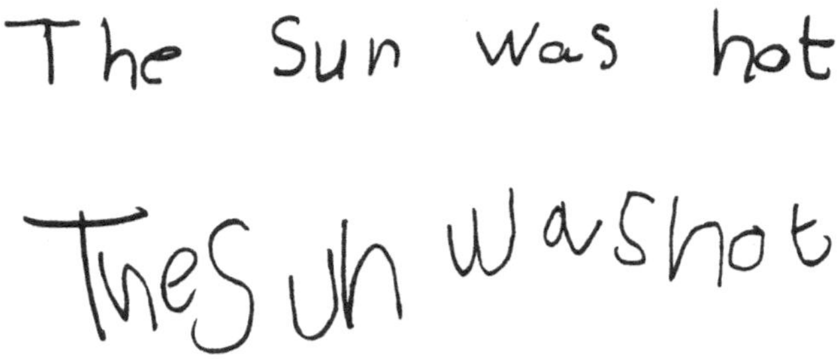

(52 secs)

(24 secs)

Spina bifida Boy A (above): Age 7·7 years; mean WISC FS IQ 91. Non-reader.
Spina bifida Boy B (below): Age 9·0 years; mean WISC FS IQ 86. Reading age 11·3 years.

Both these boys have hydrocephalus controlled by a valve and similar mean WISC Full Scale IQs but there the resemblance ends. The first boy, heavily handicapped, chairbound most of the time and a non-reader, has a WISC Verbal IQ of 79 but a performance IQ of 97 and as the extract above shows, good writing ability. The other was the most mobile boy in the sample and gets about slowly without a walking aid. He is also a fluent reader. However his WISC Verbal IQ of 97 and performance IQ of 86 are almost a reversal of the other boy's scores, and as this example shows he has a marked handwriting problem.

Helping children with writing difficulties

The research findings discussed here suggest that many children with spina bifida and hydrocephalus (and possibly also some of those without hydrocephalus although this was not investigated) are likely to have handwriting difficulties. The main factor accounting for these problems is, we suggest, impaired hand and fine finger movement control resulting from the neurological deficits (discussed in chapter 1) associated with hydrocephalus and/or the Arnold-Chiari malformation. Thus pre-writing activities which improve motor control, eye–hand co-ordination and tactile perception are all very important for spina bifida children.

Although poor motor control is probably the major problem, poor perceptual and visuo-motor difficulties almost certainly contribute to many children's difficulties in making the correct spatial judgments involved in the spacing and alignment of the letters and words on the page and here systematic training can help. Frostig and Maslow (1973), for example, suggest that a child with difficulties in spacing words should place the index finger of the non-writing hand at the end of the word and leave the same amount of space before writing the next word. 'Usually', they state, 'this exercise is necessary for only a short time before the child acquires the habit of correct spacing.' It is, therefore, well worth while isolating a particular facet of a general writing problem, and then carrying out a very specific plan of remediation.

More important than this, however, is the broad implication of all our findings on writing skills, that this is likely to be a problem area and that, therefore, spina bifida children should be quite systematically *taught* to write. Children who are not taught to write are likely to regard handwriting as if it were a pattern-copying task. They will copy letters and words as if they were patterns, using whatever idiosyncratic movements they find necessary and will be concerned mainly with the visual discrimination aspect of the task. Certain teachers follow this approach to writing, giving the children some training in making visual discrimination and then expecting writing to follow without much teaching being necessary.

This approach will not be the most effective way of helping children with spina bifida. They are likely to need much more systematic teaching of handwriting, in which particular hand and arm movement patterns are emphasized, with the child being encouraged to attend to the 'feel' of the movements he is making and short movement sequences gradually being incorporated into longer ones. Later, materials are described which may be of interest to teachers who want a systematic scheme to follow. Many spina bifida children are left-handers and for this reason alone may need some guidance when beginning to learn to write; teachers of these children will find Margaret Clark's booklet (1974) on teaching left-handers extremely useful.

Because of poor motor control many spina bifida children may not enjoy the usual pre-writing activities such as modelling, painting or drawing as much as activities which make fewer demands on motor skill and hand–eye co-ordination. It will then be even more important than usual to ensure that the children are motivated to want to learn to write and that when they do reach the stage of writing proper this is done in a situation which has meaning and purpose for the child.

If it is clear that even after systematic training a child does have a marked writing problem, for instance still writing very slowly, then a teacher can help in two important ways. Firstly, the writing demands made on the child can be reduced. Teachers can and usually do lower the standards for acceptable handwriting, particularly for older children when time pressures (for instance in a test) are imposed. Teachers can also often reduce the amount of written work that has to be done. In number work, for instance, the child may be overburdened by the sheer mechanics of copying out the sums. If practice in computation is the aim, teachers could consider using mimeographed sheets where only the answers have to be filled in, or could write out the questions rapidly themselves, or ask parents or an assistant to copy the examples and let the child fill in the answers.

Secondly, teachers can try to ensure that alternative forms of expression are, from an early age, made available to the child, since it will be very discouraging for him if attention is focused all the time on what he finds difficult. If his written work is slow and poor, a teacher should give him the chance to express himself orally or even to record his compositions on a tape-recorder. In the case of older children, attempts to improve handwriting may reach the point of diminishing returns; it may be wise to accept that further improvement is unlikely and to consider other modes of expression. It might increase the self-confidence and the competence of many spina bifida children if they were given instruction in typewriting from quite an early age and certainly once they have reached their teens. While typing may present some difficulties because of poor motor co-ordination, poor spatial memory or difficulties in sequencing motor activity, many handicapped children with writing difficulties (for example cerebral-palsied children) have found typing more motivating than writing partly because it is a grown-up activity, partly because although progress may be slow it should be possible eventually to produce a professional-looking piece of work.

Additional classroom problems at the secondary level

Many of the new problems which face spina bifida children in secondary schools have to do with their social, emotional and sexual life and are discussed in chapter 10. As regards their school-work, the subjects they are most likely to have difficulty with are those for which visuo-perceptual, visuo-motor and motor skills are necessary. Children with spina bifida and hydrocephalus who were able to compensate for such difficulties at the primary level may find them interfering with progress at the secondary level, particularly in mathematics (especially geometry), the sciences and geography, since map-making and map-reading, the making of diagrams, the handling of lab equipment in science and constructional work in mathematics all require good visual spatial skills and good eye–hand co-ordination. Handwriting difficulties may also persist in many children and hold back progress as more and more written work is required.

Since so many spina bifida children will, on leaving school, depend heavily on driving their own cars for mobility it is particularly important that time and thought is given to the teaching of map-reading. At present many spina bifida teenagers leave school unable to read maps, or feel so unsure of their ability here that they simply do not use their cars outside the immediate neighbourhood. It is best that this skill is taught early on, and that the child is later encouraged to map read from a wheelchair as he goes out with his parents in his own locality, and later in a car when being driven by someone else, so that by the time he learns to drive he is fairly compentent in this respect.

Games and PE

Teachers, particularly those in ordinary schools, are frequently anxious about the child's participation in physical activities at school. They often have no information about how far a child can and should participate and so tend to be over-cautious, particularly if the child is heavily handicapped and normally uses a wheelchair or if he has a valve. Clearly, teachers require first of all much more specific information about the nature of the child's disabilities. Sometimes sufficient information is obtained from the parents but sometimes it is clear that a talk with someone with medical knowledge is needed so that a teacher can get specific information (for example about the valve), and also reassurance that what she is doing or plans to do will not endanger the child.

The second type of help which teachers require is very practical suggestions about what the children can do in physical education. The physiotherapist can be helpful here and if the child is attending a hospital for physiotherapy she can be invited to visit the school to advise the teacher. Another potential source of advice is the local special school. Contacts between staff of special and ordinary schools are still uncommon but it is important that they are developed further and special schools usually welcome requests of this kind for advice. Useful suggestions on physical activities for handicapped children can also be found in a booklet published by the DES (1971a).

The section which follows is addressed particularly to teachers in ordinary schools with spina bifida children in their classes. Most of the material presented here was kindly provided by Alan Brown (1974, personal communication) a lecturer at the Physical Education Centre of the University of Newcastle-upon-Tyne and has already appeared in the Teacher's Booklet produced by the Association for Spina Bifida and Hydrocephalus (1975).

Alan Brown points out that the major aims of physical education for physically handicapped children should be: (a) to provide enjoyment and satisfaction (the latter only stemming from successful achievement); (b) to teach the child enough gross perceptual-motor and spatial skills to participate successfully in active and creative recreational activities in school and in his own leisure time; (c) to provide opportunities for physical development and to increase the fitness level of the children within the limits of the disability (in the case of spina bifida children this will be largely the development of the shoulders, upper limbs and trunk); and (d) to provide the child with the opportunity for more normal psycho/social development through the medium of recreation and group play. While these are the main aims improvement in other areas should also result from a good physical education programme, for example there should be improved body awareness.

The relative importance of each of these aims will vary according to the physical status of each child but for all spina bifida children physical education is a vital part of their total education and the teacher must look for ways of actively involving spina bifida children according to their abilities. Dependent upon the site of the lesion many spina bifida children, states Alan Brown, may achieve arm and shoulder girdle strength which is far beyond normal if they have been exposed to activities based on weight-bearing from the arms. He suggests that climbing and heaving activities are a must for these children to allow for overcompensatory development of the unaffected musculature and older children should take part in upper body weight-training programmes during normal indoor lessons. When planning programmes which make considerable physical demands on the child, teachers should of course ask the child's physiotherapist or the school doctor for advice.

Since incontinence is often a problem the teacher must know whether the child has been fitted with a urine-collecting appliance. In such cases he should not roll around the floor or put pressure on the bag in any way; however children often best appreciate these limitations themselves. Waterproof undergarments are now available commercially which allow spina bifida children to go swimming without embarrassment. Teachers should consult parents and obtain medical advice (in particular from the physiotherapist) about this but in general spina bifida children should be taught to swim. The child will (at least at first) require individual supervision and good support (e.g. inflatable water-wings): many schools encourage the mother to come and help with swimming and welfare assistants are also helpful here, particularly as it may take a long time to dress the child afterwards.

The specific visuo-perceptual, visuo-spatial and visuo-motor problems which were discussed earlier may hamper the performance of some spina bifida children, especially in the acquisition of ball skills. Without an adequate repertoire of basic ball skills such children will be excluded from many group games with their peers and it is critical that they are exposed to simple forms of ball play from an early age. The major problems which interefere with the learning of these skills are the sensory and motor organization problems mentioned above, poor hand control (a key factor), poor balance even in a sitting position and lack of gross locomotor ability which will limit the space in which the child can operate successfully.

Teachers need to assess the extent to which each of these potential difficulties is operating for any particular child and then select play material according to the child's ability and modify it according to his disability. It is also suggested that more direct and formal teaching methods than would normally be used can be most successful in the early learning stages of ball skill practice. Where spina bifida children are in ordinary classes it will often be necessary for the teacher to simplify the activities so that the children not only participate but become successful. Success in simplified performance is most important to motivate such children to continued practice. The following principles may be useful as guidelines for teachers of spina bifida children to simplify the presentation of motor activities.

(a) Ball flight can be modified to simplify the perceptual problems in catching and striking skills. A ball in flight must be assessed in three dimensional space whereas a ball which is rolled along the ground must be assessed in only two dimensions – speed and direction. Bouncing balls are simpler to track visually than balls in the air.

(b) Larger balls are considerably easier to catch or hit than small balls for children with severe perceptual and/or visuo-motor problems. The use of a large ball simplifies the motor performance which becomes more of a gross motor skill using the arms than a manipulative skill using the hands only.

(c) Multicoloured play balls are easier to track against the normal gymnasium background by children with visuo-motor disabilities.

(d) Light plastic bats and thin-handled play bats simplify the motor aspects of striking skills.

(e) Spina bifida children in a normal class can be restricted to a definite place or position on court in many group and team games, for example net position in volleyball and badminton.

(f) In certain team games such as cricket or rounders, a team-mate can act as a runner for the handicapped striker.

(g) Minor rule changes can be made for spina bifida children taking part in a normal game, for example in cricket the type of bat and the type of bowling service could differ.

(h) During indoor games lessons based on group games spina bifida children should be allowed to take full part within the limits of their locomotor ability.

(i) In gymnastic lessons they should be actively encouraged to use any apparatus which stimulates the use of unaffected body areas, particularly where wall-bars, trapeze, climbing frames and ropes are available in primary schools. Again, when the child is using apparatus, individual supervision will usually be needed, at least for young children, and an ancillary helper may be essential.

In secondary schools the very least that can be done for spina bifida children is that they should be taught to umpire and referee matches for their peers. They can thus be made to feel that they are making a positive contribution in a variety of sporting activties and this is an avenue towards social acceptance in this field where personal active performance may not be possible. Brown points out that there are currently at least three badly disabled men on the Minor Counties Cricket Umpires list for 1974 who are accepted as experts at the highest level.

Teaching spina bifida children: principles, programmes, supportive services and training

General Principles

Teachers often ask whether any specific training programmes are available for helping children with learning difficulties of the kinds discussed in this chapter. Programmes have proliferated in recent years, especially in the United States. However, although certain programmes may be helpful they are less important than the 'normal' skills possessed by an 'ordinary' trained and experienced nursery, infant or junior school teacher.

There are a number of general principles which may help teachers to apply the skills they already have in the most effective way, to the advantage not only of spina bifida children but also of other children with learning problems.

(i) Many of the learning difficulties which spina bifida children may encounter can, to a considerable extent, be ALLEVIATED BY EARLY TRAINING OR REMEDIATED. Nursery and infant teachers in particular should ensure that from as early an age as possible the children practice the relevant skills underlying the three Rs in an appropriate and motivating manner. Even spina bifida children who are considerably retarded can make surprising improvements if teachers maintain a balanced approach, on the one hand understanding the child's particular difficulties, on the other being careful not to use a disability as an excuse for lack of achievement.

(ii) Children having trouble should be identified AS EARLY AS POSSIBLE, and teachers should watch out for those who seem restless, distractable, forgetful, who miss the point of questions and explanations, and who seem to have difficulty in keeping up. Early difficulties should not be allowed to drag on, so that the child falls more and more behind, and develops a feeling of inferiority. Unfortunately, this is particularly likely to happen in the case of handicapped children, partly because the teacher does not know what to expect, and may accept a low level of performance, and partly because of the common attitude of 'let's give-him-a-bit-longer' (i.e. before seeking appropriate help).

(iii) Once specific difficulties have been identified A SYSTEMATIC PLAN OF REMEDIATION should be drawn up. Special schools are geared towards the giving of individual help. Ordinary schools by and large are not, and it will be more difficult to decide how best to use the resources (in terms of staffing and time) available. For those spina bifida children whose learning difficulties are not very severe (IQs of about 80 or 85+) it may be quite possible to provide sufficient extra help by making only minor adaptations in the classroom programme, particularly if the children's difficulties are spotted early on. Regular INDIVIDUAL help should be given wherever possible, even if only for a very short time each day. Some schools have remedial teachers on their staff; in others an interested Head sees children several times a week for individual work. Usually the task falls on the class-teacher but even if a spina bifida child gets only ten minutes a day of individual help this may, for many children, be sufficient, if the teacher is clear about her objectives. Later the question of supportive services for teachers is discussed, but teachers in doubt about how best to help the child should not hesitate to seek for help with a plan of remediation and should make full use of such sources of advice as the school psychological service, advisory teachers or perhaps a local special school. This will be particularly necessary in the case of those spina bifida children who do have marked learning difficulties, that is, children with valves and IQs below about 80. At present most of these children are placed in special schools or classes but where this is not the case a teacher is likely to need (and should request) back-up services as early on as possible.

(iv) Having identified those activities in which a child experiences difficulty, the teacher should try to break the activity down into SEPARATE STEPS, and teach these parts separately. Once this has been done, they can be combined gradually. Often it will be necessary to start the child on activities usually given to younger children. Sometimes it is useful to teach THROUGH ALL THE SENSES, for example getting the child to move his finger along cut-out letters which he is required to copy will add the sense of touch and movement to that of vision. SIMPLIFICATION OF TEACHING MATERIALS also helps, particularly if figure–ground discrimination problems are suspected or if the child is easily distracted by irrelevant stimuli on the page. Teachers should always try to EXPLOIT A CHILD'S STRONG POINTS when giving help in weaker areas. Spina bifida children often have good language skills and like to verbalize. It may help the child to verbalize what he is doing in number work, or verbalization might also be used in the teaching of handwriting. The important thing is to be sure that the child actually relates what he is saying to what he is doing. Since it is discouraging for the child if attention is always focused on what he has difficulty in doing, he needs plenty of opportunities to use those skills he does have.

(v) It is particularly important to ensure that spina bifida children are WELL MOTIVATED and see the relevance of what they are doing, since they tend to be rather passive. Teachers can use the fact that these children are generally sociable and outgoing, and enjoy having duties which make a definite contribution to the class and can try to give them tasks which are not only interesting but which also require that the child practises skills in which he is weak. For example, a child can be asked to make a map of the classroom, or a class list, or be made responsible for putting the date on the blackboard or recording the names of those absent.

(vi) DISTRACTABILITY hinders the progress of many spina bifida children. Teachers often accept this as inevitable: in fact distractable behaviour can be modified if the teacher has a SYSTEMATIC STRATEGY for tackling it. First the goal must be decided on. This might be quite modest, for example to get a child to concentrate on a number work assignment on his own for a definite period of time, say five minutes. Second (and this will depend on the age of the child), the child himself must know the goal, must feel it is his goal, not just the teacher's, and must also know what the 'reward' will be. Third, within the specified period non-attending behaviour must not be reinforced. If the child tries to communicate with the teacher when he is working on something he is supposed to know how to do, he must be ignored, not reprimanded (as this will only give him the attention he wants). Fourth, the desired behaviour should, if possible, be reinforced immediately in a way which has been planned and agreed with the child beforehand, taking into account what sort of things this particular child really *does* find rewarding. This might be a star on a chart, a 'good' in his book, verbal praise, or for older children some future reward, for instance permission to carry out a favourite activity later in the day with the child in the meantime being given a concrete token such as a star.

What is essential is that teacher and child should be clear about the goal and that the reinforcement of desired behaviour is systematic, immediate and meaningful to the child. Gradually, it should be possible to increase the demands made of the child in terms of time-span and the type of activities during which attentive behaviour is required. Reinforcement can then be given less frequently with social rewards (e.g. praise) gradually replacing concrete rewards. Presland (1974) has provided a generalized scheme which a teacher might follow in working out a behaviour modification programme for an individual child presenting problems in the classroom, and teachers with distractable children should find this article useful, as well as Cook's article (1975) about courses on behaviour modification techniques for remedial and special school teachers.

Special programmes

In the preceding paragraphs it was emphasized that learning difficulties can to some extent be prevented by giving the children systematic early training in the subskills underlying the three Rs. These include motor skills (especially hand control) as well as basic 'cognitive' skills, that is the perceptual spatial and visuo-motor skills discussed in chapter 5. Teachers must first identify the subskills necessary for, let us say, successful reading or writing: second, identify any deficiencies in these subskills; third, give the child the necessary training and drill in each of these subskills and fourth, help him to integrate the component subskills in a smooth efficient manner. Fifth, the teacher needs to ensure that these skills generalize to other tasks, in other words the newly learned skill must be shown to apply in a large number of different situations.

The value of programmes, whether they are ordinary classroom programmes devised by the individual teacher or programmes published for special categories of children, lies in the fact that they provide for the teacher a systematic and structured approach. Most of them incorporate the ideas of programmed learning, that is they are based on the propositions that learning involves frequent active participation by the learner, that he is reinforced for successful activity, and that his response to the programme should be successful most of the time.

Tansley (1967) has written in detail about such programmes and Wedell (1973) in his book *Learning and Perceptuo-Motor Disabilities* also gives a useful critical summary of some programmes (pp. 74–80, 108–11). He points out that programmes fall into two main categories: those 'aimed at the improvement of specific skills (for example the discrimination of reversed figures) as ends in themselves' and 'programmes which, while aimed at more general behaviour or educational adequacy are more particularly directed at skills which are presumed to underlie behavioural adequacy. These programmes imply that improvement on the specific skills will transfer to the "target" behaviour', for example that training aimed at improving figure–ground discrimination will bring about gains in reading attainment. Attempts to evaluate the effectiveness of such programmes in terms of gains in actual attainments have been comparatively few and the findings have on the whole been disappointing. Despite this there is still, as Mann (1971) notes, a great deal of dangerously uncritical acceptance of such programmes.

One of the best known programmes currently used by teachers of children with learning difficulties is the one devised by Marianne Frostig and her colleagues (Frostig and Horne, 1964). Frostig has postulated the existence of five main kinds of perceptual abilities, and has drawn up training programmes, consisting of work sheets with paper and pencil exercises, designed to improve performance in each of these areas. If a child does enough of these exercises improvements on the Frostig Test have been shown, but there is no clear-cut evidence that these improvements generalize to other tasks unless, as Frostig herself says, teachers deliberately train children in how to apply these skills.

Unfortunately, this has not usually been done and the value of the Frostig training programme has, as a result, been questioned. Certainly, familiarity with Frostig's worksheets could suggest to imaginative teachers how to prepare their own materials for the training of these skills and how to utilize classroom activities such as making maps, diagrams, scale drawings or work in nature study or art to help children to improve and apply their perceptual and spatial skills. However, unless used in this imaginative way the Frostig programme does little more than give isolated training of 'areas' of perception and is, in addition, very expensive.

A programme which is being used with some success in ordinary and in special schools is one by Haskell and Paull (1973) called *Training in Basic Cognitive Skills*. It consists of twenty-eight booklets for children to use, the aim being that higher level skills relating to perception, concept formation and abstract reasoning should be developed through a carefully graded approach. Although the programme is intended for normal 2–6 year olds the authors point out that older backward or handicapped children may benefit from it, and it compares very favourably in price with other programmes. Certainly it offers the teacher a systematic and structured basis on which to build her pre-three Rs classroom programme which can be adapted to individual children's needs. It is not a substitute for the teaching of reading (or numbers) but rather an integral part of a reading programme or approach to the three Rs within a classroom.

These authors have also produced a series of booklets called *Training in Motor Skills* which may be very helpful to children with motor problems. The booklets contain systematic and graded exercises designed to provide children with an opportunity to practice eye–hand co-ordination and control in the form of pre-writing skills. Starting with a straight line through a wide 'road', the exercises progress through curves and angles to following dotted-line patterns which finally lead to the formation of single letters of the alphabet. As mentioned earlier, children with spina bifida need to be specifically *taught* to write, and these booklets provide a useful introduction.

Supportive Services for Teachers

Teachers in special schools usually have available quite a comprehensive range of back-up services for dealing with medical, social, educational or psychological problems. These sorts of services are generally much less available to teachers in charge of special units or classes in ordinary schools, while in this respect the teachers of 'special' children who have been placed in ordinary classes are worst off of all.

In the last chapter we noted how the teachers of the spina bifida children in the GLC survey who had been placed in ordinary schools would have liked more information, as would the majority of teachers in Anderson's (1973) study of disabled children in ordinary schools. They were often unclear about what spina bifida and hydrocephalus really were and about 'what sort of things are likely to go wrong'. They frequently wanted straightforward technical information about, for instance, incontinence appliances, the ileal loop operation, the question of loss of sensation and the working of the shunt system. Closely allied to these were questions about what the child could and could not do and should and should not do, especially in relation to physical activities. A talk with a doctor or someone else with the required professional expertise could often very easily have answered their questions and alleviated their anxieties but the doctor and class-teachers rarely met. Teachers' requests for medical information are almost always channelled through the head and this in itself, coupled with the fact that teachers have little free time in school, means that the wish for information is often never voiced. When it is, the 'confidentiality' of medical information is still sometimes quoted as valid reason for not giving teachers the information they really want and need.

The findings of other studies have been strikingly similar. For example, Holdsworth and Whitmore (1974b) in their study of children with epilepsy in ordinary schools 'were disturbed to discover that discussion between teachers and school doctors was the exception rather than the rule'. Teachers were rarely given and rarely sought specific advice about the handling of a child's seizure and 'no less surprising was the number of occasions on which the teacher had not been told of a child's epilepsy by the school doctor'.

The only real answer to this problem is that it should be made a matter of routine practice that when a disabled child is placed in an ordinary school the staff of that school, in particular the head and class-teacher, should be given full information about the child's physical condition. When the new assessment procedures described earlier (p. 192) become very widely used the teachers should then have more information. However, in cases where a teacher is likely to feel particularly anxious, information should be given by the medical officer concerned in person, and should be followed up by a further visit to the school and class-teacher after the child has been in school for some weeks, or sooner if requested. The medical officer should also be willing to write to the hospital on behalf of the school if any particular problem arises. The medical officer is not always the most appropriate person to give information to the school, although he should always have the responsibility for ensuring that this is done. Sometimes the health visitor is, if she has been closely involved with the child, the best person to give the teachers the advice they need.

Close contacts between teachers and the parents of spina bifida children in ordinary and in special schools are also very valuable. While parent-teacher relationships are often very good, sometimes greater understanding on each side is needed of the anxieties of the other person. Teachers, for example, need to realize how difficult it is for the parent of a handicapped child to steer a middle way between taking adequate precautions for the safety of the child on the one hand, and encouraging him to be independent on the other and should beware of too rapidly labelling parents as 'over-protective'. The mother, on her part, may not always realize the extent of a teacher's apprehension about taking responsibility for a severely handicapped child when she has thirty-five other children to look after. At the other extreme, she may feel so pleased to have got her child into an ordinary school and so reluctant to bother the teacher or cause trouble that she does not raise problems her child is having which should be raised. Misunderstandings can also easily arise regarding the progress a child is or is not making. If a child is progressing only very slowly a teacher may not wish to make this clear to the parent and may offer only vague reassurances such as 'he's doing fine'. This is not helpful in the long term and it is part of a teacher's responsibility to help the mother to come to a realistic appreciation of the child's level of functioning in any particular area. Open days can be very helpful here as the teacher can direct the mother's attention to work done by children of the same age.

Teachers who are worried about a child's lack of progress may need back-up advisory services. This is true not only of teachers in ordinary schools but also of those in special schools, many of whom have had no special training yet on arrival are expected to be able to deal with a class of children with a multiplicity of complex problems. A teacher of a child presenting real learning difficulties may have already done all that was suggested earlier in this chapter but may still see few signs of progress. At this stage or when planning a remedial programme, every teacher should be able to call on a source of expert help. This might be a trained remedial teacher within the school, the School Psychological Service or an adviser in special education, depending on the resources available. Too often this sort of help is not available, or, at best, months pass before the teacher gets the help she needs. The inadequacies in the remedial services and the pressure on them and on the School Psychological Services are well documented (cf. DES, 1971). In areas where greater numbers of handicapped children are being placed in ordinary schools there have been some promising developments such as the appointment of advisers in special education with special responsibility for disabled children in ordinary schools, but at the time this book is being written expansion of services seems unlikely. More could be achieved if better use were made of the specialist knowledge which is already available within an area through, for instance, in-service training.

Another problem is that teachers often do not ask for special help. For example, Holdsworth and Whitmore (1974a) found in their study of epileptic children in ordinary schools that of those children who were 'frankly failing in their education' only 60 per cent had been referred to an educational psychologist. The reluctance of some teachers to seek out help actively may in some cases be because prior experience has shown that such help will not be forthcoming, and sometimes because the teacher does not know what to expect of the child and may be satisfied with a very slow rate of progress. But it is also the case that since requests for help must be channelled through the Head, teachers wrongly but very naturally feel that it is an admission of failure which may be held against them to have to 'admit' that they cannot cope alone. This will only be resolved if it is made absolutely clear from the start to class-teachers with 'special' children that supportive services do exist and are there to be used.

Training teachers

The training of teachers of handicapped children is one of the questions which the Warnock Committee Enquiry is currently concerned with and only a few points will be made here. A major point is that the preparation of teachers for work with children with learning difficulties cannot be met only by the small number of existing one-year advanced courses. More needs to be done during the initial training years and much more offered (as a number of LEAs are now doing) in the way of intensive in-service training courses.

Surveys such as the one carried out in the Isle of Wight (Rutter *et al.*, 1970) and the DES survey of slow learners in secondary schools (1971b) make it quite clear that nowadays all teachers are likely to find children in their classes who are in some way handicapped and this should be made clear to teachers during their initial training. The head of one college's special education department, D. N. Thomas, recommends (1975) that there should be a general introduction to children with learning difficulties during initial training. At this stage it is important that the approach is a very positive one. The information given 'should make the listener feel secure by sounding certain, by offering solutions [to classroom situations] by presenting understandable explanations and by reducing anxiety in other ways'. In his own college, experienced teachers attending a one-year in-service course in the education of handicapped children are brought face to face in small group seminar situations with second- and third-year students in initial training. Although the students do attend mass lectures they can subsequently discuss specific problems with qualified teachers (who are, temporarily, also students) in an informal manner, a system which is mutually satisfying.

The lack of specialist advice for teachers in ordinary schools to draw on has already been noted. However, a recent survey carried out in the ILEA indicated that even where advisory services of many kinds are available, they do not appear to be meeting teachers' needs (Tuckett, 1976). One problem seems to be that teachers often leave colleges of education without knowing, except in the most general terms, exactly what back-up services are available, and there is a strong case for ensuring that teachers are given much more specific information about such support services and time to investigate these.

Short, in-service training courses run by local authorities on specific problems can be very valuable, and more trained and experienced special school teachers need to be given the time and opportunity to lead seminars or workshops at such courses. A DES survey (1971b) of slow learners in secondary schools suggested that opportunities provided by LEAs for in-service training are not always full utilized. One problem is that teachers are often reluctant to ask heads for secondment on such short courses held during school hours when they know that other teachers will have to cover classes for them. The value of 'releasing' a class-teacher must be recognized, particularly in the case of special school teachers, and a number of local authorities do in fact close their special schools or classes for perhaps half a day each term to enable the staff to attend. Teachers in ordinary schools with physically handicapped pupils should also be informed of the LEA's programme of in-service training and helped to attend wherever possible. Some voluntary bodies also provide courses; the Spastics Society, for example, runs in-service training residential weekends at Wallingford College, Berkshire. The programme is not confined to cerebral-palsied children and recently courses have been available specifically for teachers of spina bifida children in ordinary or special schools.

References

Anderson, E. M. (1973), *The Disabled Schoolchild: A Study of Integration in Primary Schools*, Methuen, London.

ASBAH (1975), *Children with Spina Bifida at School. A Booklet for Teachers and Students*, Publ. ASBAH.

Ball, M. (1975), 'Investigation into the reading abilities and related perceptual abilities of spina bifida children', unpublished report submitted for Masters degree in Child Development, University of London.

Brown, A. (1974), personal communication.

Burton, L. (1975), *The Family Life of Sick Children*, Routledge and Kegan Paul, London and Boston.

Chapman, J., Lewis, A. and Wedell, K. (1970), 'A note on reversals in the writing of 8 year old children', *Remedial Education*, 5, pp. 91–4.

——, and Wedell, K. (1972), 'Perceptuo-motor abilities and reversal errors in children's handwriting', *Journal of Learning Disabilities*, 5, pp. 321–5.

Clark, M. (1974), *Teaching Left-handed Children*, University of London Press.

Cook, J. (1975), 'Easing behaviour problems: an example', *Special Education*, 2 (1), pp. 15–17.

Cope, C. and Anderson, E. M. (1977), *Special Units in Ordinary Schools. An Exploratory Study of Special Provision for Disabled Children.* Institute of Education, London.

Daniels, J. C. and Diack, H. (1960), *The Standard Reading Test*, Chatto and Windus, London.

Davie, R., Butler, N. R. and Goldstein, H. (1972), *From Birth to Seven.* The second report of the National Child Development Study, Longmans, London.

DES (1971a), *Physical Education for the Physically Handicapped*, HMSO, London.

——, (1971b), *Slow Learners in Secondary Schools, Education Survey 15*, HMSO, London.

Diller, L., Gordon, W. A., Swinyard, C. and Kastner, S. (1969), *Psychological and Educational Studies with Spina Bifida Children*, Project No. 5–0412, Washington, US Department of Health Education and Welfare, US Office of Education.

Frostig, M. (1966), *Manual for the Marianne Frostig Developmental Test of Visual Perception*, Consulting Psychologists' Press, Palo Alto, California.

——, and Horne, D. (1964), *Frostig Program for the Development of Visual Perception – Teachers' Guide*, Fellett Publishing Co.

——, and Maslow, P. (1973), *Learning Problems in the Classroom*, Grune and Stratton, New York.

Galperin, P. (1957), 'An experimental study in the formation of mental actions', in Simon, B. (ed.), *Psychology in the Soviet Union*, Routledge and Kegan Paul, London.

Gulliford, R. (1969), *Backwardness and Educational Failure*, NFER, Windsor, Berks.

Haskell, S. H. (1972), *Arithmetical Disabilities in Programmed Instruction. A Remedial Approach*, C. C. Thomas, Illinois.

——, and Paull, M. E. (1973), *Training in Basic Cognitive Skills*, Educational Supply Association, Harlow, Essex.

——, ——, (1973), *Training in Motor Skills*, ESA, Harlow, Essex.

Hendrickson, L. N. and Muehl, S. (1962), 'The effect of attention and motor response pre-training on learning to discriminate "b" and "d" in kindergarten children', *Journal of Educational Psychology*, 53, pp. 236–41.

Holdsworth, L. and Whitmore, K. (1974a), 'A study of children with epilepsy attending ordinary school, I: their seizure patterns, progress and behaviour in school', *Developmental Medicine and Child Neurology*, 16 (6), pp. 746–58.

——, ——, (1974b), 'A study of children with epilepsy attending ordinary school, II: information and attitudes held by their teachers', *Developmental Medicine and Child Neurology*, 16 (6), pp. 759–65.

Jones, C. H., Leith, G. N. and Gulliford, R. (1966), 'Programming: an aspect of reading readiness', Research Report, National Centre for Programmed Learning, University of Birmingham.

Mann, L. (1971), 'Perceptual training revisited', *Rehabilitation Literature*, 32 (11), pp. 322–7, 335.

Neale, M. (1966), *Neale Analysis of Reading Ability*, Macmillan, London.

Pless, I. B. and Pinkerton, P. (1975), *Chronic Childhood Disorder – Promoting Patterns of Adjustment*, Henry Kimpton, London.

Presland, J. (1974), 'Modifying behaviour now', *Special Education*, 1 (3), pp. 20–2.

Riding, R. J. and Shore, J. M. (1974), 'A comparison of two methods of improving prose comprehension in educationally subnormal children', *British Journal of Education Psychology*, 44 (3), pp. 300–3.

Rutter, M., Tizard, J. and Whitmore, K. (eds.) (1970), *Education, Health and Behaviour*, Longmans, Harlow.

Schonell, F. J. and Schonell, F. E. (1957), *Diagnosis and Remedial Teaching in Arithmetic*, Oliver and Boyd, Edinburgh.

Stollard, J. (1975), personal communication.

Tansley, E. (1967), *Reading and Remedial Reading*, Routledge and Kegan Paul, London.

Tew, B. and Laurence, K. M. (1972), 'The ability and attainment of spina bifida patients born in South Wales between 1956–62,' *Developmental Medicine and Child Neurology*, Supplement 27, pp. 124–31.

Tew, B. J. and Laurence, K. M. (1975), 'The effects of hydrocephalus on intelligence, visual perception and school attainment', *Developmental Medicine and Child Neurology*, Supplement 35, pp. 129–34.

Thomas, D. N. (1975), 'The teacher and the handicapped child', ch. 14 in Loring, J. and Burn, G. (eds.), *The Integration of Handicapped Children in Society*, Routledge and Kegan Paul, London.

Tuckett, I. (1976), personal communication.

Vernon, P. E. (1971), *Arithmetic-Mathematics Test Manual* (Decimal Edition), NFER, Windsor, Berks.

Wedell, K. (1973), *Learning and Perceptuo-Motor Disabilities in Children*, John Wiley and Sons, New York.

4 The child and the adolescent in Society

9 Behavioural, emotional and social problems of children and adolescents with spina bifida

The literature on the behavioural, emotional and social problems of disabled adults and children is now extensive and varied. The psychological implications of disability have been discussed by sociologists (e.g. Goffman, in *Stigma*, 1963), psychologists (e.g. Wright, 1960) and the disabled themselves (Hunt, 1966). Research on the emotional and social adjustment of disabled children has been reviewed by Kellmer Pringle (1964) by Dinnage (1970, 1972), by Pilling in a useful series of annotated bibliographies (1972, 1973a and b, 1974, 1975) and, very comprehensively, by Pless and Pinkerton (1975).

Several important points are suggested by these accounts. First, disabled children, particularly those with central nervous system disorders, tend to be more vulnerable to psycho-social disturbances than their able-bodied peers. Second, children with varying disabilities tend to experience the same kinds of problems, that is few if any disabilities are associated with specific patterns of disturbances. Third, however, particular disabilities may have special features which cause problems not shared by other disabled children. Incontinence, for example, raises social and emotional problems for many spina bifida children whereas for other disabled children problems might be raised by impaired communication or facial disfigurement or a life-threatening illness. A fourth less obvious point is that children with mild or a moderate degree of disability seem to be as vulnerable, psychologically, as the severely disabled, perhaps because such children may be trying particularly hard to keep up with their 'normal' peers. The actual degree of disability may thus be much less crucial than the fact that a child may feel 'different' from his peers and is liable to be treated by them as different when in fact his basic emotional needs for security, affection, acceptance in a social group, achievement and recognition are identical to theirs.

A final very important point is that a disabled child's psycho-social problems are rarely caused directly by the disability but rather by his own reactions and the reactions of society to it. While a child's reactions will be influenced by his personality and by his level of emotional maturation at that point in time, they will also be strongly affected by the reactions of society, including his parents, teachers and, especially in adolescence, his peers. Burton (1975) puts this point very well: 'When one considers the development of any chronically sick child . . . one is assessing behaviour which results not only from the disease but more especially from the whole amalgam of social experiences, hardships, anxieties and evasions which surround it.' Research findings suggest consistently that the most crucial factor in the child's adjustment is likely to be his parents' reaction to the disability, and their way of coping. If they worry about it, so does he. If they are ashamed, he will be sensitive too. If they regard it objectively, he will be more likely to accept it as a fact. Unfortunately parents of handicapped children still tend to have few opportunities to discuss their feelings about the disability and the effects upon their management of the child.

In this chapter we concentrate on problems which need to be given special consideration in the case of spina bifida children although most of these will apply equally to children handicapped in other ways. The first half of the chapter is about pre-school and primary school children, while the second half deals with the emotional and social problems of adolescents, in particular with the problems of depression and of social isolation as well as with the question of how disabled teenagers can be provided with information about the nature of their handicaps and with help and guidance in coping.

Pre-school and primary school years

General emotional development

Spina bifida children vary a great deal in their emotional and behavioural development but certain patterns of behaviour do seem fairly common, especially in those with hydrocephalus. As babies they are described as friendly and socially responsive. They are usually even-tempered although sometimes irritable in strange situations and over-sensitive to certain noises, and they tend to vocalize a lot. In the pre-school years many continue to give the impression of being happy and sociable. Beneath this apparent contentment, however, problems can already be noticed. It was observed in the GLC study and by other researchers that spina bifida infants tended to be very passive and failed to display the intellectual curiosity usually shown at this age when toys were placed in front of them. Taylor comments (1959) on the 'under-current of anxiety' which starts to become evident, particularly when the children suspect any pressure.

Little systematic research has been done into the nature and extent of behaviour disorders in young spina bifida children but some data for the three year olds is available from the GLC survey and this can be compared with data from Richman *et al.* (1975) on non-handicapped children of this age. The mothers were questioned about the child's behaviour in a number of areas, including eating and sleeping problems, temper, worries and fears, and it was noted whether any difficulties were mild or severe. On the whole the spina bifida children showed no more disturbance than did the non-handicapped children in Richman's sample, at least as far as these were perceived by the mothers.

Since many young spina bifida children spend frequent and sometimes long periods in hospital (see chapter 1) the effects of this upon emotional development must be considered. It is well established that the hospitalization of a young child, especially between the age of eighteen months and three years, can result in profound emotional disturbance which may show itself in the ward and when he returns home. Since the main reason for the disturbance is the separation of the child from his mother, his reactions will be affected by whether or not his mother can stay in hospital with him or can visit frequently. The child's experience of pain will also colour his reactions.

In the GLC survey mothers were asked about the effects of hospitalization. The main finding was that this appeared to be a greater source of stress for the parents and the sibs than for the handicapped child himself. The comparative absence of anxiety about hospitalization may have been because the survey was carried out in a city where much more frequent visiting by parents was possible than is the case for parents living in rural areas, although it is also possible that since most surgery is carried out on limbs where the child has no feeling he does not associate the hospital with painful procedures. Certainly much of the content of the imaginative play of pre-school and older spina bifida children is dominated by what appears as an almost obsessive interest in hospitals, doctors and nurses.

The anxiety noted in many pre-school spina bifida children may increase during the primary school years. Sometimes these anxieties seem to be related to academic work, where the children begin to sense their limitations and become unhappy when pressed. The children may become more cautious, moody and apathetic, one reason for this change being that they can no longer depend on their verbal ability alone since, at primary school, motor and perceptual skills become increasingly important.

Until recently, most of the evidence about the emotional and behavioural problems of spina bifida children of primary school age came from observations made in the classroom or clinic but more systematic research evidence is now becoming available. The GLC survey provides information about 6 year olds from behaviour questionnaires filled in by their teachers. The questionnaire used was one devised by Rutter (1967) for 7–13 year olds (and later modified for 5–7 year olds) and used in the Isle of Wight Study (Rutter *et al.* 1970). It consists of a series of behavioural descriptions and the teacher completing the scale has to note whether the description 'certainly applies', 'applies somewhat' or 'does not apply'. Children scoring above a certain cut-off point on this scale (9 or more points) are then said to show a 'behaviour disorder', although this does not in itself imply psychiatric disturbance.

Full details of the findings are shown in Appendix F, and details for selected items are shown in Table 9.1 below.

Table 9.1 *Percentage of 6 year old spina bifida children and controls scoring on selected items of deviant behaviour on the Rutter teacher questionnaire*

		Spina bifida children	
Behaviour	*Controls* (*N*=48)	*No valve* (*N*=39)	*Valve* (*N*=86)
Restless	18·7	28·2	34·8
Irritable, touchy	10·4	12·8	23·2
Can't settle to anything	25·0	25·6	41·8
Fearful of new things	31·2	25·6	48·8
Resentful of correction	12·5	20·5	30·2
Unresponsive, apathetic	12·5	20·5	26·7
Not much liked	16·7	7·6	13·9
Solitary	25·0	23·0	33·7

These findings showed that the children with valves tended to have somewhat higher scores (mean deviance score = 6·5) than those without valves, whose rate of behaviour disorder overall was similar to that of the controls (mean for both groups = 4·6). When individual items of behaviour were considered the spina bifida children with valves were reported as being more restless, irritable and unable to settle to anything than the controls and on items measuring fearfulness or nervousness they also appeared to show more disturbance. Two other items on which both groups of spina bifida children showed up poorly compared to the controls were the 'resentful of correction item', which presumably reflects their general immaturity, and the 'unresponsive and apathetic' item. However, there were no striking differences between the groups on items reflecting anti-social behaviour. Very few children were reported as 'not much liked by other children'.

Data on the same teacher scale was obtained from Anderson's study (1975) of 7–10 year olds with spina bifida myelomeningocele and hydrocephalus. Overall, only three out of twenty-six children (11 per cent) showed a behaviour disorder (i.e. scored above the cut-off point) the mean average score being 3·4. When individual items of deviant behaviour were looked at 'poor concentration' was found to be the problem affecting the largest proportion of the spina bifida group (56 per cent) followed by 'fearfulness', especially of new things (33 per cent). Very few children scored on items indicative of anti-social or aggressive behaviour.

The findings from these two studies suggest that two kinds of problems characterize spina bifida children of this age: concentration difficulties and anxieties of different kinds. In contrast, anti-social behaviour appears to be comparatively rare, although Fulthorpe (1974) reports that some of the boys in his study of thirty-three 8–15 year olds with spina bifida showed 'marked symptoms of aggressiveness and assertiveness'.

Overall we still know very little about the extent of psychiatric disturbance in spina bifida children. The Rutter teacher questionnaire only provides information about behaviour perceived as deviant by the teachers within the school. High scores on this scale do not automatically imply psychiatric disturbance: conversely, a child who is psychiatrically disturbed will not necessarily make a high score on the teacher scale. It is therefore possible that the rate of actual psychiatric disturbance in spina bifida children with hydrocephalus is higher than our findings have indicated. In a recent study of 5–15 year olds carried out by Seidel and his colleagues (1975) the incidence of psychiatric disorder (assessed by questionnaire and interviews) was found to be twice as high (24 per cent) in neurologically abnormal children (who were either cerebral-palsied or hydrocephalic) as in children with physical disorder not involving the brain (12 per cent); they, in turn, show a higher incidence of psychiatric disorder than children in the general population (Rutter *et al.*, 1970). This finding, which replicates earlier findings in the Isle of Wight Survey (Rutter *et al.*, 1970), suggests that children with spina bifida and hydrocephalus are probably more *at risk* of developing psychiatric disturbance than are those without valves, or non-handicapped children. However, as Seidel *et al.* (1975) stress, three-quarters of the children with neurological abnormalities were not disturbed, and whether or not psychiatric disorders actually develop 'probably depends on much the same psycho-social variables which are important in non-handicapped children'.

Specific behavioural and emotional difficulties

(i) *Distractability.* Most accounts of research with hydrocephalic children as well as reports from teachers suggest that distractability is a major problem. In their study of spina bifida children Tew and Laurence (1975) asked teachers to estimate the length of time the child was usually able to concentrate on basic school subjects: the average time reported for the controls was 18 minutes and for the children with valves only 9 minutes. In Anderson's study (1973) of disabled children in ordinary primary schools 17 of the 19 children with spina bifida (90 per cent of the group) were rated by teachers as having poor concentration compared to only 43 per cent of the disabled children without neurological involvement and 36 per cent of the non-handicapped children.

Distractability is characteristic not only of hydrocephalic children but of children with other kinds of neurological abnormalities. Such children often react continuously to inessential stimuli which may be visual, auditory or tactile; they may also have difficulty both in focusing attention and in maintaining it on the relevant stimulus. Many spina bifida children seem particularly liable to be distracted by auditory stimuli.

The cause of the attentional problems of hydrocephalic and other neurologically abnormal children is not clear. Many workers have suggested a causal link between attentional problems and neurological impairment. One commonly held theory is that the neurological impairment is such that the child has not the normal ability to filter out or inhibit irrelevant incoming stimuli. In this respect children with neurological abnormalities may function like younger normal children: Turnure (1970) for instance has shown that extraneous distractors have a more detrimental effect on the performance of younger than of older children but that normally by the age of about $6\frac{1}{2}$–$7\frac{1}{2}$ years children are much less likely to be distracted by irrelevant cues.

However, attentional problems do not necessarily result from neurological abnormalities only. In the case of spina bifida children a number of other factors may also be important. One is that a spina bifida child may, from quite an early age, have been given toys which were unsuited to his level of functioning, perhaps because of difficulties in manipulation or perception. Activities which are too demanding do not usually hold a child's attention for long and he fails to develop the ability to concentrate. In this respect the work of Moyer and Gilmer (1954, 1955) on the attention span of young normal children is interesting. They designed a set of toys until each toy reached its maximum 'holding power' and then, under conditions of minimum distraction, tested the attention span of 426 children between 18 months and 7 years old. They found that age was much less important than the stimulus material and its 'drawing-power'; even children as young as 18 months could concentrate for relatively long periods of time (up to half an hour) with one toy if they had the right toy.

More recently Sen (1967) has investigated the effects of different distractors (e.g. background noise, conversation, words) on tasks requiring verbal responses, her subjects being young mentally retarded adults. Although they were more likely to show distractable behaviour than normal adults, the most significant factor was the level of difficulty of the task, that is, the more difficult the task, the greater the effect of the distractors. Task difficulty may thus contribute to distractability in spina bifida children.

Social factors may also play a part. Spina bifida children often depend heavily in the early years upon adults, both at home and in hospital, to meet their physical needs. It thus becomes important for the child to pay attention to the visual and verbal cues given out by adults, and for him to develop ways of gaining their attention. Children may become more sensitized to 'social' stimuli than to the stimuli present in the toy or the book, and never actually learn to pay attention for long to any one activity. Adults may inadvertently reinforce inattentive and inappropriate behaviour by smiling or cuddling or praise, and fail to reward the child for actually concentrating on a task.

(ii) *Impulsivity.* Great individual differences can be observed in the way in which children attempt to solve problems. Some seem to try to get through the task as quickly as possible, others take a more organized approach. During the 1960s psychologists became increasingly interested in these different strategies or 'cognitive styles' and the research in this area has been thoroughly reviewed by Kagan and Kogan (1970) and by Santostephano (1969).

Kagan himself has been particularly interested in distinguishing between 'impulsive' and 'reflective' behaviour. For this purpose he devised a Matching Familiar Figures Test (Kagan, 1965) in which the child has to select from an array of six pictures, all variations on a 'standard', the one which is identical to the standard. Depending mainly upon the time taken to reach a decision, the children can be categorized along an impulsivity-reflectivity continuum. As may be expected, significant positive correlations are usually found (e.g. Drake, 1970) between impulsive behaviour and the number of errors made. Data obtained by Kagan and his colleagues indicate that response-latencies (i.e. decision times) increase and errors decrease with age. There is also evidence (e.g. Lore, 1965; Schwebel 1966; Zucker and Stricker, 1968) that economically and socially disadvantaged children tend to be much more impulsive than middle-class children, unless taught to stop and reflect.

Our own observations have suggested that many children with spina bifida and hydrocephalus act impulsively rather than reflectively. Anderson (1975) used Kagan's test and another similar but simpler matching test to investigate this and found that the majority of the spina bifida children fell into the 'impulsive' rather than the 'reflective' or in-between category. If teachers, parents and others are aware that spina bifida children tend to tackle problems in an 'impulsive' way they can go on to consider how best to change such behaviour. Meichenbaum and Goodman (1971) describe an experiment in which impulsive 7–9 year olds who had been placed in a special class because of behaviour problems such as hyperactivity and poor self-control and/or low intelligence were trained to talk to themselves while carrying out a variety of tests. The goals of the training procedures were 'to develop for the "impulsive" child a cognitive style or learning set in which the child could size up the demands of a task, cognitively rehearse and then guide his performance by means of self-instruction, and when appropriate reinforce himself'. This training did result in an increase in self-control and in better test performance.

The results of this and other studies suggest that children can be trained in more effective ways of tackling problems and that systematic training of this kind could help many spina bifida children to make better use of their abilities.

(iii) *Passivity and lack of motivation.* Passivity and impulsivity/distractability do not obviously go hand in hand yet teachers, researchers and others working closely with spina bifida children frequently comment on the children's apathy and passivity. Passivity can be observed very early on and the unusual lack of interest in toys shown by infants in the GLC study has already been commented on.

Passive behaviour has also been noted by Dorothy Hodges (1974) an organizer of playgroups for spina bifida children: 'Restricted mobility means that the child cannot release his feelings by running, jumping, or other energetic movements. Long periods in hospital and the anxious care of adults on whom he must depend also control his freedom in this respect. In his attempts to deal with his experiences he generally learns to inhibit emotions he considers dangerous or painful particularly anger . . . and so becomes passive, apathetic, obedient and "good".' One important function of pre-school playgroups, believes Hodges (1974), is to create conditions under which the children (and their parents who have also learned to control their normal feelings of grief, anxiety and anger) can express their feelings and learn to 'let themselves go'.

Loss of motivation and passivity may also occur if the intellectual demands made on a child by his teachers are either too low or too high. Sometimes teachers and parents may expect too little of the child, and give indiscriminate praise. The result is often that the child becomes satisfied with poor performance too. Handicapped children who are being tested often make comments such as, 'I'm doing well, aren't I' or 'I'm a clever boy', often quite inappropriately, whereas non-handicapped children of the same ability level rarely make such remarks unless they are very young. On the other hand boredom and apathy can also result when a task is too hard, and therefore unrewarding. Non-handicapped children who experience constant failure rapidly learn to 'give up', often coupling this with aggressive anti-social behaviour. Spina bifida children who give up are more likely to show withdrawn, passive behaviour, but this should not occur if they are given the right kind of stimulation by parents and teachers at the right time.

(iv) *Fears and anxieties.* The research findings reported earlier suggest that considerable fearfulness and anxiety may underlie the outwardly easy-going sociable behaviour of spina bifida children. This is, of course, true of many other handicapped children. Burton (1975), for example, found that unforthcoming and unreactive behaviour (where the child is afraid of new tasks and strange situations and is timid with people) was common in children with cystic fibrosis.

Fearfulness can take several forms. A fear of failure may mean the child refuses to attempt a new task or requires much encouragement and constant reassurance that he is doing all right. Fearfulness in new situations is also common: a child for example, may refuse to go on an expedition with the rest of his class. One reason for this is that he may not know how he will cope physically and it often helps to spend considerable time describing in advance (as one may to a younger child) the sequence of events. As Burton (1975) comments about children with cystic fibrosis or asthma, 'sick children seem to develop a special and understandable defensiveness in order to ward off occurrences which might prove stressful for them'.

Apart from specific anxieties, many spina bifida children probably have unexpressed feelings of anxiety of a more general kind about themselves. Ineichen (1973), a social worker, states that while working with a group of pre-adolescent spina bifida children she 'picked up a lot of feelings of anxiety and inferiority . . . Many have an envy, almost a fantasy, about their normal peers, thinking of them as perfect. Children showed their stress by withdrawal, dependency and exploitation of their handicap and I wonder whether they have learned to suppress any anger they feel.'

Because spina bifida children tend to 'cause no trouble' in school teachers may wrongly assume an absence of emotional stress when the child probably has anxieties which it would be helpful for him to be able to express. Burton's study of children with cystic fibrosis is relevant here. She comments on the fact that the parents, coping as they were with the heavy duties of the child's daily care, had little energy left for worrying about his emotional feelings concerning his handicap. As a result, only 32 per cent of the school-age children (all but two still at primary school) felt able to talk over their illness worries with anyone. When the subject was sympathetically broached by the interviewer they were glad to speak of their feelings and 65 per cent of the group expressed a fear of being hurt, 50 per cent of being ill, and 47 per cent of going into hospital, while 58 per cent said the illness made them sad and 36 per cent said it worried them. There is of course, a crucial difference between children with cystic fibrosis and spina bifida in so far as the former are much more likely to become seriously ill. However, the children's growing appreciation of their physical limitations, increasing self-consciousness about being 'different' and apprehensions about the future are probably very similar.

Social Problems

(i) *Incontinence.* Incontinence, a major if 'invisible' handicap for a very large proportion of spina bifida children, is likely to give rise to both emotional and social problems. It might be expected that those children whose incontinence has been reasonably reliably controlled by the wearing of a urinary appliance or by a urinary diversion (referred to hereafter as 'continent' children) would have fewer emotional and social problems than those who were often uncontrollably wet or soiled ('incontinent' children), but the small amount of evidence we have so far suggests that this is not so and also that boys and girls may react differently to having to depend on urinary appliances.

Fulthorpe (1974), for example, found no significant overall differences in the Bristol Social Adjustment Guide scores of 12 incontinent and 21 continent spina bifida children attending a residential school for physically handicapped children. However, the findings differed considerably according to the sex of the child. The boys who had been made continent by the fitting of a urinary appliance tended to show 'unforthcoming' social behaviour while the incontinent boys were more forthcoming, and Fulthorpe suggests that the wearing of a penile bag may emphasize feelings of being different and become an increasingly acute problem as the boy grows older. In contrast, the girls who had had urinary diversions were significantly better adjusted than the incontinent girls, who showed marked symptoms of anxiety, inferiority and inadequacy and were easily disheartened and upset. The girls, thinks Fulthorpe, may have been more aware than the boys of the social problems likely to arise from their incontinence and that this may have fostered 'feelings of inadequacy and apprehensiveness'. However, since the number of children in Fulthorpe's study was small and they were all drawn from one residential special school, his findings may not apply to spina bifida children in general and more information is needed on this important question.

Large numbers of spina bifida children who are incontinent are now placed in ordinary schools. In chapter 7 the special physical arrangements which might be required were discussed: here the question of social acceptability is considered. A major issue for the child, his parents and his teacher is whether or not the other children should be told about his problem. When a child starts off in an infant class it is comparatively easy to give the rest of the class a simple explanation about why he is still wearing nappies or why he goes off with a welfare assistant regularly, and they usually accept this, with perhaps only occasional mild teasing. It is much more difficult to decide how to handle the problem when an older child joins an ordinary class, and in such a case the class-teacher, the parents and, depending on his age, the child himself will need to discuss as early on as possible whether and, if so, how to explain the problem to the rest of the class.

Often a child's peers (apart from perhaps one or two close friends) do not know about his incontinence. In such cases children may be extremely anxious lest the fact that they wear special appliances is discovered. Teachers often do not realize that almost all spina bifida children, in whatever kind of school, are deeply ashamed of their incontinence. They can help, firstly, by ensuring that the children have toileting privacy. In an ordinary school this might mean putting a lock on a toilet door or allowing a spina bifida child to use the staff toilet. Children, and even their parents, are often reluctant to bring this problem to the attention of the staff: it is up to the Head and the class-teacher to discuss with the mother the most suitable arrangement.

Secondly, the child must know who the adult is who knows of this problem, and to whom he can go for help. The class-teacher should always be informed about a child's incontinence and how he copes, although the person responsible for helping the child will generally be a welfare assistant, who should regularly ask the child's mother if he has mentioned any problems. If problems do arise the assistant should get to the heart of the problem with the mother as soon as possible, and the latter should always be notified if there has been an accident. If the toileting arrangements are adequate there is no need whatsoever for a child to be smelly in class; however bags do sometimes leak and the child, because of loss of feeling, may not know that he is wet or dirty.

On the whole the little evidence there is (e.g. Anderson, 1973; Tew, 1973) suggests that incontinence does not give rise to major social problems in school, although individual instances of teasing or of other problems arising from incontinence are sometimes reported by parents, teachers or the children themselves (e.g. Welbourn, 1975; Scott *et al.*, 1975).

(ii) *Friendships.* The extent to which a disabled child is accepted by his peers seems to depend more on personality factors and on intellectual level than on the severity of the physical handicap. Qualities which make children attractive as friends include social-emotional characteristics ('friendliness', 'fun to be with'), expertness ('being bright', 'having good ideas about how to do things'), 'associational' characteristics (having common interests) and, least important, physical prowess. A spina bifida child may have less chance than his peers of developing these qualities. Since his physical prowess is impaired his main interests, especially if he is a boy, may differ from those of other children, while lack of experience coupled sometimes with perceptual and visuo-motor problems may mean that he is not good at playing games or making things. He may thus have to rely more on his ability to get along well with people if he wants to make friends. If a child has been treated by his parents or other adults or siblings as being younger than he really is, he may well appear immature or 'babyish' to other children, although this is much less likely to be the case if he has had pre-school experience.

Attempts have been made to measure the 'social maturity' of spina bifida children, but one problem here is that the main scales used for this purpose (the Vineland Scale of Social Maturity, Doll, 1947; and the Manchester Scales of Social Adaptation, Lunzer, 1966) contain many items which depend on a child's physical status (e.g. ability to dress himself, go to the shops or to the park alone): since these will be impossible for a severely physically handicapped child, his scores may be somewhat misleading. The few studies which have been made (Tew, 1973; Fulthorpe, 1974) show that spina bifida children deviate on these scales very markedly from non-handicapped children. Tew (1973) suggests that this poor social performance may partly reflect 'over-solicitous attitudes on the parts of parents and older siblings, denying the handicapped child the opportunity to acquire social skills', and some evidence for this was found in the GLC survey.

A child learns to develop social skills through regular social contacts with other children. While there is an increasing awareness of the importance of these contacts in the pre-school years (chapter 6), social contacts must also be actively fostered throughout the primary and secondary years wherever the child is at school.

Most spina bifida children who attend ordinary schools fit in well socially (Anderson, 1973; Hicks, 1975) and parents and teachers frequently comment on how such placement helps the child to grow up. However a child may need help in doing so from his teacher, and it is valuable if she can meet him before he starts school, either at home or in a pre-school or nursery group, so that she can get some idea from her own observations and from talking to his mother and teacher both about his physical problems and his level of social and emotional maturity. A teacher may also want to plan, along with the mother, how she will introduce a child into the class. Many teachers find it helpful to give the class a little advance information both about the condition itself and about what sort of help is and is not needed. Books about disabled children such as Camilla Jessel's *Mark's Wheelchair Adventures* (1975) may be useful. Seating arrangements may help to determine friendships and the child's seating partners should be selected carefully.

In trying to help handicapped children in their social development teachers need to consider the behaviour of the handicapped child's peers and of the child himself. Teasing has to be watched for, especially in situations where the children are not closely supervised. Less obvious is the opposite danger, that the non-handicapped children will be over-solicitous. It is not always enough to encourage the handicapped child to do all he can for himself: it may also be necessary to explain to the other children what things a child can do or is learning to do for himself and why it is important that he is allowed to, and here the teacher's own behaviour will provide an important model for the class.

Children are often more sensitive about being left out than is apparent and it is important that spina bifida children should participate actively in all that goes on. While the child needs to experience both failure and success, failures must be balanced by successes and it will help the child in his peer relationships if he can attain an average or above average level of competence in some area which he enjoys and which is valued by his peers, particularly if this is something he can continue in his holidays and after he leaves school.

Non-handicapped children should not be expected to make allowances all the time for demanding, or socially inappropriate or unattractive behaviour in the spina bifida child. He, too, has to learn certain social skills and must be helped by his teachers to modify behaviour which the other children may correctly perceive as assertive, self-centred, withdrawn or babyish. Laing (1975) has suggested that slow learners are often deficient in social techniques and need to be taught social skills, 'in particular . . . those who are segregated from the others in special classes or special schools'.

Children attending special schools need as many opportunities as possible to mix with their non-handicapped peers. Many special schools encourage children to join in out-of-school groups such as scouts or guides, but there is still great scope for the development of closer links between children in special and ordinary schools. Loneliness and boredom in the school holidays can be a major problem. Ineichen (1973) has found a great demand for holiday groups in pre-adolescent spina bifida children and she reports on a very successful scheme in Bristol where sixteen severely handicapped spina bifida children attend a holiday group for one day each week. The group was run by a team consisting of an occupational therapist, social worker, nursery nurse, local youth leader and non-handicapped teenagers, the aims being 'the development of independence, responsibility, meaningful relationships and purposeful expression through group activities and discussion'. Discussion with the children and their parents indicated the need for more arrangements of this kind.

Adolescence

Handicapped teenagers have been a neglected group. As Younghusband *et al.* (1970) point out in *Living with Handicap*, 'There is a surprising failure to recognize the acute problems of isolation from their peers that confront many of the more seriously handicapped adolescents, who face, often without the chance to satisfy them, the normal urges of young people for companionship, relations with the opposite sex, sport, enjoyment of leisure pursuits, travel, spending money, achievement, and the prospects of their own future home and family. We think it urgent that the needs of adolescents who are handicapped should receive more systematic study and that greater effort should be made to meet them.'

With comprehensive early treatment of spina bifida not becoming common practice until the early 1960s, it is only now that large numbers of spina bifida children are reaching adolescence. The little evidence available suggests that their needs and problems are very much those described in the extract above. Before considering any specific problems, however, one important general point needs to be emphasized. This is the need for spina bifida teenagers, like all teenagers, to develop *personal independence* so that they can become separate individuals, apart from their parents and other people. This is something which is very difficult for a handicapped teenager to achieve, particularly when he is heavily dependent physically upon his parents or other adults, and in their study of adults with spina bifida Evans *et al.* (1974) note that 'some . . . who have survived, perhaps only because of the competence and determination of their mothers are still under their mother's domination'. Likewise, although the group of spina bifida teenagers interviewed by Dorner (1976) felt that they had reasonably good relationships with their parents, the most common complaint was that parents were 'too protective' or did too much for them.

There is a particular problem for teenagers attending residential schools or institutions which Doherty (1973) the warden of a centre for young cerebral-palsied adults states clearly. He refers to the 'paternalistic' attitudes of institutions which are otherwise modern and enlightened, above all to the 'assumption that the staff know best . . . whereas the handicapped residents are inexperienced, immature . . . incapable of sensible decisions and choices'.

Even if physical dependence is to some extent inevitable, parents can foster 'independence of spirit . . . by enabling and encouraging the young people to make choices and decisions for themselves' (Morgan 1972). Elizabeth Robertson (1972) makes a very similar point in her study of limb-deficient children: 'Independence is a state of mind rather than a series of physical skills, and with the handicapped child it is the mother's attitude which counts in the end.' A cerebral-palsied psychologist, asked to advise the parent of a similarly handicapped teenager on the question of independence, puts the point well (Richardson, 1972) '. . . if you really love your daughter then the best thing you can do for her is to prepare her for the outside world . . . Don't hide her from things, don't shelter her from things, and most importantly, encourage her . . . and give her a sense of responsibility.'

However, even when parents do assist teenagers in this way, problems are still likely to arise and below three important and closely related problem areas are discussed, these being the question of depression, of social isolation and finally of the needs of spina bifida teenagers for much more information and counselling about their own physical and sexual development than they are at present receiving.

(a) *Depression*

The extent to which depression exists among handicapped teenagers is rarely openly acknowledged. Freeman (1970), for example, writing of cerebral-palsied adolescents, refers to Christy Brown's comment (1955) that 'instead of coming to a better understanding of my handicap as I got older, I only became more troubled and bitter'. He suggests that feelings such as these are probably more common than is generally recognized and that 'the mistrust of the adolescent for grown-ups and our tendency to concentrate on the physical, intellectual and perceptual aspects of brain damage tend to limit our awareness of these reactions'.

Recent interviews with spina bifida adolescents and their parents carried out by Stephen Dorner (1975, 1976) endorse this view. Dorner's group consisted of 63 families with spina bifida teenagers and the data presented here comes partly from the parents (usually the mothers) and partly from 46 of the teenagers themselves. These teenagers (21 boys and 25 girls) ranged in age from 13 to 19 years (mean age 16·4 years) and all were living with their families in Outer London or the South of England. 30 per cent of the group had minimal or mild handicaps, 32 per cent moderate multiple handicaps, and 38 per cent severe multiple handicaps, the girls, in general, being more handicapped than the boys. Half of the group had left school and were either engaged in further or higher education (7), in employment (10), or at home (6).

One of the problems investigated was the extent of depression. According to the parents, as many as 66 per cent of the adolescents had had definite and recurring feelings of misery over the past year compared with a figure of 41 per cent for normal 14½ year olds in the Isle of Wight study (Rutter *et al.*, 1976). 31 per cent of the girls and 15 per cent of boys had had persistent feelings of hopelessness and/or suicidal ideas over the past year. In contrast to the high incidence of depression there was a striking absence of anti-social problems such as aggressive behaviour.

When the adolescents themselves were interviewed a very similar pictured emerged, and it also became clear that teenagers often withheld their feelings of depression from their mothers 'whom, rightly, they saw as vulnerable' (Dorner, 1975). Each adolescent was asked whether he sometimes felt miserable and unhappy to the extent of being tearful or wanting to get away from it all, and 85 per cent reported having felt like this. Girls were more likely than boys to report frequent misery (56 per cent compared with 19 per cent), although almost as many boys as girls had sometimes felt miserable. Half the girls but less than a quarter of the boys had felt on some occasion that life was not worth living, while only one boy but nearly one quarter of the girls (compared with 8 per cent of 14½-year-old girls in the Isle of Wight study (Rutter *et al.*, 1976) had had suicidal feelings.

In the few other studies in which the emotional problems of spina bifida teenagers have been investigated in any systematic way the findings are very similar. In Sheffield where Lorber and Schloss (1973) studied social and emotional problems in fifty-eight 14–22 year olds with spina bifida myelomeningocele, depression was the most common problem, followed, according to the parents, by sullenness, temper tantrums, needless worry about health, nail-biting and disobedience.

All adolescents have major adjustments to make but for those who are severely disabled many extra stresses will be present so that it is not surprising that the incidence of depression is so high. In adolescence social status and feelings of competence are derived to a considerable extent from participation in group activities, particularly physical activities such as sports, athletics and dancing. Lack of mobility will make it difficult, first, for a teenager with spina bifida to reach the place where these activities go on, particularly in the holidays, and, second, for him to take part in them. Often the situation may be exacerbated by protective attitudes on the part of the family, and rejecting or indifferent attitudes on the part of non-handicapped peers, who at this stage are often acutely conscious of differences, and disabled children may find themselves neglected by former friends for whom group membership and group identity have become very important.

Wright (1960) has emphasized the importance of physique in adolescence particularly in establishing one's sexual role and identity. 'Physique becomes evaluated in terms of rigid standards in sex appropriateness' and the handicapped adolescent will have, like other adolescents, 'an intense interest in all matters that have to do with the establishment of status as a man or woman'. A teenager who is confined to a wheelchair or who only walks with difficulty, in whom obesity may be an increasing problem and who also has to cope with the physical and emotional strains of having a urinary appliance may experience enormous doubts and feelings of inadequacy about his or her sexual identity. This is likely to be particularly true of boys, who may in fact be impotent. Even if the teenager's self-confidence has been fostered by support and encouragement from family or school, he or she is likely to have great difficulty in expressing his sexual identity through normal social (including sexual) relationships with a member of the opposite sex.

These are not the only extra stresses for the disabled teenager. At this stage he (and perhaps his family too) may, for the first time, be trying to come to terms with the fact that he will not be 'cured'. He cannot, like many teenagers, look forward with any degree of confidence to independence on leaving school, to marriage, or to the certainty of employment. When school-leaving does come, particularly if he has been in the sheltered child-centred environment of a special school, it may come as a shock to find that the hitherto apparently intense adult interest which has accompanied him throughout his school days 'will evaporate rapidly' (Morgan, 1972).

(b) *Social isolation*

All these stresses will contribute to feelings of depression in the spina bifida teenager but the one which is most consistently present (and which could be ameliorated) is social isolation. In Dorner's study (1976), no significant association was found between depression and mobility problems or between depression and overall severity of handicap; there was however an association for the girls but not for the boys (who were less isolated) between misery and social isolation, 10 out of 13 isolated girls admitting to feelings of misery compared with only 4 out of 12 non-isolated girls.

The problem is very much one arising *outside* school hours. Within school or college (whether this was an ordinary establishment or a special one) all but 4 of the 46 teenagers interviewed said that they had had real friends. 19 out of 46 admitted to being teased at school but only 5 had been seriously distressed by this and neither teasing nor bullying were related to the kind of school attended.

Outside school, however, the problem of social isolation was marked. Approximately half of the teenagers in the study were judged to be severely socially isolated, the criterion for this being that the teenager had not been visited at home or gone out with friends of his own age for at least one month prior to the interview, or, if he attended a residential school, that he had had no peer contacts over the last holiday. Dorner (1975) comments that it was common to find cases where complete absence of peer contacts outside school extended over much longer periods than a month, and there were a few teenagers who had never visited friends in their homes and had never been visited themselves. Social isolation outside school or college was much more likely to occur if the teenager attended or had attended a special school or college: only three out of eighteen (16 per cent) of those attending ordinary schools/colleges said that they had no friends compared to sixteen out of twenty-eight (57 per cent) of those attending special institutions.

Dorner points out that 'one cannot conclude from this that being at special school in itself leads to isolation at home since one difference between children at ordinary and at special school is the severity of mobility problems and these are closely associated with social isolation'.

However he also notes that all four teenagers with significant mobility problems who had been at ordinary schools had at least one friend outside school compared to only six out of the eighteen special school attenders with similar mobility problems.

Although the association between social isolation and mobility problems was a very marked and highly statistically significant finding (and one which has also been reported by Ingram *et al.*, 1964 for cerebral-palsied children) there was a clear difference in Dorner's study (1975) between the girls and the boys. This was that although the boys were more mobile they were as likely to be socially isolated as were the girls. Dorner suggests that the reason for this is related to whether the boy wore a urinary appliance. Boys whose mobility problems were only moderate, rather than severe, were more likely to be isolated if they wore a urinary appliance than if they did not, and although the numbers were small, those with penile bags were more likely to be isolated than those who had had a diversion. Mobile girls who wore appliances were not, however, likely to be isolated. These findings tie in quite closely with Fulthorpe's findings (p. 249).

Summing up, it seems that those teenagers whose social contacts were likely to be most limited were, firstly, those whose mobility was severely restricted, whether they were boys or girls, and, secondly, among the more mobile children, boys who needed to rely on urinary appliances, especially penile bags.

The findings of Dorner's study in London and south-east England and of the Lorber and Schloss study (1973) of adolescents and young people with spina bifida in Sheffield (where 3 per cent of the group were reported as having no friends and 80 per cent as never going out) are depressingly similar. They also raise two major questions: why these teenagers were so isolated and how their situation could be improved.

Reasons for social isolation. Almost certainly the social isolation of these teenagers arises from several factors rather than from a single one, with physical, social and emotional factors all playing a part. On the physical side, access to buildings and transport are key factors. Architectural barriers make most youth clubs, libraries, cinemas, coffee bars and other places where young people normally meet either inaccessible or extremely difficult for a person in a wheelchair to enter. Transportation is equally important since access to and within buildings is irrelevant if a handicapped person has no means of getting to them from his home (see also p. 261).

Social factors must also contribute to the adolescent's difficulties. Richardson (1972) has published an interesting verbatim report of a session at which three people with cerebral palsy discussed their problems and experiences. Placement in special schools was seen by the participants as contributing to the difficulties they encountered later on in their social relationships with non-handicapped peers, the early lack of contact leading to feelings of strangeness and anxiety on both sides. They also mentioned that attendance at a special school makes it less likely that a handicapped teenager will have close neighbourhood friends or non-handicapped friends.

Another group of factors often contributing to the social isolation of handicapped teenagers are those connected with their own attitudes to themselves and with the attitudes of their families. Sometimes a handicapped youngster (or adult) does not take advantage of opportunities to mix with his peers because of his own anxious or shameful feelings about his handicap. Kathleen Evans and her colleagues (1974) found that the adults with spina bifida who they interviewed had many such anxieties. 'These were often expressed in such phrases as: "Will your handicap make you undesirable as a friend or marriage partner? If you get a girl friend when do you tell her about your urine bag? Are men potent? Can women conceive and bear a child? Might a child also have spina bifida? Is it fair to a child to have a parent in a wheelchair? Can a man with a serious disability ever provide for a wife and family?" Such anxieties may prevent the making of friendships, and some patients, particularly the housebound and unemployed, are isolated and lonely.'

Dorner, too, in his interviews with handicapped teenagers (1976) found that those boys who were mobile were often reluctant to go out with their peers because of anxieties connected with the wearing of a urinary appliance. This was also 'a serious pre-occupation in their aspirations towards the opposite sex'. For example one boy who had had a urinary diversion and currently had a girl friend had been unable to bring himself to tell her about it as he had been rejected because of it when he had told a previous girl friend.

Although all but one of the 46 teenagers interviewed by Dorner (1976) expressed an interest in the opposite sex, very few (5 out of the 21 boys and 8 of the 25 girls) had ever had a heterosexual friendship, and at the time of the study only 4 of the boys and 2 of the girls currently had a boy or girl friend.

Often it is not only handicapped teenagers' feelings of insecurity about themselves but also the attitudes of their parents which contribute to their isolation from their peers. Many non-handicapped teenagers have to be encouraged to take part in peer-group activities and handicapped teenagers may need even more encouragement. Unfortunately, and very understandably, parents and other adults often have ambivalent feelings about encouraging independent behaviour. This is illustrated in an extract from a conversation (Richardson, 1972) between the parent (W.W.) of a handicapped 17-year-old cerebral-palsied girl and a counselling psychologist (S.D.) herself severely handicapped by cerebral palsy. The parent is asked whether she feels that her daughter could attend a summer holiday camp with non-handicapped teenagers.

> W.W. 'She has problems. I don't think – I don't know, she might be able to. But I'd be a little, as a parent, I'd be afraid to put her out there because she can't do everything on her own, and if you go to a regular camp you have to do everything on your own.'
> S.D. 'It fits in with what I said before. That's an attitude I think is perpetuated by . . . the people who work in the handicapped world. That if we go into the normal world, who is going to help if you need help . . . The normal world is very ready to help us, and I think that family saying that they don't know what to do for us or how to handle us, I think that's a laugh . . . some people are bunglers, but you tell them, "I need this kind of help" and the normal world does help. I do a great deal of travelling round the country and I need a lot of help. The best thing I do is feed myself. Frankly, the rest needs a lot of help and people are eager to help me.'

Reducing social isolation. Since the reasons for the social isolation of handicapped teenagers are multiple it follows that any attempt made to improve the situation must be made on a number of fronts and some suggestions are made below.

(i) *Access.* There is considerable awareness in this country of the importance of making buildings accessible to the disabled and this awareness must extend to recreational facilities used by young people. In any area groups of parents of the disabled, or of disabled people themselves, or of others concerned about the welfare of the community could usefully make a survey of local facilities from the point of view of access and, where necessary, put pressure on local authorities for the required modifications. The situation should improve in the future since, under the British Standard Institution Code of Practice (Access for Disabled to Buildings, 1967) which was made law under section 8 of the Chronically Sick and Disabled Act, 1970, wheelchair access to new buildings must be put in at the design stage.

(ii) *Transport/mobility.* Many spina bifida teenagers have enormous problems in getting to places of recreation, to friends' houses and eventually to training or work. For every severely handicapped pupil receiving secondary education, in whatever type of school, there should be someone in the school responsible for discussing systematically with the pupil and his family how mobility in his home and neighbourhood can best be achieved, taking into account actual local conditions, and then for drawing up a mobility training programme. In some respects special schools are in a better position to do this, although for the child attending a local school it will be easier to relate such a programme to the geography of the neighbourhood. The handicapped pupil must know, well before he leaves school, how he can best get about his neighbourhood without having to rely solely on his family and that he has had supported practice in actually doing this. If he is so handicapped that he cannot be mobile on his own, then statutory or voluntary help on a regular basis should be made use of but the teenager must know how to obtain this help himself. Although it may be very difficult to arrange this, pupils should be given driving instruction before they leave school if this is to be their main means of outdoor transport and some schools are making imaginative attempts to do this. It takes courage for a disabled person to drive unaccompanied, especially in busy city traffic. The supportive framework of the school will help a teenager to overcome his fears, and those who are timid can see how their more adventurous friends are managing. After leaving school it may be more difficult to undertake an activity that is basically very frightening. As noted earlier, many young people with spina bifida will need extra training in map-reading if they are to venture far from home.

(iii) *Local contacts with non-handicapped and handicapped peers.* In many recent reports (e.g. Scottish Education Department Report, 1975) it has been strongly recommended that practical steps should be taken to increase contacts between children in special and ordinary schools. This would certainly be an important step towards combating the social isolation of many young handicapped people, although such contacts do need to be carefully prepared for by the staff and pupils of both kinds of schools.

Often a handicapped teenager's social isolation does not become fully apparent until he has left school. School staff, in particular the staff of special schools (who usually recognize that it is part of their responsibility to foster the pupil's social development), could do more to help the pupil and his parents to find out what youth clubs and other groupings of young people do exist in his own neighbourhood. They could then give the teenager more encouragement to join a particular club as well as practical guidance in working out with him how he sets about this and how he will get there.

There are also clubs for disabled people but it is often the case that older handicapped children (and adults) go through a stage of development during which they want to have nothing to do socially with their handicapped peers. Evans and her colleagues (1974) found this sort of reaction in adults with spina bifida and in the extract below (Richardson, 1972) a psychologist with cerebral palsy looks back at his feelings on this question.

> When I graduated from special school, I said 'Thank God, no more handicapped people'. And I slipped into college. The first year I didn't have any friends. My parents said, 'Why don't you invite the old high-school friends?' I said 'No, I'm not going to be associated with handicapped people anymore. I'm finished with that.' The second year I was getting lonelier and lonelier . . . so I said 'Hey, what's the matter with handicapped people? You're one of them yourself.' Then I started to join organizations for handicapped adults . . . and realized that I was missing a good bet. I was disregarding a whole mass of people for foolish reasons.

(iv) *Group support for handicapped teenagers.* While many handicapped teenagers may identify strongly with their non-handicapped peers and may wish to have non-handicapped friends, there is also a great need for groups to be set up (perhaps by the Social Services Department on a neighbourhood basis) where teenagers with spina bifida and other handicaps similar in their effects can meet to express their feelings and discuss mutual problems. It might also be helpful occasionally to invite similarly handicapped adults to such groups, as many handicapped teenagers might be helped by the chance to talk over a particular problem with an adult who offers a 'coping' model.

The experience of one of us has shown that a group run specifically for young handicapped people (aged 15–25) is greatly welcomed and enthusiastically received, provided that it is coupled with a real attempt to give factual information on relevant subjects, for example on the neurological basis of the condition, the possibilities of parenthood, how to make a claim for social security, and how to discover what evening classes are available locally. Any *social* activities, however, should be undertaken in conjunction with the non-handicapped. Non-handicapped young people who are included in discussion groups can help to demonstrate that becoming an adult holds problems even for the able-bodied and that many of the difficulties experienced by handicapped young people are shared by all adolescents. Groups run on a local basis could build up information over time about the accessibility of buildings, availability of suitable clubs, how best to deal with local transport services, and so on. In addition, the disabled young people would gradually build up a network of local contacts and so become more involved in neighbourhood activities. Local branches of Phab (an organization specifically for physically handicapped and able-bodied young people) are now beginning to grow and anyone interested in forming a local group to help handicapped young people should contact Phab national headquarters (see Appendix I).

(c) *Physical and sexual problems*

Knowledge about the general physical condition. Discussions with spina bifida teenagers reveal that they often do not have a clear idea of what spina bifida and hydrocephalus really are, or of the reasons for the surgical procedures which they have been subjected to. This was a very clear finding in two recent research studies with spina bifida teenagers (Scott *et al.*, 1975; Dorner, 1976). Scott *et al.*, interviewed twenty adolescents aged between 12 and 16 years, and found that only two 'felt that they had a good understanding of their condition'. One 16-year-old boy, for example, 'said that he was born with a lump on his back and when the surgeon cut it off his legs became paralysed'. When asked about their urinary diversions, none of the adolescents were satisfied with the reasons given for having surgery, even though all but one had specifically asked their mothers: most 'felt it had something to do with improving their urinary function but were vague as to how this came about'.

The findings in Dorner's study (1976) were similar. Of the forty-six adolescents interviewed only four had a good understanding of the nature of spina bifida and eight an adequate understanding (e.g. 'I'm paralysed from the waist downward because my nerves are damaged at the base of my spine'.) There were twenty-four whose understanding seemed limited (e.g. 'your spine is unjoined. I don't know why it stops you walking. I'd like to know more') while the other ten were unable to give any description of the condition.

It was clear from both these studies that the teenagers wanted to know more. Scott *et al.* (1975), for example, refer to one boy who said he had asked his mother in the presence of a careers officer exactly what was the matter with him, saying that if other people had the right to ask questions about him he had the right to ask questions too. Studies of children handicapped in other ways (e.g. Feinberg *et al.*, 1974; Burton, 1975) show that this lack of information on the part of young people about their own handicaps is the rule rather than the exception.

Why has this situation arisen? Part of the problem is that it is probably assumed that parents will inform their children about the nature of their condition and explain why surgery is necessary. The Scott *et al.* study (1975) made it clear that in the case of urinary diversion operations the parents themselves had little understanding of surgical procedure and none had discussed the operation and its implications with their children. Remarks such as 'she was too young' or 'how could I explain when I didn't really understand it myself' were typical, and as Pless and Pinkerton (1975) point out, this lack of understanding is true of parents with children handicapped in many different ways.

It is not only the parents who are responsible for their children's lack of understanding about their condition. Both medical and care staff often continue to treat an adolescent as a child by excluding him from conferences and decisions which affect him. Information is probably not deliberately withheld, but rather it has been nobody's particular responsibility to ensure that teenagers have a chance for full and unhurried discussions with a consultant or expert about the nature of their condition and about the procedures associated with its management. Even if consistent efforts have been made to explain the condition to the child, as he grows older adolescence will change his awareness of himself and will give rise to new feelings about the handicap and fears for the future. Thus Scott *et al.* (1975) recommend that as the child gets older 'the focus should move from the parent to the child', giving him 'the opportunity to ventilate feelings, dispel ignorance and ask those questions which he thinks to be important. Privacy is essential for this purpose.' The better informed a disabled person is about his handicap and about the procedures which will enable him to live as healthily and as normally as possible, the more likely he is to have and to feel that he has some degree of control over what happens to him.

Sex and marriage. One aspect of the teenager's understanding of himself which has been particularly neglected is his sexual development. Until recently, discussion of the sexual needs of handicapped adults and young people has been minimal (particularly where the handicap is congenital), and it is not surprising that many misconceptions exist. This is illustrated in the following quotation which introduces Ann Shearer's excellent report (1972) on public and professional attitudes towards the sexual and emotional needs of handicapped people.

> 'Sex isn't really something that comes up here at all. They're too bound up in themselves to bother about relationships with other people.'
>
> 'Of course we want to get married, yes, and have children as well. Don't you see, we have to? Just because we're handicapped, it doesn't mean that we haven't got the same rights and feelings as everyone else.'

The first speaker is the warden of a home for physically handicapped people, the second a girl in the same home, half of one of six couples whom, she says, feel the same way as she does.

The situation is slowly beginning to change, and in this respect the Swedish Central Committee for Rehabilitation (SVCR) have taken a lead by setting up, in 1971, a special working party led by Inger Nordqvist to look at the social and in particular the sexual problems of handicapped individuals. The ultimate aims of the working party are to achieve a situation where a mature person can, regardless of handicap, (a) himself assume responsibility for his own sexual life, (b) obtain information on how to function sexually in spite of his handicap, and (c) acquire greater opportunities for outgoing contacts and be in a better position to choose a marriage partner. Similar developments are taking place in some other European countries (Lancaster-Gaye, 1972) and a recent development in this country has been a survey carried out by the National Fund for Research into Crippling Diseases of the sexual problems of the disabled (Commitee on Sexual Problems of the Disabled (Stewart, 1975). In the USA a major centre of research is at the University of Minnesota Medical School where workshops on sexual and attitude counselling provide education and training to disabled adults and to professionals from a variety of backgrounds who work with the disabled; in addition, a great deal of useful material has been published from this centre (e.g. Cole *et al.*, 1973; Cole, 1975; Mooney *et al.*, 1975).

(i) *Information and views held by disabled teenagers.* Handicapped teenagers frequently have little knowledge about normal sexual development, and even less about sexual development as related to their own particular individual situation. Not only is little in the way of sex education given in many schools for handicapped children but, in addition, the restricted social contacts of handicapped teenagers mean that they have much less chance to 'pick up' such information than do many of their non-handicapped peers.

In this country very little research has been done on this question, but in Sweden Bergstrom-Walan (1972) describes an investigation organized by the Swedish Central Committee for Rehabilitation into the knowledge of and attitudes towards sex among physically handicapped adolescents who attended special schools, some as day pupils, most as boarders. Seventy-five pupils aged from 16 to 25 from three different institutions for the physically handicapped in Sweden took part in the study. A major aim of the investigation was to find out what the pupils felt their main information needs to be. There was a marked demand for more sex education and for chances of discussion, especially (a) about the ethics and values, as well as the norms of sexual relationships and (b) about technical information and aids, including in particular information about contraceptives.

Research findings in this country coupled with personal experience (Spain) in discussion groups with spina bifida teenagers make three things clear. Firstly, teenagers with spina bifida have had little ordinary sex education and, with few exceptions, no personal counselling. Secondly, they feel a strong need for counselling. Thirdly, such counselling must encompass not simply the facts of sexual development as related to a particular individual's condition but also the opportunity to discuss the implications of these facts for relationships with the opposite sex and also for marriage and procreation. Findings in an American study (Feinberg *et al.*, 1974) of teenage boys with exstrophy of the bladder and complete epispadias (a severe congenital anomaly of both urinary and sexual functions) were remarkably similar.

In this country, Dorner's study (1976) showed that the main concern expressed by spina bifida boys was about whether they could be potent. The girls were much more preoccupied with the question of marriage and the great majority said that they thought a lot about whether they could have children and wished to do so. While some had discussed this with a doctor few had done so in detail and most had simply been told that there was probably no physical obstacle to their conceiving. Genetic counselling had either not been given or had been ineffective, since most girls denied that there was an increased risk that their child would have spina bifida or anencephaly, nor had the question of the girl's capacity for caring for a baby adequately been considered. Overall, of those teenagers who definitely hoped to marry, about half thought they would be able to have children, including a number of boys and girls with urinary and locomotor problems. Findings on the marital status of adults with spina bifida (Evans *et al.*, 1974) suggest that the aspirations of many of these teenagers are unlikely to be fulfilled: in her study only one in eight of the spina bifida men with a moderate or severe disability had married and just under one in three of the moderately severely disabled women.

(ii) *Attitudes of parents.* Most disabled teenagers find it difficult or impossible to discuss their anxieties about sex and marriage with their parents. A study carried out by Bloom (1969) in the USA indicated that many such parents felt 'embarrassment, inadequacy and reluctance in discussing the sexual aspects of life with their child. Often implied but unstated was horror at the thought of their child having sexual relationships, getting married and producing children', although, comments Bloom, 'we know that handicapped persons do date, do marry and do have children.' In this, as Shearer (1972) points out, the attitudes of parents resemble very closely public attitudes towards the sexuality of handicapped people.

Parents often behave as if their handicapped adolescent was a sexless individual. Tew (1974) in an ongoing study of spina bifida children in South Wales suggests that 'there is evidence that the parents of children who have had surgical treatment for urinary diversion see this as a castrating procedure and appear to deny the realities of sexual development'. Undoubtedly another major reason underlying the tendency for the parents continuing to treat the adolescent as a child rather than a young man or woman is that they want to give him 'security' and they are understandably reluctant to expose him to possible bitter disappointments.

(iii) *The provision of counselling to disabled teenagers.* The question of who should provide counselling and emotional support on problems related to sexual development, to marriage and to procreation is a crucial one. In the Swedish study discussed earlier (Bergstrom-Walan, 1972), the majority of the adolescents felt that this person should be a visiting expert and not one of their regular teachers or nursing staff, and a very similar view has been expressed to one of us by spina bifida adolescents in this country.

This is probably a view which most of the staff of special schools and institutions would share. As Nordqvist (1972a) points out, it is difficult emotionally for teachers and nursing staff to deal with such questions. The staff may be afraid of arousing false expectations among the pupils about their future sexual lives and anxious to protect pupils from being hurt by their own experiences; they are also afraid lest parents blame them for discussing these matters. In the Swedish study Nordqvist (1972b) found a very widespread reluctance on the part of the staff of special schools to undertake either the responsibility for the sexual education of their pupils or the responsibility for discussing and trying to solve the problems of individual pupils. The general opinion was that the responsibility for these matters should lie with 'experts' from outside the institution. Attitudes such as these are not only held by teachers: many doctors also feel that counselling on sexual functioning is not part of their responsibility.

Even when teachers or others are competent and willing to discuss normal sexual development, and where they can see the need to encourage adolescents to have normal experiences, risking rejection and disappointment if needs be, they are unlikely to have specialized knowledge about a particular handicapped individual's sexual potential. This is hardly surprising since even among gynæcologists or the medical staff of rehabilitation centres there is still comparatively little known about the sexual functioning of those with paraplegia resulting from trauma to the spinal cord, and even less about those (including spina bifida adolescents) with congenital lesions of the cord.

These findings have two main implications. First, there is clearly a need for seeing that every spina bifida teenager, whether in an ordinary or special school, has available the opportunity of discussing sexual and related problems as they affect him personally with an informed counsellor. Who this should be will depend partly upon how services are organized in a particular area as well as on the relationships with particular adults which a teenager has already developed. Scott *et al.* (1975)

suggest that counselling would ideally be done 'by a doctor who has developed a relationship of trust built up over a long period of time' and who is 'sufficiently familiar with the total problem to be able to give factual information as well as emotional support'. Certainly someone must take the responsibility for ensuring that teenagers with spina bifida are given the opportunity to discuss sexual and related problems and the best person to do this is probably the consultant pædiatrician. However, he would not necessarily do the actual counselling himself but might arrange for another professional with training in counselling techniques to do so, himself acting as a source of factual information. The counsellor might be a social worker or a person with experience in working with disabled young people: there are also now a number of psychiatrists with expertise in counselling non-handicapped people over sexual problems whom it might be possible to approach for help. SPOD (see Appendix I for address) can also be contacted for advice on counselling. As we indicated earlier, there is, in addition to individual counselling, clearly a place for group discussions led by an experienced counsellor between teenagers who share similar problems.

Second, however, although counsellors with special expertise would be invaluable, all those who work with disabled teenagers should be prepared to shoulder part of the responsibility for helping teenagers with personal (including sexual) problems, since otherwise they may well get no help at all. One major function of the schools will be to ensure that disabled teenagers are, like other teenagers, provided with information about normal sexual development. Here it is helpful if teachers can inform parents in advance about what the teaching will cover to prevent them from feeling that they have been kept out of things.

In addition, however, the training of teaching and care staff at special schools (especially residential schools) with pupils in their teens should include information about normal sexual development, information about the sexual needs and abilities of handicapped people, and simple training in counselling techniques. SPOD hopes to be able to provide training of this kind. Disabled teenagers need sympathetic adults to talk to, and if an adult without special training is approached by a teenager with problems he can do a great deal to help if he shows that he is not frightened or put off by a discussion of sexual problems; if he realizes that disabled teenagers can 'take it' and that they find it more helpful to talk with someone who is sensitive but honest rather than someone who is evasive or who uses euphemisms because afraid the teenager will be hurt; if he sanctions a disabled teenager's expression of sexual feelings, and appreciates that sexual competence may be very important to him as well as the quality of his relationships with the other sex; and if he talks about sex in a multi-problem context, that is, as one of several related problems which disabled teenagers are trying to come to terms with. At the end of a talk of this kind the adult should offer the teenager the opportunity to discuss the matter again, or, if he feels unable to handle the problem, should suggest that the teenager sees someone with more knowledge and himself take the responsibility for arranging this. This means, of course, that the staff of schools and institutions where there are disabled adolescents should know who they can go to for more specialized help (for example, the pædiatrician or social worker) and should liaise closely with this person.

References

Anderson, E. M. (1973), *The Disabled Schoolchild: A Study of Integration in Primary Schools*, Methuen, London.

——, (1975), 'Cognitive and motor deficits in children with spina bifida and hydrocephalus with special reference to writing difficulties', unpublished Ph.D. thesis, University of London.

Bergstrom-Walan, M. B. (1972), 'The problems of sex and handicap in Sweden: an investigation', ch. 7 in Lancaster-Gaye, D. (ed.), *Personal Relationships, the Handicapped and the Community*, Routledge and Kegan Paul, London.

Bloom, J. L. (1969), 'Sex education for handicapped adolescents', *Journal of School Health*, 39, pp. 363–7.

Brown, C. (1955), *My Left Foot*, Simon and Schuster, New York.

Burton, L. (1975), *The Family Life of Sick Children*, Routledge and Kegan Paul, London.

Cole, T. M. (1975), 'Sexuality and the physically handicapped', in Green, R. (ed.), *Human Sexuality. A Health Practitioner's Text*, Williams and Wilkins, Baltimore.

——, Chilgren, R. and Rosenberg, P. (1973), 'A new program of sex education and counselling for spinal cord injured adults and health care professionals', *International Journal of Paraplegia*, August 1973, pp. 111–24.

Dinnage, R. (1970), *The Handicapped Child. Studies in Child Development Research Review, Vol. I*, Longmans, London.

——, (1972), *The Handicapped Child. Studies in Child Development Research Review, Vol. II*, Longmans, London.

Doherty, E. E. (1973), 'The young adult and his desire for integration', ch. 20 in Loring, J. and Burn, G. (eds.), *The Integration of Handicapped Children in Society*, Routledge and Kegan Paul, London.

Doll, E. A. (1947), *The Vineland Social Maturity Scale*, Educational Test Bureau, Minneapolis, Minn.

Dorner, S. (1975), 'The relationship of physical handicap to stress in families with an adolescent with spina bifida', *Developmental Medicine and Child Neurology*, 17 (6), pp. 765–76.

——, (1976) 'Adolescents with spina bifida – how they see their situation', *Archives of Diseases in Childhood*, 51, pp. 439–44.

Drake, D. M. (1970), 'Perceptual correlates of impulsive and reflective behaviour', *Child Development*, 2 (2), pp. 202–14.

Evans, K., Hickman, V. and Carter, C. O. (1974), 'Handicap and social status of adults with spina bifida cystica', *British Journal of Preventive and Social Medicine*, 28, pp. 85–92.

Feinberg ,T., Lattimer, J. K., Jeter, K., Langford, W. and Beck, L. (1974), 'Questions that worry children with exstrophy', *Paediatrics*, 53, pp. 242–7.

Freeman, R. D. (1970), 'Psychiatric problems in adolescents with cerebral palsy', *Developmental Medicine and Child Neurology*, 12, pp. 64–70.

Fulthorpe, D. (1974), 'Spina bifida: some psychological aspects', *Special Education*, 1 (4), pp. 17–20.

Goffman, E. (1963), *Stigma: Notes on the Management of Spoiled Identity*, Prentice Hall, New Jersey.

Hicks, J. (1975), Personal communication.

Hodges, D. (1974), *The Child with a Chronic Medical Problem. An Annotated Bibliography*, NFER, Windsor, Berks.

Hunt, P. (ed.), (1966), *Stigma: The Experience of Disability*, Geoffrey Chapman, London.

Ineichen, R. (1973), 'Towards co-ordinated care of spina bifida children', *Social Work Today*, 4 (11), pp. 321–4.

Ingram, T. T. S., Jameson, S., Errington J., and Mitchell, R. G. (1964), *Living with Cerebral Palsy*, Clinics in Developmental Medicine, 14, Spastics Society/Heinemann, London.

Jessel, C. (1975), *Mark's Wheelchair Adventures*, Methuen, London.

Kagan, J. (1965), 'Reflection-impulsivity and reading ability in primary grade children', *Child Development*, 36, pp. 609–28.

——, and Kogan, N. (1970), 'Individual variation in cognitive processes', in Mussen, P. (ed.), *Carmichael's Manual of Child Psychology* (3rd edition), Wiley, New York.

Kellmer Pringle, M. L. (1964), *The Emotional and Social Adjustment of Physically Handicapped Children*, occasional publications, no. 10, NFER, Slough, Bucks.

Laing, A. F. (1975), 'Social skills for slow learners', *Special Education*, 2 (1), pp. 27–8.

Lancaster-Gaye, D. (1972), *Personal Relationships, the Handicapped and the Community*, Routledge and Kegan Paul, London.

Lorber, J. and Schloss, A. L. (1973), 'The adolescent with myelomeningocele', *Developmental Medicine and Child Neurology*, 15, Supplement 29, pp. 113–14.

Lore, R. K. (1965), 'Some factors influencing the child's exploration of visual stimuli', doctoral dissertation, University of Tennessee.

Lunzer, E. A. (1966), *Manchester Scales of Social Adaptation*, NFER, Windsor, Berks.

Meichenbaum, D. and Goodman, J. (1971), 'Training impulsive children to talk to themselves. A means of developing self-control', *Journal of Abnormal Psychology*, 77 (2), pp. 115–26.

Mooney, T. O., Cole, T. M. and Chilgren, R. (1975), *Sexual Options for Paraplegics and Quadruplegics*, Little, Brown, New York.

Morgan, M. (1972), 'Like other school-leavers?', ch. 26 in Boswell, D. M. and Wingrove, J. M. (eds.), *The Handicapped Person in the Community*, Tavistock, London.

Moyer, K. E. and Gilmer, B. V. H. (1954), 'The concept of attention spans in children', *Elementary School Journal*, 54, pp. 464–6.

——, ——, (1955), 'Attention spans of children for experimentally designed toys', *Journal of Genetic Psychology*, 87, pp. 187–201.

Nordqvist, I. (ed.), (1972a), *Life Together – the Situation of the Handicapped*, Swedish Central Committee for Rehabilitation, Bromma 3, Sweden.

——, (1972b), 'Sexual problems of the handicapped: the work of the Swedish Central Committee for Rehabilitation', ch. 8 in Lancaster-Gaye, D. (ed.), *Personal Relationships, the Handicapped and the Community*, Routledge and Kegan Paul, London.

Pilling, D. (1972), *The Orthopaedically Handicapped Child. Social, Emotional and Educational Adjustment: An Annotated Bibliography*, NFER, Windsor, Berks.

——, (1973a), *The Child with Cerebral Palsy. An Annotated Bibliography*, NFER, Windsor, Berks.

——, (1973b), *The Child with Spina Bifida. An Annotated Bibliography*, NFER, Windsor, Berks.

——, (1974), *The Child with a Chronic Medical Problem. An Annotated Bibliography*, NFER, Windsor, Berks.

——, (1975), *The Child with Asthma. An Annotated Bibliography*, NFER, Windsor, Berks.

Pless, I. B. and Pinkerton, P. (1975), *Chronic Childhood Disorders – Promoting Patterns of Adjustment*, Henry Kimpton, London.

Richardson, S. (1972), 'People with cerebral palsy talk for themselves', *Developmental Medicine and Child Neurology*, 14 (4), pp. 524–35.

Richman, N., Stevenson, J. E. and Graham, P. J. (1975), 'Prevalence of behaviour problems in 3 year old children: an epidemiological study in a London Borough', *Journal of Child Psychology and Psychiatry*, 16, (4), pp. 277–87.

Robertson, E. (1972), 'Follow-up study into the functional abilities at home and at school of multiple limb deficient children', report obtainable from Children's Prosthetic Unit, Queen Mary's Hospital, Roehampton, London.

Rutter, M. (1967), 'A children's behaviour questionnaire for completion by teachers: preliminary findings', *Journal of Child Psychology and Psychiatry*, 8, pp. 1–11.

Rutter, M., Graham, P., Chadwick, O. F. D. and Yule, W., (1976), 'Adolescent turmoil, fact or fiction?', *Journal of Child Psychology and Psychiatry*, 17, pp. 35–56.

——, Tizard, J. and Whitmore, J. (eds.), (1970), *Education, Health and Behaviour*, Longmans, London.

Santostephano, S. (1969), 'Cognitive controls and cognitive styles: an approach to diagnosing and treating cognitive disabilities in children', *Seminars in Psychiatry*, 1 (3), pp. 291–317.

Schwebel, A. I. (1966), 'Effects of impulsivity on performance of verbal tasks in middle and lower class children', *American Journal of Orthopsychiatry*, 36, pp. 13–21.

Scott, M., Roberts, M. C. C. and Tew, B. J. (1975), 'Psychosexual problems in adolescent spina bifida patients with special reference to the effect of urinary diversion on patient attitudes', paper given at the annual meeting of the Society for Research into Spina Bifida and Hydrocephalus, Glasgow, 25–28 June 1975.

Scottish Education Department (1975), *The Secondary Education of Physically Handicapped Children in Scotland*, HMSO, Edinburgh.

Seidel, U. P., Chadwick, O. F. D. and Rutter, M. (1975), 'Psychological disorders in crippled children. A comparative study of children with and without brain damage', *Developmental Medicine and Child Neurology*, 17, pp. 563–73.

Sen, A. (1967), 'Factors affecting distractability in the subnormal: an experimental investigation', unpublished doctoral dissertation, University of Hull.

Shearer, A. (1972), *A Right to Love?*, Spastics Society/National Association for Mental Health, London.

Stewart, W. F. R. (1975), *Sex and the Physically Handicapped*, National Fund for Research into Crippling Diseases, Springfield Road, Horsham.

Taylor, E. M. (1959), *Psychological Appraisal of Children with Cerebral Defects*, Harvard University Press, Cambridge, Mass.

Tew, B. J. (1973), 'Spina bifida and hydrocephalus: facts, fallacies and future', *Special Education*, 62 (4), pp. 26–31.

——, (1974), 'Spina bifida: family and social problems', *Special Education*, 1 (2), pp. 17–20.

——, and Laurence, K. M. (1975), 'The effects of hydrocephalus on intelligence, visual perception, and school attainment', *Developmental Medicine and Child Neurology*, Supplement 35, pp. 129–34.

Turnure, J. E. (1970), 'Children's reactions to distractors in a learning situation', *Developmental Psychology*, 2 (1), pp. 115–22.

Welbourn, H. (1975), 'Spina bifida children attending ordinary schools', *British Medical Journal* 1, pp. 142–5.

Wright, B. (1960), *Physical Disability – A Psychological Approach*, Harper & Row, New York.

Younghusband, E., Birchall, D., Davie, R. and Kellmer Pringle, M. L. (eds.) (1970), *Living with Handicap*, National Bureau of Co-operation in Child Care, London.

Zucker, J. S. and Stricker, G. (1968), 'Impulsivity-reflectivity in preschool headstart and middle-class children', *Journal of Learning Disabilities*, 1 (10), pp. 578–84.

10 After school: prospects for further education, training and employment

Introduction

The authors of the Tuckey Report (a follow-up survey of handicapped school-leavers published in 1973), make the point that the 'generous outlay of money and effort on the education of handicapped children until the age of 16 and sometimes beyond . . . should obviously be followed by an equally generous provision of further education, of training and of opportunities for employment, according to ability'. In fact, 'extraordinary little', as they put it, is known about what actually happens to school-leavers and the evidence there is indicates that provision for the handicapped after school compares very poorly indeed with provision for school-age children.

Too often, those who had responsibilities towards the school-age child, whether as teachers, psychologists, pædiatricians, social workers or even researchers, see their roles as over once the teenager leaves school, and in contrast to the efforts they made on behalf of the schoolchild display comparatively little interest in what happens to him afterwards. There would seem to be a strong case for teachers in special schools or in special units in ordinary schools to monitor what happens to their leavers, not only so that the school can continue to provide some support if necessary to the leaver and his family, but also so that the relevance and effectiveness of the 'curriculum' (in its very widest sense) can be reviewed regularly and discussed in the light of what happens to the leavers. This may be done more in the future: at least one special-school head we know has designated a staff member to follow up the leavers.

Most books about handicapped children reflect this situation and fail to discuss, except in the briefest way, the world which the handicapped school-leaver enters. One reason for this is that very little material is available about what happens to disabled leavers in general and spina bifida leavers in particular. What we have tried to do here is, firstly, to outline the main types of provision or placements available for disabled school-leavers, secondly, to review the research findings about what actually happens to these leavers, thirdly, to look at the issues specifically in relation to spina bifida, and, finally, to make a number of suggestions about how the situation for spina bifida and other disabled leavers may be improved.

1 Types of provision available for handicapped school-leavers

When a handicapped teenager leaves school, which in the majority of cases is at 16+ although sometimes later, there are four main avenues he may follow. First, he may go straight into open or sheltered employment (and many leavers from special schools wish to do this). Second, he may continue his education either in higher/further education or in some sort of specialized training or in a combination of these. Third, he may find diversionary employment in a centre provided by the local authority social services department or at home. Fourth, he may simply remain at home doing nothing.

Open and sheltered employment

Employment may be 'open', where the leaver competes for a job on the open market, or sheltered. Sheltered employment facilities exist for those so severely handicapped that there is no suitable work available for them on the open market, or for those who cannot work on equal terms with the able-bodied. Three main groups of people provide sheltered workshop facilities: some of the voluntary associations for the handicapped, local authorities and Remploy, an independent non-profit making company which aims to provide work under sheltered conditions for those so severely disabled that it is unlikely that they would otherwise be able to obtain employment. According to Glanville (1974) whose study has provided much useful material for this chapter, there are about eighty-seven Remploy factories in this country employing 8,000 disabled people: although these factories offer a wide range of work, what may be available to a particular individual depends very much on where he lives.

Further education and/or training

More than half the population of disabled leavers from special schools are likely, at the present time, to go on to some sort of further education or training either before they find employment or, less commonly, in conjunction with it; for those leaving ordinary schools no statistics are available. The main types of provision which can be included under the umbrella of further education/training are very varied but include: (a) higher education, for example at a university or college of education; (b) full-time or part-time further education, usually in a college of further education; (c) specialized residential courses providing assessment and/or training; (d) assessment and training in Employment Rehabilitation Centres (formerly known as Industrial Rehabilitation Units); (e) day centres and training centres. In addition to these types of provision, comparatively small numbers of leavers may receive some further education in the form of occasional classes run by the local authority, or home tuition.

(a) *Higher education.* While some of those with spina bifida meningocele and a mild degree of disability may go on to higher education, it is unlikely that this will be appropriate for more than a small minority of those with myelomeningocele and associated hydrocephalus since, as we discussed in chapters 5 and 8, these children tend to be of low average or below average ability and attainments. For those who are able to benefit from higher education but are very severely disabled the Open University has a great deal to offer, 600 handicapped students being registered in 1973.

(b) *Further education.* A much greater proportion of spina bifida leavers will, on the other hand, benefit from further education, in some cases in ordinary courses, in others in courses geared towards the needs of the handicapped (or those disadvantaged in other ways) although not exclusively for them. Until recently, few courses of the latter type were available but an increasing number of courses (educational, vocational or recreational) are now becoming available for those with a wide range of handicaps, including, in a few areas, the severely subnormal (e.g. Sanders and Watson, 1975). At the same time a number of FE colleges are establishing much closer links both with special and with ordinary schools.

A few FE colleges have been unusually imaginative. In London, for example, Kingsway-Princeton College began by taking a particular interest in partially-sighted students, and Brixton in the hearing-impaired. At Brixton this interest has been extended to leavers handicapped in other ways. At present, in addition to seventy-four severely hearing-impaired students there are about 125 students handicapped in other ways and the college has established close links with twenty-five special schools in south London. Contact is made with senior pupils from these schools at least a year before they leave so that all know about the college (some also visit it) and about the wide range of courses available. Brixton has no special facilities (e.g. no lift) but over the years a willingness on the part of the staff to accept handicapped students and considerable expertise in helping them has been developed and the Principal believes that there is no reason why other colleges of further education could not increase their numbers of handicapped students. Some are in fact doing so, but the situation varies enormously from one college to another.

One scheme which has aroused great interest is the Work Orientation Unit at the North Nottinghamshire College of Further Education; a full account of this scheme has been given by Hutchinson and Clegg (1975). The unit, set up in 1970 to provide courses for handicapped school-leavers who were not yet ready to be placed in a work situation, now has 110 students (including 43 who are physically handicapped, a number of them by spina bifida) and 12 specialist staff. Its objectives are (a) to provide vocational education based firmly on the needs both of the individual student and of industry within the student's locality, (b) general education ranging from advanced study to remedial treatment to improve basic skills and (c) a wide variety of recreational and educational courses. The development of self-confidence and self-reliance is also emphasized.

Before being assigned to courses, careful assessments are made of each student's work skills and of his work personality. After assessment three levels of courses are available in the broad areas of engineering, construction, business studies and management, general studies, catering, dress/fashion, retail trades and hairdressing, the average length of course being two years. Level I students are seconded full-time from the work orientation unit to other departments within the college; Level II students are seconded for part of the time for vocational education and recreational education while remaining in the unit for general education; Level III students receive both their vocational and general education in the unit but are seconded from it for recreational education. A major feature of the college is a 'work experience' scheme designed to give those students able to work outside the college in open or sheltered employment at least one day a week during term time at a place of employment. For those unable to work outside the college a similar scheme operates inside.

Reference must also be made to the first national college of further education for the physically handicapped to be administered by a local authority, Hereward College in Coventry (described by Lowe, 1973). This is a residential college catering for 100 physically handicapped students. All do a one-year foundation course with a business studies, engineering, GCE (arts) or GCE (science) basis. After this some are referred to ordinary FE colleges or to higher education, others complete academic/vocational courses at Hereward and others do linked courses given partly at Hereward and partly at other Coventry colleges, in particular an ordinary FE college on the same campus. A marked trend at Hereward has been the need to cater for much larger numbers of severely handicapped students than was originally anticipated, and also for increasingly large numbers of applicants of below average intellectual ability, both these trends presumably reflecting the fact that larger numbers of the less handicapped and/or more able leavers are being absorbed into ordinary FE facilities.

(c) *Residential courses.* A number of residential courses for handicapped leavers are available in colleges set up by voluntary bodies. These are comparatively few in number, and sometimes specialized according to handicap. Some offer further education leading to vocational training, some both further education and vocational education and some are 'open-ended' that is students may go on to higher education. Assessment may be included at the beginning of the course, while a few residential courses have been set up solely for assessment purposes. Residential courses of possible interest to spina bifida leavers are listed in Appendix H.

(d) *Employment Rehabilitation Centres.* These used to be called Industrial Rehabilitation Units and were set up, initially, for adults who had been hospitalized because of the onset of physical or mental illness and needed a period of rehabilitation before returning to work. However, Glanville (1974) reports that this pattern has been changing. In 1971–2, for example, there was a fall to 65 per cent in admissions of people with recent sickness or injury and a rise to nearly 30 per cent of those with long-standing disabilities. In 1971, those with spinal injuries formed the second largest group of people attending the centres (next to those with psychoneurosis). A few ERCs now offer alongside their normal courses special assessment and work experience courses for school-leavers, but in general, with the exception of the specialized ERCs run by the Spastics Society, they do not provide vocational training.

(e) *Day centres and training centres.* Day centres for the physically handicapped and training centres for the mentally handicapped provide for only a small number of school-leavers. In many little training is offered, their main function being to provide diversionary occupation and social contacts for people who might otherwise be very isolated. As these are often older people the centres may not be very helpful even in providing social contacts for teenagers and thought needs to be given as to how they can be made more suitable and enjoyable for young people. In some centres special training is given to those considered able to benefit and this can lead on to sheltered work and eventually to open employment.

2 The current situation for handicapped school-leavers

It is very difficult to present an accurate assessment of the current situation for disabled school-leavers because this can change quite rapidly according to the general economic situation in the country. The employment prospects of handicapped leavers have to be looked at within the wider context of current employment prospects for able-bodied leavers and for disabled adults, and in periods of recession both these groups are particularly vulnerable.

Figures for disabled school-leavers are hard to come by and most surveys have involved quite small numbers. A valuable recent report is the Scottish Education Department Survey (1975) of physically handicapped pupils leaving special schools in Scotland in 1973. 51 per cent of the leavers went straight into employment, 21 per cent into sheltered workshops and work centres, 11 per cent into training courses and 2 per cent only to FE colleges, while 2 per cent were in hospital at the time of the survey, and 13 per cent were unemployed. The authors of the report comment on the surprisingly high proportion of those who found jobs immediately after leaving special school: interestingly, very similar figures come from a much larger survey carried out of leavers from special schools in England (Tuckey *et al.*, 1973) where figures for placement in employment (50 per cent) and in sheltered workshops (23 per cent) were identical to the Scottish ones. However, since the first job taken up by a leaver is often unsuitable, these figures may be somewhat misleading.

The Tuckey survey was set up in 1968 under the sponsorship of the DHSS, DES and Department of Employment 'to investigate the range, availability and suitability of the facilities for further education, training and employment of handicapped school-leavers'. From a total of 7,094 children (covering the whole range of handicaps) expected to leave special schools in the year 1968–9 a sample of 1,700 was selected for further study, about whom basic information was obtained from the schools. In the end, 788 were included in the follow-up study carried out in 1971, 247 of these being physically handicapped leavers. Information about this group was obtained from careers officers, the young people themselves, their parents and, where applicable, their employers.

A number of changes have occurred which date the Tuckey survey findings. One is that the population of the special schools is altering and their leavers tend to be more handicapped both physically and intellectually than hitherto, another that employment prospects for all leavers are currently much poorer than when the survey was published. On the other hand, prospects of disabled leavers obtaining higher or further education or training are slowly improving. Despite such changes a number of the findings are still relevant.

As regards employment, 64 per cent of the leavers interviewed had done some paid work since leaving school 18–24 months earlier, three-quarters of these in open and a quarter in sheltered employment. Some had gone straight into employment and some had had some training or further education first. The Tuckeys comment that 'on the whole . . . head teachers were more pessimistic about employment potential than was found to be justified', and careers officers tended to rate the chance of a leaver obtaining open employment rather higher than the head teacher. However, the seemingly high employment figures conceal the fact that many leavers underwent a long and anxious period before finding employment and also that periods of employment are often interspersed with long periods of unemployment. The major reasons for leaving a job, especially the first job, appeared to be either that the work was too demanding or, in a number of cases, because the pay was poor.

Turning next to further education and training, the most striking finding in the Tuckey Report was the discrepancy between the proportion of those leavers who were considered by their teachers as suitable for further education and/or training and the very much smaller proportion who actually received it. Problems of access and transport (see chapter 9) are partly responsible, but Glanville (1974) and Morgan

(1975) go to the heart of the difficulty when they refer to the lack of further education courses suitable for physically handicapped leavers of below average potential. A similar point is made in the Scottish Report (1975) where it is suggested that in any one year approximately 38 per cent of leavers from special schools will be capable of taking ordinary further education courses, although not all will wish to do so, but that the majority of the leavers (about 60 per cent) 'may well find formal further education courses too exacting'. Increasing numbers of FE colleges are, however, providing 'ordinary' courses geared to the needs of disadvantaged or less-able students but whether or not such courses are available to a particular handicapped leaver will depend on where he lives.

Overall, three main sorts of further education provisions will be required for disabled students. Firstly, there is no doubt that many leavers will wish to attend ordinary FE colleges. Some of this group will benefit from more formal courses, others will be better suited to courses geared to the needs of the less able.

Secondly, there appears to be a need for an extension of the kind of provision exemplified by the Work Orientation Unit at North Nottinghamshire FE College, that is, a form of rather more specialized further education which combines vocational training and 'social education' in its widest sense, which is closely geared both to the abilities of the handicapped students and to the requirements of local industry and which, finally, is an integral part of an ordinary college of further education. For many leavers who are severely handicapped by spina bifida and hydrocephalus, this type of provision would seem particularly useful.

Finally, a relatively small number of severely disabled students will find their requirements met best by residential colleges such as Hereward which specialize in the needs of physically handicapped students, while at the same time maintaining contact with local FE colleges. However, over the past few years there has been a growing dislike among handicapped leavers of leaving home for further education and training; apart from this, most handicapped leavers prefer to have further education and training alongside their able-bodied peers so that the demand for this very specialized sort of provision is unlikely to increase.

Both the Scottish Report and the Tuckey Survey make it clear that there are substantial numbers of leavers, especially those both physically and mentally handicapped, who are neither able to obtain further education/training, nor employment. One voluntary agency with particularly relevant experience of coping with this situation is the Spastics

Society. Morgan (1975) reports, for example, on a survey carried out by the Society of 348 cerebral-palsied young people who had left the Spastics Society's residential schools between 1966 and 1973. Only 10 per cent of the ESN leavers had had any form of continued education or training compared to 80 per cent of those of average ability and an equally wide discrepancy was found in the placements of these two groups in employment and in occupation centres. However, only 14 per cent of the total group of 348 were not occupied in 'reasonably satisfactory ways outside the home' for at least three days a week. At the same time many of these young people, especially those of low ability, continued 'to depend on their parents for all their social contacts'.

3 The situation for spina bifida school-leavers

In the preceding section a number of points were made about physically handicapped school-leavers in general, but how much do we know specifically about spina bifida leavers? As yet very little, since it is only now that those who have had comprehensive early treatment are approaching school-leaving age. However, we have tried in this section to discuss particular problems facing young people with spina bifida where employment is concerned and to draw together the fragmentary information which does exist about what happens to this group when they leave school.

Specific problems

The many factors which may contribute to the difficulties of spina bifida school-leavers in finding employment can be grouped into physical factors, factors related to general intellectual ability and to specific aptitudes, and social and personality factors.

The two major physical problems are impaired mobility and incontinence. Peter Large, in a thorough discussion of outdoor mobility problems of the disabled (Large, 1974) notes that in Buckle's survey (1971) of handicapped and impaired people in Britain, two in five of the 291,000 unemployed impaired people under retirement age gave difficulty in travelling as their reason for not working. Large points out that for a variety of reasons public transport will never be suitable for all and that 'for many of the most severely disabled the private car (or van) is and will remain their sole means of mobility outdoors'. In their study of adults with spina bifida cystica Evans *et al.*, (1974) also comment on the fact that those capable of work 'may not be able to get there. Those who wear calipers and special shoes may have long waits for supplies and repairs .... There may be a delay in the delivery of the standard three-wheeler invalid cars. Some who get invalid cars give them up because they are afraid to drive them, find them too cold or cannot get them started.' The recommendations made in chapter 9 (p. 261) about learning to drive are thus very important in the context of employment.

Access to and within the place of work can also be a problem and housing difficulties also often restrict the choice of employment: if more residential provision were available (hostels, flatlets and residential centres of all kinds) in areas with good employment prospects a leaver would not be tied, as he usually is, to finding work within reach of his home.

Incontinence is the other main physical problem. This raises difficulties both of a practical kind (e.g. the necessity for adequate toileting facilities at the place of work) as well as of a social nature. Clearly satisfactory toilet management is essential both if the teenager is going to secure employment in the first place and if he is going to keep it.

The second group of problems are those relating to intellectual difficulties and to aptitudes for particular types of employment. In chapter 5 differences between children with and without hydrocephalus were noted. These differences were reflected in a study of the aptitudes of adolescents with spina bifida carried out by Parsons (1972). Fifty-nine adolescents took part, twenty with spina bifida and no hydrocephalus, three with hydrocephalus only and thirty-six with spina bifida and hydrocephalus. Sixteen of the group could walk unaided while forty-three needed calipers or wheelchairs. However, Parsons stresses that the young people in his study had been born before early treatment was given: they tended not to have a severe degree of hydrocephalus (only one third of the hydrocephalics had shunts) and were probably less handicapped intellectually than many of those now approaching school-leaving age.

Parsons used a battery of standard aptitude tests to look at skills in four main areas: (a) clerical skills, (b) spatial ability, (c) mechanical comprehension and (d) manual dexterity, these being the sorts of skills needed in many of the jobs usually available to disabled people. In the case of the non-hydrocephalics performance was below average on all the tests except for mechanical comprehension, although these teenagers were in the normal range of intelligence. However, the situation was much worse for the hydrocephalics whose performance was poor on all the tasks, with especially marked difficulties in tasks requiring visuo-spatial skills and manipulative ability. For example, on the manual dexterity task only four (10 per cent) of the hydrocephalics were average in their performance, five low average and the others (over 75 per cent) very poor indeed. The problem was not one of understanding the task but of carrying it out with precision and at high speed. For both groups performance was best on the mechanical comprehension tests which was untimed. On the clerical skills test Parsons notes (both for hydrocephalics and non-hydrocephalics) that the teenagers did make accurate responses but failed 'because they could not complete enough items in the required time'.

The main implications of Parsons's findings is that most spina bifida school-leavers (whether or not they have hydrocephalus but especially the latter) will, particularly in view of their motor (manual) and spatial difficulties, need quite a long period of training in order to reach their full work potential. Even though it should be possible to bring about considerable improvements in speed with training, the sort of work which will suit many leavers is likely to be work in which accuracy is more important than speed and where a high degree of manual skill is not required.

The third group of factors affecting the employment prospects of any handicapped (or non-handicapped) person are those relating to level of social maturity and personal adjustment: these factors, as Mary Greaves (1972) has pointed out are generally more important than the severity of disablement.

In their study of adults with spina bifida Evans and her colleagues (1974) comment on the striking differences they found in the attitudes of adults to their handicaps. 'At one end of the scale are the highly motivated and energetic; they are challenged by their handicap and determined to succeed in spite of it.' The examples they quote include a man who is the warden of a hostel for alcoholics and a man who manœuvred himself daily about five miles across London traffic in a hand-propelled invalid chair to university. Several individuals in this group 'have a good knowledge of statutory and voluntary sources of help, and are able and willing to help others.' At the other end of the scale are those who are 'less . . . resilient, sometimes embittered, frequently apathetic, and often with a dominating parent.' Examples are a young man who since his urinary diversion has not had the courage to go back to work and stays at home to do the housework while his mother works'; and a young woman 'who is doubly incontinent, has not been persuaded to have a diversion, has never worked, and rarely goes out though she is pretty and intelligent'. Few of this group know how to get what help is available and many state emphatically that they do not wish to join groups of disabled people.

The present position of school-leavers and adults with spina bifida

Information about what actually happens to school-leavers with spina bifida is available from only a few studies. The Association for Spina Bifida and Hydrocephalus is carrying out a survey (1976) of young people with spina bifida aged from 16 to 24 years who attended the spina bifida Combined Clinic at the Children's Hospital, Sheffield, while data is also available from Dorner's study (1975) about the placement of those who had left school. It must be remembered that these young people were all born before 1960, that is, before modern methods of surgical treatment had been introduced, so that they tend to be a less disabled group than those leaving school now. Comparatively few of the leavers in Dorner's study, for instance, had valves.

The findings from these studies are summarized in Table 10.1 below: what is particularly striking is that about one in four of the young people in each study had no employment or occupation outside the home (although in a minority of cases this was from choice).

Table 10.1 *Placement of leavers with spina bifida (From Dorner 1975 and ASBAH 1976)*

<table>
<tr><th></th><th colspan="2">ASBAH Survey</th><th colspan="2">Dorner's Study</th></tr>
<tr><th>Type of placement</th><th>N</th><th>%</th><th>N</th><th>%</th></tr>
<tr><td>Open employment</td><td>17</td><td>20·4</td><td>13</td><td>39·4</td></tr>
<tr><td>Full-time FE/Training</td><td>13</td><td>15·7</td><td>7</td><td>21·2</td></tr>
<tr><td>Sheltered employment</td><td>14</td><td>16·9</td><td rowspan="2">5</td><td rowspan="2">15·2</td></tr>
<tr><td>Day centres</td><td>17</td><td>20·4</td></tr>
<tr><td>Not working</td><td>22*</td><td>26·5</td><td>8</td><td>24·2</td></tr>
<tr><td>Total</td><td>83</td><td>100·0</td><td>33</td><td>100·0</td></tr>
</table>

* Four of these were not working because of illness.

The only other relevant findings are for adults with spina bifida cystica, although they comprise a somewhat different population from today's spina bifida school-leavers, both as regards the nature of their handicaps and their school and training experiences. A smaller proportion of them are severely disabled and have hydrocephalus than is true of today's teenagers, while a larger proportion than would probably be true today lacked both an adequate education (many only had home tuition) and any sort of vocational training.

The larger of the two studies which have been published (Evans *et al.*, 1974) was of 202 adults with spina bifida cystica who had attended the Hospital for Sick Children, Great Ormond Street, before 1954. Nearly half of them (mostly with uncomplicated meningocele) had no serious disability and were leading normal lives but there were 47 men and 58 women with a serious disability. Of these men about one-half were working regularly but one-third had never worked at all, while of the women one-half worked regularly or were active housewives but about a quarter had never worked at all. Details are shown in Table 10.2 below.

Table 10.2 *Occupations of spina bifida adults with a serious disabililty (From Evans et al., 1974).*

	Men	*Women*
Office worker (secretary, typist, clerk)	14 } 24	14 } 19
Other jobs	10 }	5 }
Full-time students	5	—
Active housewife	—	13
Sheltered workshop	3	—
Off sick	1	4
Unemployed	14	22

Although many of those who were working regularly had had initial difficulties in getting work, once it was obtained they found employers and co-workers mostly sympathetic and helpful. Office work provided the most frequent occupation and the authors comment that 'though the qualifications for entry are high, the civil service, banks and local authorities seem able to look after disabled workers particularly well'.

In the other study (Beresford and Laurence, 1975) the present placement of 51 adults living in South Wales was investigated. Of particular interest was the placement of 20 people with 'moderate' handicaps (walking with aids and partially continent or continent only after operation) and 16 with 'severe' handicaps (i.e. chairbound, and/or totally incontinent). 16 of the 20 with moderate handicaps were in 'normal occupations' (14 in open employment and 2 housewives) and 8 of the 16 with severe handicaps (6 in open employment, 1 housewife and 1 full-time student) and as in the Evans *et al.* study half of those employed were in office jobs.

A few important points emerge from these studies. Firstly, it is encouraging to see that about half of those with moderate or severe handicaps are coping well in open employment in spite of, in many cases, an inadequate education and an absence of vocational training.

Secondly, these studies indicate that 'office work' of some kind may offer reasonably good prospects for employment to many of those without severe hydrocephalus. It can, of course, be very dangerous to think of one kind of work as being particularly 'suited' to a person with a particular disability as this may mean that only lukewarm attempts are made to discover what a particular teenager really wants to do and has the potential to do. At the same time, it would be foolish to ignore the fact that this is a potentially important area of employment. The Training Services Agency has recently published an interesting discussion paper on vocational preparation for young non-handicapped people (1975) in which the point is made that the provision for specific training for clerical or commercial work is still very limited. The basic skills required (literacy and numeracy) are developed at school, while 'teaching in the more specifically clerical and commercial skills such as shorthand, typing, and book-keeping is also provided in the education system'. However, little training is available in other skills required 'like those involving interaction with people (customers and colleagues), knowledge of matters dealt with, efficient use of the telephone, etc.' it is suggested that one reason for the lack of clerical training is 'the common practice in offices of dividing up the work to be done into its component parts, to the point where it requires little ability and consequently minimal training. The work thereby becomes less demanding – and, for many, less satisfying.'

As Mary Greaves points out (1972), it is assumed too often that if a disabled person has a job all is well, while 'the fact that the disabled person is limited in his choice of work is too easily overlooked'. The better the initial training the more likely it is that a young adult with spina bifida will have both some degree of choice in the kind of office jobs he or she does and also greater and more varied responsibilities within that job.

A third point arising from these surveys is that quite a substantial number (15 per cent in the Evans *et al.* study, 1974) had frequent periods of unemployment. Mary Greaves (1972) commenting on the Buckle report (1971) emphasizes the 'striking' correlation between unemployment and lack of qualifications, by far the largest proportion of those who were unemployed having no qualifications or skills.

The final extremely important point to come from the spina bifida surveys is that a large number of adults with moderate or severe disability had never been employed. In the Evans *et al.*, study (1974), for example, about one-third of this group had never been employed and 'will never be able to lead independent lives in the sense of being able to be both financially self-supporting and able to care for their own physical needs'. The proportion of young spina bifida adults falling into this category is likely to increase as larger numbers with severe handicaps leave the schools and for them the question of sheltered employment and or diversionary provision has to be raised. Mary Greaves (1972) makes the point that sheltered work is often boring and poorly paid (because the workshops are competing in the open market for work), and goes on to raise questions which have considerable relevance for many severely handicapped spina bifida leavers as well as for those disabled in other ways. For example, should occupation centres, which are divorced from any pretence at productivity and are largely remedial, be extended? Should firms be encouraged through incentives to employ some of those now placed in sheltered workshops? Is every use being made of the available aids and appliances? Should we be more imaginative in our training?

4 Preparation for school-leaving

Two important aspects of this question are considered here. The first can be described as 'preparation for work', that is, all the things that can be done while a teenager is still at school to maximize his chances of finding a satisfactory placement (whether in employment or in further education or vocational training) as soon as possible after he leaves. The second is 'education for living': this has already been touched on in the previous chapter but also needs to be looked at in the context of school-leaving.

(i) *Preparation for work*

If they are to settle successfully in employment all young people need adequate information and guidance about the possibilities open to them and also some understanding of what life at work will be like. For a handicapped teenager the transition from school to work is likely to be particularly stressful, especially if he has come from the protective environment of a special school. Often too, before a placement is made the leaver has a long period of waiting at home during which he may become increasingly despondent and less motivated to do anything outside his home. At the time of writing many non-handicapped leavers are experiencing a similar situation.

Whether or not the leaver finds a suitable placement depends very much on what is done before he leaves school. At this stage the key people are the handicapped pupil himself, his parents, certain members of the school staff (usually the careers teacher, if there is one, the Head and the class teacher) and the local authority careers officer. In some districts there is now a specialist careers officer with responsibility for the handicapped. All these people may be involved in the preparation for school-leaving although their roles will be different. The careers officers, and particularly the specialist ones, have been trained in giving vocational guidance, know what is available in further education and employment and act as consultants to careers teachers. The careers teacher will be primarily concerned in giving the pupils information about the different openings available and in collecting together the school reports and other information required by the careers officer. However, many special schools do not have careers teachers, while those in ordinary schools may not be well equipped to help a handicapped pupil.

Many secondary schools now provide specific careers education for pupils in their third year at secondary school. This can include group discussions, outside speakers and films. Some schools also arrange visits to places of work or to colleges of further education under such schemes as work observation courses, work experience courses or linked courses. Work observation courses involve visits to employers' premises, the purpose being more to help familiarize pupils with working life rather than as a guide in making career choices. Work experience courses, in which the pupil actually gets some experience of work (e.g. one day a week) while still at school, are less common as they raise problems of organization and supervision but some have been arranged, both by special and ordinary schools (e.g. Holland and Paine, 1975). Linked courses enable young people at school to spend time at a college of further education and give them some insight into the work environment and the range of occupations open to them on leaving school, thus easing the transition from school to work and there has been a considerable development of such courses both in ordinary and special schools.

Improvements of this kind have, however, been very uneven: in the case of ordinary schools it was pointed out in a recent DES survey

(1973) that for pupils aged 14 plus less than half the schools provided careers education for all pupils and 28 per cent did not provide it at all.

Whatever the situation within a particular ordinary school, it is suggested by ASBAH (1975) 'that the careers officer's attention should be drawn to the needs of handicapped pupils about a year earlier than those of the rest of the class'. There are a number of good reasons for doing this. The careers officer may want to meet the pupil and also his parents several times to discuss his work aspirations; if group visits are being arranged to places of employment special preparation may have to be made regarding access to and within the buildings for the handicapped pupil. Wherever possible the handicapped pupil should participate in the existing preparation programme in an ordinary school and make as wide-ranging visits as possible. Inevitably this will mean that a severely handicapped pupil will meet situations which will be discouraging, for example places where part of the building is inaccessible to him. While he should not be protected from such experiences he must not be left with the impression that there is no place for him in the world of employment and the careers officer should discuss constructively with him and his parents the sort of work he can or might be able to do or the ways in which problems he has encountered can be overcome.'

In special schools a careers education department is likely to be much more geared to the needs of individual pupils. It may include information about and visits to sheltered workshops, employment rehabilitation units and day centres as well as to places of open employment, with generally, only two or three pupils going on each visit. There is a danger that visits made by special-school pupils are so carefully planned and the places visited so carefully selected that these pupils get a less realistic view of the employment world than those from ordinary schools, and again it is important that the pupil has the opportunity to visit a wide variety of places, not just the type of place (e.g. sheltered workshop) where it is thought a particular pupil is most likely eventually to settle. Conversely, it is also sometimes the case, as is pointed out in the Scottish Report (1975), 'that some potential students (i.e. in further education) are not aware of the opportunities that are open to them. It may be that they or their advisers feel that the challenge would be too great. *We recommend*, therefore, that all physically handicapped pupils in special schools should have their attention drawn to the type of courses which their abilities would enable them to pursue in further education. *We would also recommend* that the special schools should take steps towards more formal liaison with further education colleges.'

The careers officer's main function is to act as co-ordinating agent between school and employment or other settlement, before, during and after further education. Before he can give any vocational guidance he will need to know as much as possible about a particular pupil and should try to meet the school's careers teacher as well as obtaining written information from him. For spina bifida pupils at ordinary schools he will probably also need more detailed medical and psychological reports than those usually provided for leavers. Problems of co-ordination may arise for pupils in residential schools; normally the local careers officer sends all the relevant information to his colleagues in the home area so that the leaver can be interviewed at home in the holidays with his parents, when the recommendations made by the school and careers service can be reviewed in the light of the employment opportunities available in the home area.

Whether the leaver is attending an ordinary school or a day or residential special school it is essential that these preparations should begin early on, preferably at the beginning of the third year of his secondary school life, particularly since, as is pointed out in the 1975 ASBAH booklet, 'it takes a careers officer some considerable time to get to know a handicapped pupil, to assess his abilities and personality as well as the practical effects of his disabilities, and to win his confidence and that of his parents'.

A recent inquiry carried out by Queen Elizabeth's Foundation for the Disabled suggested that many problems arise for disabled leavers because the assessment of the leaver's potential had been inadequate. This meant that pupils were often directed into unsuitable courses of training or employment in which they either failed to succeed or failed in the long run to realize their full potential. Whichever is the case, the result is similar: disappointment and frustration. As a result of this inquiry a multi-disciplinary centre for the total assessment of physically handicapped school-leavers was set up at Banstead Place, Surrey, in 1974. It has to be recognized that for many pupils the decisions about placement made at school-leaving age will not and should not be a final one and that further assessment within the place of work or in a training or further education establishment will be needed.

(ii) *Education for living*

A school's responsibilities towards its leavers does not lie simply in working closely with the specialist careers officer. Schools can do a great deal more to prepare their pupils, on the lines suggested in *Living with Handicap* (Younghusband *et al.*, 1970) where it was recommended that 'the school curriculum, especially in the last years, should give due consideration to the need for preparation for life after school, particularly personal independence, social relationships and pre-work experience'.

In the previous chapter some of the ways in which the school could help the teenagers towards personal independence and in their social relationships were discussed. Other aspects of 'education for living' which will clearly affect a leaver's employability are the extent to which education in personal hygiene and self-care have been given. In the case of spina bifida teenagers, for example, toilet management will be of crucial importance; also, since paraplegic individuals are prone to pressure sores, it is essential that the child should learn to move regularly in order to change the points of maximum pressure, and the relevance of establishing regular habits of these kinds to later employability needs to be discussed with the teenager. In the Scottish Report it is suggested that another function of the school is, as part of the curriculum, to give each pupil a sound knowledge of the aids and equipment which are available to him as an adult and also exactly how to obtain these so that he will be able to assess in a realistic way the extent to which he can achieve independence at home, at work and in travelling to work. This means that he will need to be given information about organizations such as the Disabled Living Foundation, the Disablement Income Group and others (see Appendix I). As mentioned earlier, teenagers also need to be taught while still at school about the services available under the Chronically Sick and Disabled Persons Act, about the Attendance and Mobility Allowances and about how to claim benefits for themselves. This is something which could be done in special schools in a civic studies course. However, the close co-operation of the social worker would be needed in planning such courses, since teachers are unlikely to know in detail exactly what is available. It would also be important for the teacher involved in such a course or, if there is one, the social worker to explain to parents the importance of teaching teenagers about these facilities and of encouraging them to assume as much responsibility as possible themselves for claiming and using them.

It is often assumed that these different aspects of education for living will be part of the curriculum of a special school – in fact this is not usually the case. The Scottish Committee in their visits to schools for the handicapped found only one school in which education for living was an established part of the curriculum and recommended that much more should be done in this area.

Another major area in which schools could do more to prepare for life after school is in the use of leisure. For non-handicapped people the amount of time available for leisure is increasing. For the handicapped, especially for those with severe handicaps whose employment prospects are poor, or whose jobs may be particularly monotonous, as well as for many others who may have long periods of unemployment, leisure activities will be even more important. They will serve to equip handicapped pupils with similar skills to the non-handicapped, thus making social contacts on an equal basis easier to achieve.

In many special schools clubs of various kinds and after-school activities are encouraged, but often these spring up in rather an *ad hoc* way. While this is not necessarily a bad thing, more thought is needed about what sorts of leisure activities are, for a particular group of children, likely to be enjoyed and continued in adult life. For example, more attention could be paid to music education for children with spina bifida, some of whom could become competent performers on a variety of instruments and most of whom count listening to music among their leisure-time interests. Sporting activities, including swimming, can be very important after school, both in providing opportunities for mixing with the non-handicapped and also because obesity is often an increasingly great problem for those who have left school.

Disabled teenagers often do not know where or how they can continue with leisure-time interests after leaving school. Perhaps part of the final year curriculum could involve project work in which, under the teacher's guidance, and where possible with his family's help, the leaver could find out what leisure-time pursuits, recreational facilities and clubs are available in his home neighbourhood.

5 Follow-up and supportive services for those who have left school

Surveys of handicapped leavers suggest that too often the months or years immediately after leaving school constitute a period of great uncertainty for a young handicapped person. He may be in and out of jobs, he may wait months for plans for training or further education to be finalized, or he may have finished his training but be unable to find employment; if he has a job he may, like many of his non-handicapped peers, have great difficulty in adapting to working life and in understanding and accepting the discipline of the work-place. These problems are becoming increasingly common among non-handicapped young people; for the handicapped person, they are likely to be very much harder to cope with, not only because he may have spent most of his life in the sheltered highly supportive environment of the special school, but also he is unlikely to have friends in his neighbourhood facing similar problems with whom he can share his anxieties. He may rapidly become isolated at home, frustrated and bitter. The situation will also have changed regarding his medical supervision: in theory he is no longer the responsibility of the pædiatric department but it is often not clear who is responsible for his medical supervision. Evans *et al.* (1974), for example, found that some of the adults with spina bifida in their study who had had urinary diversions in childhood had had no hospital treatment as adults and that the doubly incontinent needed more expert help than they were at present getting.

It would thus seem essential that the leaver should have available to him follow-up service in three main areas: firstly, with the practicalities of finding a placement, whether this is for training or education or in employment as well as in settling in, secondly, continuing help both as regards his welfare needs (accommodation, transport, etc.) and his emotional needs, and, thirdly, continuing medical supervision.

A major problem is that it is often almost impossible to identify exactly who has responsibility for a particular leaver since after leaving school handicapped young people may, depending on their situation, be either the responsibility of the LEA or the social services department, or the Employment Services Agency or a voluntary agency.

It is suggested here that three people should play key roles. Firstly, in every special school a member of staff should be appointed to follow up the leavers. This could be a special member of staff or one of the teachers of the leavers' class. There would be two main benefits from such a system. The leaver himself and his parents would know they had a continuing link with the school and that there was someone there whom they could approach if difficulties about placement arose and if no one else seemed to be able to help. The school would get extremely valuable feedback about what happened to each leaver which could be used in planning the curriculum.

Secondly, each leaver and his family should in the two years prior to school-leaving build up a close contact with the local careers officer, preferably a careers officer specialized in the placement of handicapped leavers. The careers officer should be recognized as the co-ordinator in the team involved in any placement decision. His responsibility will not only include seeing that the young person is appropriately placed immediately after leaving school but also ensuring that he finds a suitable placement after a period of further education and training. In cases where a young person is not thought to be employable and therefore becomes the responsibility of the Department of Social Services rather than the Employment Services Agency, it is the careers officer who should take the responsibility for effecting the change-over and making quite sure that the social services department is aware that the change-over has been made.

Thirdly, each leaver should have an identified local social worker (this was recommended in the Tuckey Report) whose function should be to work closely with the careers officer in ensuring that the total welfare and emotional needs of the young person were being met. Some special schools have social workers attached. While they may be able to give valuable help before the young person leaves school, they should, before he leaves, hand over responsibility to his local social worker if this has not already been done.

Most of the problems which have been discussed here are problems which will be faced, although usually in a less acute form, by a great many non-handicapped leavers. It is not only disabled leavers, for example, who 'want employment but are unaware of the discipline, speed and sustained effort demanded by most jobs' (Ingram *et al.*, 1964, writing of cerebral-palsied leavers). Disabled and able-bodied leavers alike face the prospect of jobs which are repetitive and boring with no prospects of developing into anything more interesting. For both groups careers education and careers guidance is often quite inadequate and for both the facilities for vocational training 'are profoundly unsatisfactory' (TSA, 1975). Young people from ordinary as well as from special schools leave school without an adequate grasp of the skills of literacy and numeracy, but resist a return to an educational environment which they associate with school. Improvements in induction training in a new job are needed by all young people. Disabled and able-bodied leavers alike may become embittered by long periods of unemployment. That these problems do exist for many able-bodied leavers is made very clear in the Training Services Agency's recent paper on vocational training (1975) and their proposals for improving this situation are of great relevance to many disabled leavers.

References

ASBAH (1975), 'Survey of young people with spina bifida', unpublished report from the Education Training and Employment Officer, ASBAH, London.

Beresford, A. and Laurence, M. (1975), 'Work and spina bifida', *New Society*, 32, pp. 75–6.

Buckle, J. (1971), 'Work and housing of impaired persons in Great Britain', Part II of *Handicapped and Impaired in Great Britain*, HMSO, London.

Department of Education and Science (1973), *Careers Education in Ordinary Schools*, DES Survey, 18, HMSO, London.

Dorner, S. (1975), 'The relationship of physical handicap to stress in families with an adolescent with spina bifida', *Developmental Medicine and Child Neurology*, 17 (6), pp. 765–6.

——, (1976), 'Adolescents with spina bifida – how they see their situation', *Archives of Diseases in Childhood*, 51, pp. 439–44.

Evans, K., Hickman, V. and Carter, C. O. (1974), 'Handicap and social status of adults with spina bifida cystica', *British Journal of Preventive and Social Medicine*, 28, pp. 85–92.

Glanville, R. A. (1974), 'The education, training and employment of the handicapped school leaver', unpublished M.Ed. thesis, University of Reading.

Greaves, M. (1972), 'Employment of disabled people, *British Hospital Journal and Social Services Review*, 15 January 1972, pp. 135–6.

Holland, P. and Paine, I. (1975), 'Experimenting with Trident', *Special Education*, 2 (4), pp. 21–2.

Hutchinson, D. and Clegg, N. (1975), 'Orientated towards work'. *Special Education*, 2 (1), pp. 22–5.

Ingram, T. T. S., Jameson, S., Errington, J. and Mitchell, R. G. (1964), *Living with Cerebral Palsy*, Clinics in Developmental Medicine, 14, Spastics Society/Heinemann, London.

Johnston-Smith, P. (1975), personal communication.

Large, P. (1974), 'Outdoor mobility: the situation today', *Physiotherapy*, 8, pp. 264–7.

Lowe, P. B. (1973), 'Two years at Hereward College', *Special Education*, 62 (3), pp. 12–14.

Morgan, M. (1972), 'Like other school-leavers', paper read at 31st National Bienniel Conference Course of the Association for Special Education held at Cardiff, July 1972.

——, (1975), 'Follow-up studies of the Spastics Society's school-leavers; 1966–1973', unpublished report obtainable from the Spastics Society, London.

Parsons, J. (1972), 'Assessment of aptitudes in young people of school-leaving age handicapped by hydrocephalus and spina bifida cystica', *Developmental Medicine and Child Neurology*, 27, pp. 101–8.

Sanders, L. and Watson, P. (1975), 'Pioneering at Park Lane', *Special Education*, 2 (4), pp. 14–16.

Scottish Education Department (1975), *The Secondary Education of Physically Handicapped Children in Scotland*, HMSO, Edinburgh.

Training Services Agency (1975), 'Vocational preparation for young people', a discussion paper, TSA, London.

Tuckey, L., Parfit, J. and Tuckey, B. (1973), *Handicapped School Leavers*, NFER, Windsor, Berks.

Younghusband, E., Birchall, D., Davie, R. and Kellmer Pringle, M. L. (eds.) (1970), *Living with Handicap*, National Bureau for Co-operation in Child Care, London.

Main findings and conclusions

Our aim in this short concluding section has been to summarize the research findings which are of particular relevance to all those working with spina bifida children and their families and to consider their implications for policy and individual practice. We felt that it would be useful to focus on the main problems at each of three stages: the pre-school years, the school years (pre-adolescent) and in adolescence. At each of these stages we have asked a number of questions which we felt to be particularly crucial, and our findings and conclusions are presented in the form of answers to these questions.

Pre-school years

1 *What sort of help is needed by families with spina bifida children and how could services to them be improved?*

Research with families with spina bifida children suggests that three main kinds of needs can be distinguished. These are, firstly, the need for information, secondly the need for advice and practical help with problems arising from the day-to-day management of the child and, thirdly, advice and support over psychological and emotional problems which may arise within the family.

The need of the parents for information and explanations is present throughout the child's life but particularly immediately after the birth of the handicapped child, when mothers often feel the diagnosis was insufficiently explained; during the weeks following the birth when the mother is often separated from the child; in the period when the mother first goes home with the baby and needs information about how to handle him and also how to tell when he is seriously ill; at all times when treatment or operative procedures are being decided on; and after operations, when advice is needed about the management of the child at home. Genetic counselling is also needed early on. At present problems arise both because the mother does not always get sufficient information, and because she does not understand fully the explanations she has been given. The situation arising after the birth of a handicapped child could be improved if a service were set up in all maternity units to ensure that the staff had been taught how to treat the parents when this situation arose, and that an adequate follow-up service was available to the mother when she and the baby left hospital, and in this context a specialist health visitor could play a particularly crucial role.

The second main need is for help and support over daily management problems. The parents, especially the mother, are faced by many physical (and often financial) strains caused, for example, by dealing with incontinence, using and maintaining appliances, lifting, transport and frequent hospital appointments. Regular support and advice is needed from hospital-based staff, health visitors and social workers, on how to minimize the problems and utilize those statutory resources which are available. Again it is suggested that this could best be achieved through the appointment of one or two health visitors in each district specializing in the care of multiply handicapped (including spina bifida) children working in close liaison with the local social workers and the hospital.

Thirdly, rearing a handicapped child often gives rise to emotional and psychological strain affecting the mother in particular but also in many cases the father and the siblings. Caring for a child continuously without relief is a source of strain – the parents may rarely be able to go out together or to take the other children out much; resentment and anxieties on the part of the siblings may occur; the mother may need advice about her relationship with the child. These problems also frequently arise for families with mildly handicapped children. The help of a social worker or counsellor should routinely be made available, especially in the early stages. In particular, the involvement of the father in the child's care should be actively fostered. Contacts with other parents in a similar situation can also be very helpful and one-to-one contacts as well as more formal discussion groups should be arranged for those parents who wish it.

2. *What can be done by the parents in the home to foster the intellectual and physical development of spina bifida children in the pre-school years?*

Two main points must be emphasized. The first is the importance of the pre-school years for the intellectual as well as the motor development of handicapped and non-handicapped children alike. Secondly, although clinicians can do a great deal for the child in the period, greater emphasis needs to be placed on the role of the parents in fostering the child's development, and professionals should pay more attention to helping parents to help the child.

Two kinds of factors may retard the development of the young spina bifida child first his physical, and in many cases intellectual impairments, and second environmental factors. Impairment of mobility is often severe: the child may have poor standing, walking and sitting balance; ocular problems, particularly squint, are common; and hand function may be impaired, especially if he has hydrocephalus. While verbal ability (apart from comprehension) may be relatively normal, perceptual and eye-hand co-ordination skills are likely to be poor. Behavioural problems, in particular distractability and passivity, may be additional problems. The child's environment may be more restricted than a normal child's so that he does not receive the same amount of stimulation. He may spend long periods on his back at home or in hospital, he may be unable to explore; his parents may find it difficult to take him out of the house. Also the environment may provide the wrong kind of stimulation, for example toys which are too difficult for him because of perceptual or motor problems.

Parents can do much to reduce these problems if they are taught to develop the following skills: (1) an understanding of normal development, (2) an understanding of their own individual child's particular problems (and this will involve teaching them to use observational techniques so that they can monitor the child's progress), (3) information about what to do both to prevent deprivation of normal experience and to provide appropriate extra experiences in those areas where his skills are poorest. Advice will also be needed about how to handle problems of distractability and passivity. Parents will need to be taught about the value of play and how to help their children to play, as well as specific advice about the kinds of play and toys needed to promote, for example, visual awareness, tactile awareness and body skills and eye–hand co-ordination.

The ideal person to give such help is an occupational therapist or psychologist, although a health visitor with special training working with these professionals could be of great help. However, the general principle is that those with the relevant expertise (who will usually be hospital-based) should place much greater emphasis on helping parents to help their children. This will pay dividends not only in terms of the handicapped child's development but in the parent's self-confidence, and will also benefit the other children in the family.

3 *What has been the experience of mothers of spina bifida children regarding pre-school education and what improvements are needed?*

Today the value of pre-school education for handicapped children is widely recognized. Mothers of spina bifida children who have attended pre-school facilities of various kinds generally report many advantages, including gains in sociability and the development of social skills, gains in emotional development, progress in motor development, an increase in the child's overall ability to play, in some cases, where specific training is given, intellectual gains, and, overall, a general preparedness for entry to school. Mothers themselves benefit from the support given by the nursery and feel less isolated: they get some relief from the constant care of the child and they gain a better understanding of the child and how to help him.

Problems are of two main kinds. Firstly, in many parts of the country there is still not sufficient provision, although the situation has improved greatly over the past decade and in some parts of the country most mothers are able to obtain pre-school placement for their children. Secondly, a great deal remains to be done to ensure that the pre-school facilities which are available really meet the needs of the child. Some spina bifida children are placed, at least initially, in special groups or classes set up for handicapped children although even there may not get any specific training. However, while a minority of children may need this specialized environment many pre-school spina bifida children can benefit from placement in an ordinary playgroup and from the contact with and stimulation of their normal peers which this offers, provided information, support and advice from hospital-based and other specialized staff is made available to the playgroup staff. At present such information and support is usually lacking. Improvements are badly needed on two fronts. Firstly, those working in pre-school facilities of different kinds need more training in the care of handicapped children. Secondly, better back-up services from advisory teachers and psychologists must be made available to the staff of ordinary pre-school facilities. Extra helpers may also be needed. While individual initiatives (e.g. the building up by a hospital-based playgroup of contacts with local community groups) can be extremely helpful, what is needed in the long term is a systematically planned liaison between the local education authority the health district and the social services department in providing early help of all kinds for handicapped children.

School-age children

4 *What is known about the intellectual development of children with spina bifida and hydrocephalus?*

Spina bifida children do not have a normal distribution of intelligence: instead their scores are skewed to the lower end of the IQ range with a peak of scores in the low average and backward range. There are marked differences between the intelligence levels of children with and without hydrocephalus. Children with spina bifida only are usually within the normal range of intelligence, while those with only a mild degree of hydrocephalus which arrested spontaneously and did not require the insertion of a valve tend to be slightly below average. However children with hydrocephalus requiring shunt treatment generally have IQs in the range of 70–90, although some will be of normal or even superior intelligence and some severely retarded.

Where there is intellectual impairment, all areas of functioning are not equally impaired, and performance ability tends to be poorer than verbal ability. Spina bifida children appear to have fairly good verbal skills, particularly as regards the acquisition of vocabulary and the development of syntax. However, their comprehension of language tends to be below average. About 20 per cent of spina bifida children show markedly hyperverbal behaviour. Although superficially fluent, their comprehension of language is often very poor and the content of what they say inappropriate and even bizarre.

The main intellectual impairments of spina bifida children, especially those with hydrocephalus, are in perceptual and visuo-motor skills. Distinguishing figure from background is difficult for many, and the children tend to be slower than normal in other perceptual tasks. Impairment on tasks requiring eye–hand co-ordination ability is evident from an early age: poor hand function is partly responsible but the children almost certainly also have impaired ability in planning and organizing their movements in space.

5 *What are the main problems arising in connection with school placement and how could the present situation be improved?*

Parents often receive inadequate help and support in finding the right placement for their child. They may not be informed early enough (if at all) of what the procedures for assessment for schooling will be, are rarely given full information about the different possibilities open to the child and a chance to visit possible special or ordinary schools, and, although the situation is now changing, often feel that they have not been sufficiently consulted. Teachers also need to try especially hard to keep in close touch with parents throughout the child's school career.

Teachers themselves, particularly those in ordinary schools, have not in the past been consulted fully enough or given enough information about the child's handicaps. Now that new assessment procedures involving the parents, psychologists, teachers and doctors are being used in many areas, the situation should improve, and the recent emphasis on the need for annual reviews of the suitability of a particular placement should also be helpful. Even so, final decisions about placement (and even then it may be for 'a trial period') should not be taken until all those involved at the grass roots level – i.e. parents, child (if old enough), head and class teacher of the receiving school – have been fully consulted, and provided with relevant information. It may also be useful to provide the non-handicapped children with information appropriate to their age about a handicapped child who is joining an ordinary class. Careful advance planning is needed at transition points in the child's education (e.g. at the move from primary to secondary school) and information must be passed from one school to another.

The decision about the type of placement most appropriate is difficult, ordinary school placement usually being favoured by disabled people themselves and by parents. Before a decision can be made the child's special educational, physical and social needs at that particular age must be diagnosed and understood clearly by all those involved, and the different possibilities in that particular area considered in the light of these needs. Incontinence coupled with restricted mobility should not preclude ordinary school placement. Decisions are more difficult in the case of children with severe physical handicaps (although provided that ancillary help and physiotherapy is made available such children can do well in ordinary schools), and most difficult of all in the case of children handicapped both physically and intellectually and thus likely to require not only special physical assistance but also special teaching help. While special school placement may seem appropriate for the latter group, the possibility of making special provision available in an ordinary school must always be considered, since the child has much to gain socially and educationally from such a placement.

There is a clear need for more special provision (in the form, for example, of special classes or specially staffed resource centres) to be made available for groups of handicapped children within ordinary schools. In addition everything possible needs to be done to foster closer links between special and ordinary schools to ensure that children in segregated schooling are not socially isolated.

6 *What kinds of learning difficulties do spina bifida children have and how can their teachers best help?*

By no means all spina bifida children have specific learning difficulties, and many children without hydrocephalus or with only a mild degree of hydrocephalus can cope intellectually with ordinary class placement. Often however, these children are retarded in their attainments. The reasons for this may include hospitalization, or the existence of emotional problems, and sometimes lowered expectations on the part of parents and teachers.

The group most likely to have learning difficulties are those with spina bifida and hydrocephalus controlled by a shunt, particularly those with IQs below 80. They may be slow in learning to read: even if they become reasonably fluent readers their comprehension may be poor. Number work is likely to cause more problems than reading: the factors contributing to this include deprivation of experience in the pre-school years and the existence of perceptual, visuo-motor and motor problems. As a result of neurological impairment writing will also be difficult for most hydrocephalic children: they will tend to be slow writers and the quality of writing will be poor. Many, too, will be left-handers or slow to develop a preference. A spina bifida child needs to be taught systematically how to write and consistent use of one hand should be encouraged from an early age.

All sensitive and competent teachers whether or not they have had special training can do much to help these children if they are given relevant information about the child and about those areas in which he is likely to have particular problems. Early identification of children having trouble is crucial and should be followed by a specific plan of remediation, with individual teaching or teaching in small groups being given whenever possible, even if only for a short time each day. The problem of distractability must be tackled by teachers early on and it is also important to see that the child is well-motivated. If the child's difficulties are not severe an experienced teacher may be able to give the child all the help needed but teachers should not hesitate to ask for specialized advice and help, if necessary from outside the school. In particular the teacher of a child who is likely to have marked learning problems should know from the outset exactly whom she can turn to for help, whether this is the school psychological service, a local special school, or an adviser for special education. What is crucial is not so much where the child is (special school, special class, regular class) as whether an assessment of his difficulties is linked to an appropriate programme of work.

We wish to emphasize most strongly the need for providing teachers with back-up services early on, rather than postponing this until the child is clearly failing. As more spina bifida children – and other learning-disabled children – are placed in ordinary schools it is becoming increasingly important for a greater part of a teacher's initial training to cover the question of handicap, and there is also a need for opportunities for in-service training to be made available to teachers.

7 *What sorts of behavioural, emotional and social problems are children with spina bifida likely to have?*

Overall, we ourselves have not found a higher incidence of behaviour disorders in spina bifida children without hydrocephalus than in non-handicapped children of primary school age. The evidence from other studies, however, is that children with a physical disability coupled with neurological impairment are more 'at risk' of becoming disturbed than children without such impairment, and this is likely to be true of spina bifida children with hydrocephalus, particularly those of low ability.

Certain specific behavioural problems do, however, seem to be fairly common in spina bifida children, one of these being distractability which can affect the child's development in the pre-school years as well as school attainments. All adults and in particular parents and teachers must be made aware of the problem and taught how to inhibit inattentive behaviour and to reinforce the child for concentrating: behaviour modification techniques have a great deal to offer here. Passivity and lack of drive is also often a problem and adults need to try to give the child the sort of activities from an early age which are meaningful to him, and which he can cope with physically and intellectually.

Fearfulness and anxiety are quite common in spina bifida children; in contrast anti-social behaviour seems relatively infrequent. Anxieties may arise because of the child's uncertainty about how he will cope with a particular situation, and much encouragement as well as clear explanations about exactly what a new situation will involve may be needed. The children also need opportunities to express their anxieties to adults.

Research findings suggest that on the whole spina bifida children get on well with their peers both in special and in ordinary schools. Incontinence does not usually give rise to major social problems in school provided that proper arrangements are made for its management and for ensuring the child toileting privacy wherever he is placed, although children are extremely sensitive about this problem. More research is needed about how to help adolescents in particular in coming to terms with this problem.

Some spina bifida children, especially those who have not attended pre-school groups and have remained very dependent on their mothers are immature socially, and teachers need to help such children to acquire those social skills which will make them acceptable as friends. Children attending special schools in particular need as many opportunities as possible to mix with their non-handicapped peers.

Adolescence

8 *What sorts of emotional and social problems do teenagers with spina bifida face?*

There is still a comparative absence of research into the needs of severely handicapped adolescents, especially those with spina bifida but what evidence there is shows that they do have severe problems, three of which appear outstanding. Firstly, there are the difficulties which young people with spina bifida have in becoming psychologically independent of their parents and other adults, secondly, the high incidence of depression in this group, and thirdly, the problem of social isolation, these last two problems probably being closely related.

Many teenagers are still heavily dependent physically upon their mothers, or, if they are in residential schools, upon other adults, and many resent this. In some cases physical dependence is inevitable but often more can be done earlier on to teach children greater physical independence especially in incontinence management. Certainly psychological independence could be fostered more than it is at present. The mother's attitude seems to be crucial and it is suggested that parents are given more systematic advice, starting as early on as possible, about the need to encourage their children to be responsible and to make their own decisions. The chance to discuss this question with other parents would also be helpful.

Research suggests that there is a very high incidence of depression in spina bifida teenagers particularly among girls. These feelings are often unexpressed and withheld from parents and other adults, and few teenagers seem to be getting any help, even when severely depressed. Many factors contribute to feelings of depression including anxieties of all kinds about the future but one which is outstanding, and where a great deal more could be done to help, is the fact that outside school hours these teenagers are often very isolated socially, substantial numbers having no contact at all with their peers. That is particularly true of those who are attending or have attended special schools partly because they tend, anyway, to be more severely handicapped and so less mobile. There is a striking association in fact between social isolation and mobility problems. However, even teenagers who are more mobile sometimes have few social contacts. This seems to be particularly true of boys who need to rely on urinary appliances, and clearly feelings of personal insecurity, shame and uncertainty about how to explain the handicap to non-handicapped peers, especially to those of the opposite sex, contribute to the isolation, loneliness and depression of these teenagers.

9 *What can be done to help teenagers with spina bifida to cope with their social and emotional problems?*

There are two main ways in which the problems outlined in the previous section can be approached. Firstly, many practical measures can be taken which will reduce the isolation of teenagers. Secondly, teenagers need help in dealing with their feelings about being handicapped, including anxieties about their sexual development and the likelihood of their being able to become parents.

Practical measures include first the question of access. Many spina bifida teenagers could attend ordinary comprehensive schools either full-time or part-time for certain activities were comprehensive schools more accessible and this also applies to colleges of further education and to many other ordinary facilities such as youth clubs. Transport is an even more crucial question and we recommend that whatever school a spina bifida teenager attends, someone on the staff should be responsible for drawing up a mobility training programme and for ensuring that before the pupil leaves school he knows exactly how he is going to get about his own neighbourhood without having to rely on his family. Priority must be given to ensuring that pupils can drive and can map-read before they leave school and this should be part of an 'education for living' programme. Teachers could also give pupils and their parents more help in finding out what youth clubs and other recreational and social facilities exist in their own neighbourhoods and could work out with them how to set about joining a particular club. Schools also need to foster the leisure-time interests of handicapped pupils so that they have common interests to share with their able-bodied peers.

Practical measures of these kinds will help to reduce isolation but there is an equal need for teenagers to be helped to come to terms emotionally with their handicaps. Here two things are important. First, teenagers need information about their handicaps and the effects of the handicap upon their functioning, including their sexual development. Second, information must always be coupled with the chance to discuss (either individually with an informed adult or in a group), the implications of this information for the teenager's future. At present spina bifida teenagers generally have little understanding of their handicaps. Their ideas of what spina bifida is are usually hazy: their understanding of operative procedures they have been subjected to often minimal. In many cases little effort is made, for a variety of reasons, either by parents or by professionals to consult older children or to explain procedures to them. Teenagers want to know more about their condition and such an understanding is a crucial first step in coming to accept their handicaps without shame. Spina bifida teenagers are, like all teenagers, very concerned about relationships with the opposite sex; they also, especially the girls, think a great deal about marriage and children so that there is a need, first, for 'ordinary' sex education and, second, for knowledge about how they will be able to function sexually in relation to their individual handicaps, as well as the possibilities for parenthood.

The opportunity to discuss these questions with an informed person must be made available to every teenager with spina bifida. While it is the school's responsibility to provide ordinary sex education, individual counselling will generally have to be given by someone from outside the school, possibly a doctor or a social worker. In addition to individual counselling, group discussions led by an experienced counsellor between teenagers who share similar problems can be invaluable.

10 *What are the prospects for young people with spina bifida of finding satisfactory placement in further education, training and employment?*

Placements available for school-leavers with spina bifida include higher education (ordinary university, Open University) further education and/or training, open employment, sheltered employment, and attendance at a day centre. It is only now that substantial numbers of those with spina bifida who have received early comprehensive treatment are beginning to reach school-leaving age: evidence from adults with spina bifida (most of whom do not have a substantial degree of hydrocephalus) suggests that many with moderate or severe physical handicaps do find open employment, office work of various kinds being the most common source of employment. However, many have initial difficulties in finding work and experience long periods of unemployment. Probably at least half and perhaps more of today's spina bifida leavers will require further education. Quite a large number of these will benefit from ordinary FE courses, including courses provided for disadvantaged or less able students. Those with severe physical handicaps and intellectual impairment arising from hydrocephalus will probably need a more specialized form of further education, closely geared to their abilities and to the requirements of local industry such as is provided in the Work Orientation Unit at North Notts FE College, and more provision of this kind is needed. A substantial number of leavers will almost certainly be too handicapped physically and intellectually to obtain open employment, even if some can benefit from further education. Present provision for this group is particularly unsatisfactory: either they attend sheltered workshops or day centres (sometimes part-time) which have usually been set up for much older disabled people, or they remain at home. The proportion of young spina bifida adults falling into this category is likely to increase in the near future and research is urgently needed into the sort of provision which will be most suitable for them.

Whether or not and how quickly a leaver finds a suitable placement will depend very much on what is done before he leaves school. If the pupil is in an ordinary school the careers officer's attention should be drawn to him about a year in advance of the rest of the class and close liaison between the careers teacher and the careers officer, the pupil and the parents is needed. Spina bifida pupils should take part in the ordinary careers education programme, and should make as wide-ranging visits as possible. Special school pupils should not only be taken to visit those places (e.g. sheltered workshops) where they are most likely to settle but should be given the chance to visit a wide variety of settings. They should also be informed about the sort of courses available to them in further education and close links between special schools and FE colleges should be built up.

Finally, it is essential that all spina bifida teenagers have available to them adequate support and help after leaving school, and should know exactly to whom they can turn. The local careers officer and an identified local social worker will have particularly crucial roles. The careers officer will be responsible for helping the leaver to find placement either immediately after leaving school or after a period of further education and training. If the leaver is not thought to be employable the careers officer should be responsible for informing the Department of Social Services that the leaver is now their responsibility. All disabled leavers should also have available to them a named social worker who will be responsible for ensuring that their total welfare and emotional needs are being met.

Postscript

Although we have written a great deal in this book about the extremely important contribution to the progress of spina bifida children which a wide range of specialists can make (including pædiatricians, orthopædic surgeons, therapists, psychologists, specially trained teachers, social workers, careers officers and others) we would like to end by placing a special emphasis on the overwhelming importance in the day-to-day management and instruction of the child of people who are *not* specialists. These will include, in particular, the parents, but also brothers and sisters, other relatives, neighbours, community play-group leaders and ordinary school teachers and staff in further education colleges. It is these people above all who need to be helped by the 'experts' to develop the skills which will enable them to help not only children with spina bifida but children with a great variety of problems.

This point has been made very clearly in a recent major project concerning policy towards 'exceptional' children in the USA in which ten federal agencies of the US Department of Health Education and Welfare took part. The findings of the project have been reported by Hobbs (1975) in *The Futures of Children*, and it is from this book that we take our final quotations. In the past, Hobbs points out (p. 223), professional efforts to help exceptional children have been focused on the individual child. The main recommendation of the project is that the major focus should, instead, be upon reinforcing and making more effective 'the normal social units responsible for child-rearing', that is, the family, the school and the neighbourhood. While 'most professional people are skilled in providing direct clinical diagnosis and treatment for the child on an episodic basis' they 'are starkly deficient in helping parents, teachers and others who must provide affection, discipline and instruction for the child year after year'.

In order that this situation is changed he recommends (p. 226), and this is our final message too, that 'specialists in child care (educators, physicians, psychologists, social workers, therapists of various kinds) must become specialists in helping parents, teachers and other primary helpers of children'.

Reference

Hobbs, N. (1975), *The Future of Children*, Jossey-Bass Ltd., London and San Francisco.

Appendices

Appendix A

GLOSSARY

Anaesthesia
Loss of feeling, naturally through damage to the sensory nerves or the brain or induced artificially through drugs.

Anencephaly
A condition thought to be related to spina bifida in which the bones of the skull fail to fuse and the underlying brain tissue is very abnormal. It is incompatible with survival.

Arachnoid
A flimsy membrane which forms part of the meninges.

Arnold Chiari malformation
An abnormality commonly found in association with spina bifida in which the structures of the lower brain stem and the cerebellum herniate or protrude downwards through the foramen magnum.

Associated movements
Movements which occur in one part of the body (usually the fingers and toes) unintentionally as a result of movements in another. It is commonly an indication of immaturity or inefficiency in the nervous system.

Autism
A condition in which a child appears not to receive visual and/or auditory stimuli in the normal way. Communication is badly affected therefore and the child is commonly very withdrawn. It is usually, though not invariably, associated with some degree of mental retardation.

Biceps
The muscles on the surface of the upper arm, on contraction of which the arm is bent at the elbow.

Bladder expression
A means of emptying the bladder by hand pressure over the lower abdomen.

Brain stem
A part of the brain near its base which helps to control basic life-support-

ing functions such as breathing, and through which nerve impulses from the body and sensory receptors pass before being processed by the cerebral lobes.

Buggy
A light-weight push-chair which can be folded up neatly, is particularly easy to carry and can be unfolded with one hand. It is produced in two sizes, known as the Baby Buggy and Buggy Major.

Calipers
Metal braces which give support to a paralysed limb.

Cerebellum
A part of the brain near its base which is particularly concerned with the fine control of movements.

Cerebro-spinal fluid
A clear fluid being produced continually within the ventricles of the brain. After circulating around the brain and spinal cord it is reabsorbed back into the bloodstream. Its function is to protect the brain and spinal cord from external shocks by providing it with an aqueous cushion, and to help to remove waste products from the brain.

Chariot
A low three- or four-wheeled vehicle in which the child sits, with back and side supports, and legs supported straight out in front. The child can manoeuvre the vehicle by turning the larger back wheels by hand. It is sometimes called a 'Chailey Chariot'.

Cranium
The skull. The bony covering surrounding the brain.

Cranium bifidum
(See *Encephalocele*)

Cystic fibrosis
A condition which produces a thickening of the mucus throughout the body, as a result of which the internal organs, particularly the lungs, may become blocked. Children with this condition are particularly liable to get severe chest infections and to have difficulty in breathing. This can be controlled if the child is treated with physiotherapy and antibiotics, but there is no permanent cure. The digestion of food may also be affected, causing diarrhoea and poor growth. Some children may lead quite normal lives but others are truly invalided. All need very careful management and many die in childhood.

Encephalitis
Inflammation of the brain, often associated with a viral infection from

which the patient may recover either fully or with some permanent handicap.

Encephalocele
A condition similar to, but much less common than, spina bifida where the abnormality is at the back of the skull (rather than in the spine). Part of the underlying brain may be abnormal. It is also called Cranium Bifidum.

Epispadias
A rare genital anomaly frequently associated with *exstrophy of the bladder.*

Exstrophy of the bladder
A rare congenital malformation occurring chiefly in boys, in which, because of the absence of part of the abdomen and of the bladder, the lower urinary tract is exposed at birth. A *Urinary diversion* may be needed.

Femur
The long bone running between the hip and the knee.

Finger agnosia
Total or partial loss of the perceptive faculty by which the fingers are distinguished from one another, by tactile or kinaesthetic sense alone, which occurs as a result of damage to a particular part of the brain.

Foramen magnum
A hole in the base of the skull through which nerves of the spinal column ascend and descend from the brain.

Hydrocephalus
A condition where too much cerebral-spinal fluid is being produced relative to the system's ability to reabsorb it into the blood-stream. It occurs frequently with myelomeningocele and less often with meningocele.

Unless it is controlled by surgery (or less commonly by drugs) it will result in a rapid growth of the head, increased pressure and brain damage in most cases. Sometimes the hydrocephalus may become controlled spontaneously, without medical or surgical intervention, and this is called 'arrested' hydrocephalus.

Hydronephrosis
(See *Renal damage.*)

Ileostomy
A surgical operation to achieve social control in patients with urinary incontinence. A small piece of the bowel (ileum) is removed from the

main part of the bowel. The ureters (tubes leading from the kidneys to the bladder) are detached from the bladder and are implanted into one end of the piece of ileum, the other end of which is brought out onto the surface of the abdomen. The urine then flows from the kidneys, down the ureters and through the piece of ileum to the surface of the abdomen where it can be collected in a disposable bag, attached to the abdomen and held in place by a small metal plate and a pelvic band. The bag is emptied through a small tap at the base.

Intra-venous pyelogram (IVP)
An investigatory procedure in which a radio-opaque solution is injected into the blood stream, following which the kidneys and ureters are X-rayed at regular intervals as their outline becomes clear during the passage of the calcium.

Kinaesthetic sense (or ability)
A term referring to the sense by which body awareness occurs through nerve receptors present in joints, muscles and tendons.

Kyphosis
A curvature of the spine in which the bones of the vertebrae project outwards forming a hump at some point along the spine.

Meninges
A name given to the membranes covering the brain and the spinal cord which protect and enclose it and which carry, among other things, the blood supply for the nervous tissue.

Meningitis
A condition in which the meninges become inflamed as a result of infection, the onset of which is characterized by restlessness, headaches, fever, vomiting, drowsiness, irritability and sometimes fits. Prolonged infection can be avoided by the use of antibiotics but some degree of permanent brain damage commonly results.

Meningocele
In this form of spina bifida the bones of the spine (vertebrae) are 'bifid' or split and some of the underlying tissues, including the meninges, are also abnormal, although the spinal cord itself is quite normal. The baby will be born with a small swelling in its back at the point where the defect (or lesion) occurs, and this can be corrected by an operation. Usually there is no damage to nerves or paralysis, but some weakness of legs, bladder or bowel may be present.

Muscular dystrophy
A progressive hereditary disorder marked by atrophy and weakness of the muscles when voluntary actions are attempted.

Myelomeningocele
This is more common than meningocele and is a more serious form of spina bifida. The vertebrae, meninges and spinal cord are all malformed and as a result the child will suffer from some degree of paralysis to legs, bladder or bowel. The severity of the handicap depends on the position of the defect (lesion) and on the number of vertebrae segments involved. In general, high (cervical) or low (sacral) defects produce less severe handicap in survivors than do lesions in the middle (lumbar or thoracic) parts of the spinal column.

Neural tube defect
A term used to cover both spina bifida and anencephaly and a few other rare related defects.

Neurogenic bladder
This term is given to a bladder which fails to function adequately in some way as a result of damage to the nerves which normally control it. In the child with myelomeningocele the nerve supply to the bladder is partially or totally affected in the majority of cases.

Paraplegia
A condition in which both lower limbs are paralysed.

Polygenic
A genetic factor which operates through the action of a number of different genes acting cumulatively rather than through only one or two genes.

Pyramidal tract
A band of nerve fibres originating in the cortex and connecting with cell bodies in the spinal cord. It plays an important part in the control of voluntary movement.

Renal damage (kidney damage)
Damage to the kidneys which may occur in spina bifida children as a result of repeated urinary infections or reflux (back flow) of urine up the ureters into the kidneys, in a bladder incapable of evacuating when full. In this case, hydronephrosis may occur in which the kidney becomes distended and the tubes within it enlarged due to the presence of urine. In time this will cause permanent damage to the kidneys and their ability to filter impurities from the blood will be greatly impaired.

Scoliosis
An abnormality of the spine, in which the spinal column is curved in a lateral direction.

Shunt
A shunt (or valve) is used to control hydrocephalus. It consists of a thin plastic tube, one end of which is placed in one of the cavities within the

brain (the ventricle) where the cerebro-spinal fluid (CSF) is formed. This is called the proximal catheter down which the CSF flows into a uni-directional valve mechanism also controlling rate of flow, which is placed under the skin behind the ear. The valve is attached at the lower end to another plastic tube (distal catheter). In the ventriculo-atrial shunt, the distal catheter is placed in the jugular vein within the neck and is threaded through it into the heart. In the ventriculo-peritoneal shunt the distal catheter enters the chest wall and is passed into the peritoneal cavity of the abdomen. In both cases this allows the excess CSF to be reabsorbed into the blood stream.

Spina bifida cystica
A term covering both meningocele and myelomeningocele where the meninges protrude through the 'bifid' (split) spinal column forming a sac or cyst filled with cerebro-spinal fluid.

Spina bifida occulta
A condition where the bones of the spine (vertebrae) are split or 'bifid' at some point but all the other underlying structures are quite normal. There may be no external change visible and the defect may be unknown, or it may be marked by a hairy patch of skin or some mark on the skin. Very rarely does this result in a malfunction of any kind, although there may occasionally be a risk of intraspinal infection.

Stoma
That part of the loop of bowel to which the ureters are attached in an ileostomy and which is visible on the abdomen. It is sometimes referred to (non-medically) as a 'cherry' because of its red colour.

Talipes
A condition in which the foot is fixed in some abnormal position as a result of muscle imbalance. It can be corrected, at least partially, by a tendon transplant which aims to make the pull of the muscles more equal. There are two main types according to the type of muscle imbalance, equino-varus and calcano-valgus.

Tendon
A bundle of fibres which attach the muscle to bone.

Triceps
The muscles at the back of the upper arm on contraction of which the arm is straightened.

Ureterostomy
A surgical operation similar to an ileostomy, but in this case the ureters are joined together and brought directly out to the surface of the abdomen, without the use of a piece of ileum.

Ureteric reflux
A condition in which the urine passes up the ureters, because the bladder fails to evacuate (empty itself) when full.

Urinal
A flexible rubber sheath fitting over the penis and attached to a disposable bag held in place by straps around the legs and waist. It is used to control urinary incontinence in males. The bag is emptied through a small tap at the base.

Urinary diversion
A method used to achieve social control of urine in incontinent patients. There are two main types, the ileostomy and the ureterostomy which are each described separately.

Valve
Strictly, that part of the shunt system which controls the direction and rate of flow of cerebro-spinal fluid. It is also used commonly as synonymous with shunt.

Ventricles
Cavities within the brain around which the nerve tissue is folded and which produce (secrete) cerebro-spinal fluid.

Ventriculogram
A diagnostic investigation in which air is pumped into the ventricles, displacing the cerebro-spinal fluid and following which the outline of the ventricles becomes visible on an X-ray. In this way it is possible to see whether the ventricles have become dilated as a result of a build-up of cerebro-spinal fluid, which would indicate whether the child was suffering from hydrocephalus.

Vertebrae
The bones of the spinal column which enclose the spinal cord.

Visuo-spatial skills
The ability to judge shape, direction and distance through visual cues.

Walking frames
The general names given to aids designed to give stability while walking is being practised. The one commonly used for spina bifida children is known as a 'Rollator'. This is a wide-based metal frame with four 'legs', the two nearest the user being mounted on small wheels. Adjustable hand-holds allow the child to gain stability while bringing the legs forward, and the frame is then advanced by pushing on the wheeled legs.

Appendix B

EXAMPLE OF HYPERVERBAL BEHAVIOUR IN A CHILD WITH SPINA BIFIDA AND HYDROCEPHALUS CONTROLLED BY A VALVE

(WPPSI Full Scale IQ 55, Verbal IQ 67, Performance IQ 50)

(Examiner's remarks and questions in italics)

CHILD I like monkeys, cos they live in zoos (*Yeh*) and when I live in the zoo I, I wasn't really scared. (*Mm. Were you?*)

There be crocodiles and things. I don't like crocodiles, or snakes, or, or, tigers (*Mm*). They're too horrible and monkeys not too horrible but they good. If, if, I, I went to the zoo my daddy said 'can I be an animal' (*Mm*). He said 'yeah' cos when I be an animal I would be a lion. Like that, and oh I be a lion. I will I wouldn't be a lion if I crawl about cos I got bad legs so I can't crawl about (*Mmm*). I can do it like this, like this in the floor, but I'm not going to be a snake so I don't like this. But I'm not Black Beauty and I can't ride. When I, when I be swimming. I go swimming when my leg's better and all go swimming. The seas came along and beat me (*Did they?*), and, and they beat me on the head. Is went they went. They went like this 'bong' and eh we and soon as I went back home, I had some tea and I went to bed and it was all dark. And it seems that funny, if it was all dark it was all dark at night. And so . . . was all dark. And my dad says 'can we goed on tour holidays tonight', and my dad said course here. We can stay one more we can stay but for about a week.

Where did you go for your holidays then?

Went to nanny's.

Where's that?

Ah Blackpool. When, when I went there I see Auntie Judith and I see Uncle Jerry and a dog and Helen and Wilfred and, and I seen only eh Sue and Iain.

What did you do?

Just play about with all the soldiers and that band. They must be in the band anyway.

Band?

Yes.

What's happening to the band?

They soldiers keep on falling down cos they all their instruments keep on damages. And as soon as I be able to play, I be a soldier one day, cos I play in the band. And . . .

What do you play in the band?

. . . And, ah ah ah, David Cassidy in the bands. Brass bands was lots of drums so I could play them. So cos I play, when I play. I just play like this then when I plays all about this then when I was doing long 'movation' and show jumping.

When you were doing what?

Long 'movation' and show jumping. And when I went show jumping I fell off my horse and I fell of the parallel bars and I hurt myself.

Did you?

Yeh, but I jumped over the parallel bars. They were all right. But the the man mended the parallel bars when I jumped.

When he jumped. I just jumped the water and it was ditched up and I did not jump.

When I did not jump I was playing a bit of footballs. I was playing Manchester United when I know the team. When I knew the teams must be coming.

He must be 'plims' in the footballs and somebody won the game must be playing (*Mm*).

Lots of footballs. When I kicked off him. And has must be playing football off the goal and I must be throwing the balls on the goal.

Appendix C

WPPSI AND *WISC* SUBTEST FINDINGS

WPPSI and/or WISC subtests	*Anderson's study: 3 matched groups of 29 children*						*Spain's GLC study*			
	Spina bifida + hydrocephalus		*Cerebral-palsied*		*Non-handicapped*		*Spina bifida children without shunts (N=40)*		*Spina bifida children with shunts (N=86)*	
	Mean	*Rank*	*Mean*	*Rank*	*Mean*	*Rank*	*Mean*	*Rank*	*Mean*	*Rank*
Information	7·5	9·0	7·3	8·0	7·1	10·0	9·6	7·0	8·1	4·0
Comprehension	7·7	8·0	9·4	1·0	8·6	7·0	8·9	9·0	7·0	7·0
Arithmetic	8·1	7·0	7·8	5·0	9·3	4·5	8·0	10·0	7·2	6·0
Similarities	8·8	3·0	8·6	4·0	7·9	9·0	9·7	6·0	9·0	1·0
Vocabulary	10·1	1·0	9·1	2·5	8·5	8·0	10·5	2·0	8·7	2·0
Picture Completion	9·6	2·0	9·1	2·5	9·3	4·5	10·2	3·0	7·5	5·0
Block Design	8·5	5·0	7·5	7·0	9·1	6·0	11·2	1·0	8·2	3·0
Pic. Arr. (WISC only)	8·2	6·0	6·9	9·0	10·3	1·5	—	—	—	—
Obj. Ass. (WISC only)	8·6	4·0	7·6	6·0	9·5	3·0	—	—	—	—
Coding (WISC only)	6·4	10·0	5·4*	10·0	10·3	1·5	—	—	—	—
Animal Hse (WPPSI only)	—	—	—	—	—	—	9·8	5·0	6·7	8·0
Mazes (WPPSI only)	—	—	—	—	—	—	9·2	8·0	6·3	10·0
Geo. Des. (WPPSI only)	—	—	—	—	—	—	10·2	3·0	6·6	9·0
WPPSI or WISC F.S. IQ	88·3 (SD=15·0)		85·2 (SD=16·3)		92·7 (SD=15·9)		99·2		82·9	
Mean Age (Yrs, Mnths)	7·8		7·9		7·11		5·10		5·10	

* Only twenty-four children were able to attempt this test.

Appendix D

EXTRACT FROM AN INTERVENTION PROGRAMME FOR USE WITH SPINA BIFIDA INFANTS

(from Rosenbaum, P., Barnitt, R. and Brand, H. L. (1975) 'A developmental intervention programme designed to overcome the effects of impaired movement in spina bifida infants', ch. 13 in Holt, K. S. (ed.). *Movement and Child Development,* Clinics in Developmental Medicine, no. 55, Spastics International Medical Publications, Heinemann, London)

Development of hand – eye skills; ideas for training in the first, second and third months

0 TO 3 MONTHS

1 VISUAL FIXATION expected to emerge and to develop significantly in first month.

Training

(a) The mother should look at the baby and smile and coo while feeding. The babies often stare at the mother during feeding.
(b) The baby is shown the bottle; visual fixation is rewarded with immediate feeding.

2 VISUAL FOLLOWING seen in second month. Horizontal following precedes vertical.

Training

(a) When fixation is well established, see 1(b), visual following (not fixation) is rewarded. Same sequence of events is carried a step further; slow, deliberate movements of objects with gradual increase in range of movement. When horizontal following is well established, vertical movement is introduced.
(b) The same thing can be done with the infant following the mother's face. Visual following is rewarded with smiling, cooing and cuddling.

3 GRASPING AN OBJECT PLACED IN THE HANDS should

occur in latter part of third month. Voluntary grasp and brief holding of an object are to be expected. (This is *not* a reflex at this stage.)

Training

(a) When the baby is relaxed and happy, with hands open, an object such as a wooden rod or ring is placed in his hands. The mother then plays at removing it, pulling the object and hand about playfully.

3 TO 6 MONTHS

4 GRASP AND PLAY WITH OBJECTS follows from 3 above. It evolves gradually and can be trained easily.

Training

(a) The baby is shown an attractive or favourite toy; as soon as visual fixation and interest are noted, the object is put in the baby's hand.
(b) The mother plays at removing the object.
(c) One now expects to see a sensorimotor link, *i.e.* the child begins to open its hands in anticipation of the object. The child is rewarded with the object only when these efforts are made.
(d) More and more active effort is expected from the baby. Arm movements towards the object are rewarded in a graded way as performance improves.

5 REACH AND GRASP follow logically.

Training

(a) When the level of achievement of 4(d) is well established, the baby's range of reaching should be extended. This is done by offering favourite toys from various positions in front of and to each side of the baby. The reward is the toy, reinforced by maternal praise.

6 MOUTHING is usually seen around the age of 20 to 24 weeks.

Training

(a) The mother is encouraged to allow the baby to feed himself. When mouthing begins, it can usually be reinforced by giving the baby dry rusks as these are intrinsically rewarding.
(b) Reaching and holding behaviours are reinforced with feeding. Babies at this age often bring both hands up to hold the bottle.

Appendix E

EXAMPLE FROM THE PARENTAL INVOLVEMENT PROJECT DEVELOPMENT CHARTS (JEFFREE, D. M. AND McCONKEY R. (1976), HODDER AND STOUGHTON, LONDON)

Section 9 Reaching

YES	(6)*Reaches and picks up small objects straightaway	NO

↓ Go to Section 10 Grasping

(5) Reaches out and grasps objects	YES	NO
(3) Manipulates objects – grasps a ring or simple play with rattle.	YES	NO
(3) Watches or follows a dangling toy moved in front of face	YES	NO
(2) Turns eye to moving finger or light	YES	NO
(1) Follows moving light with eyes	YES	NO

Go to Section 10 Grasping

Section 10 Grasping

YES	(15) Picks up small objects (e.g. small pieces of string) between finger and tip of his thumb	NO

↓ Go to Section 11 Objects

(12) Picks up objects (e.g. sweet) using finger and thumb	YES	NO
(6) Passes a toy from hand to hand	YES	NO
(6) Picks up small objects using one hand rather than two	YES	NO
(6) Begins to use thumb in grasping objects	YES	NO

Go to Section 11 Objects

* Figures in brackets indicate approximate age in months at which this skill is normally achieved.

Section 11 Objects

YES	(18) Searches actively and appropriately for a lost toy	NO

↓ Go to Section 12 Drawing

(15) Looks in correct place for toys that have rolled out of sight	YES	NO
(12) Looks for dropped toys	YES	NO
(11) Finds a toy if he sees it being hidden in a box	YES	NO
(9) Uncovers a toy if he has seen it hidden by a cloth	YES	NO
(6) Will look for toys if they roll just out of reach	YES	NO
(3) If given a toy will show some interest in it	YES	NO

Go to Section 12 Drawing

Section 12 Drawing

YES	(36) Draws a 'man' on request showing legs and head	NO

↓ Go to Section 13 Social Play

(27) Can copy a circle	YES	NO
(24) Can copy a line	YES	NO
(21) Can scribble in circles and straight lines	YES	NO
(18) Enjoys scribbling	YES	NO
(15) Starts scribbling when given pencil and paper	YES	NO
(12) When encouraged will use a pencil to scribble a little	YES	NO
(10) Holds a pencil but cannot use it to scribble with	YES	NO

Go to Section 13 Social Play

Section 13 Social Play

YES	(48) Plays co-operatively with other children, e.g. in games such as hide and seek, snap, etc.		NO
↓ Go to Section 14 Imitative Play	(30) Will join in play with one other person, e.g. chasing or kicking a ball	YES	NO
	(24) Begins to co-operate in play with other children, e.g. shares toys	YES	NO
	(21) Likes to be shown books by adult	YES	NO
	(15) Offers a toy and releases on request	YES	NO
	(12) Co-operates in games of clap-hands and pat-a-cake	YES	NO
	(11) Repeats a performance when laughed at	YES	NO
	(8) Pats and smiles at own reflection in mirror	YES	NO
	(8) Enjoys peek-a-boo	YES	NO
	(6) Enjoys being swung, lifted, etc., in play	YES	NO

Go to Section 14 Imitative Play

Appendix F

PERCENTAGE OF 6-YEAR-OLD SPINA BIFIDA CHILDREN AND CONTROLS SCORING ON SELECTED ITEMS OF DEVIANT BEHAVIOUR ON THE RUTTER TEACHER QUESTIONNIARE (FROM GLC SURVEY)

		Spina bifida	
Behaviour	*Controls* N=48	*No Valve* N=39	*Valve* N=86
Restless	18·7	28·2	34·8
Irritable, touchy	10·4	12·8	23·2
Can't settle to anything	25·0	25·6	41·8
Fearful of new things	31·2	25·6	48·8
Fussy, over particular	16·7	17·9	24·4
Tics or mannerisms	6·2	2·5	11·6
Bites nails or fingers	2·1	10·2	9·3
Complains of aches and pains	10·4	20·5	17·4
Absent for trivial reasons	4·2	7·6	8·1
Resentful of correction	12·5	20·5	30·2
Unresponsive, apathetic	12·5	20·5	26·7
Lies	8·3	10·2	12·7
Disobedient	27·1	17·9	33·7
Steals	2·1	5·1	1·1
Quarrelsome	14·6	12·8	13·9
Bullies	14·6	5·1	12·7
Damages others' property	12·5	10·2	6·9
Tears on arrival/school refusal	16·7	15·3	8·1
Not much liked by other children	16·7	7·6	13·9
Solitary child	25·0	23·0	33·7
Fidgety	27·1	30·7	29·0
Often unhappy or distressed	22·9	12·8	22·0
Worries about things	39·6	33·3	40·6
Sucks thumb	8·3	10·2	13·9

Appendix G

SOURCES OF INFORMATION ON SPINA BIFIDA, EQUIPMENT AND AIDS, BENEFITS, AND TOYS

Publications on spina bifida

Obtainable from the Association for Spina Bifida and Hydrocephalus, 30 Devonshire Street, London W1N 2EB. Tel. 01-486 6100.

Children with Spina Bifida at School by the Education, Training and Employment Committee of the Association for Spina Bifida and Hydrocephalus, 30p.

Clothing for the Spina Bifida Child by B. Webster, 15p.

Equipment and Aids to Mobility by O. R. Nettles, 25p.

The Nursery Years by M. Paull and S. Haskell, 15p.

Your Child with Hydrocephalus by J. Lorber, 15p.

Your Child with Spina Bifida by J. Lorber, 20p.

Link, the Journal of the Association, published bi-monthly at 5p per copy or on annual subscription at 75p, post paid.

Other useful publications on spina bifida include:
A Guide for Parents of Handicapped Children. This is obtainable free of charge from the Scottish Education Department, Palmerston House, 6/7 Coates Place, Edinburgh.

Help for Handicapped People in Scotland. This is obtainable free of charge from Social Work Departments in Scotland.

The Spina Bifida Baby and *Growing up with Spina Bifida*, both available from the Scottish Spina Bifida Association.

In the United States, the Spina Bifida Association of America publishes an extensive bibliography which is available, free of charge, from: The Library, Spina Bifida Association of America, P.O. Box G-1974, Elmhurst, Illinois 60126. This bibliography lists books, pamphlets and articles covering all aspects of child care and development, including education, employment, laws and social services, and schooling. It includes a list of children's fiction written especially about coping with mental and physical handicaps.

Books on aids and equipment, and achieving independence

Finnie, N. (1971), *Handling the Young Cerebral-Palsied Child*, Heinemann, London.

Forbes, G. (1971), *Clothing for the Handicapped Child*, Disabled Living Foundation, London.

Moore, G. (1972), *Teaching the Handicapped Child to Dress*, Friends of the Centre for Spastic Children, Spastics Society.

Wisbeach, A. (1974), 'Disabled child' in Wilshire, E. R. (ed.), *Equipment for the Disabled* 9, Publ. National Fund for Research into Crippling Diseases. (Other useful titles in this series include *Hoists and Walking Aids*, *Wheelchairs and Outdoor Transport*, etc.)

Organizations giving help and advice on appliances, aids and equipment, toys, etc.

Advice on appliances

Down Bros. Children's Appliance Service,
32 New Cavendish Street, London, W1M 8BU (visits by appointment) and
Church Path, Mitcham, Surrey, CR4 3UE (trained staff in attendance during office hours).
Tel. 01-648 6291
Trained staff will visit schools, hospitals or homes on request to advise on problems concerned with appliances or incontinence.

Salt and Sons Ltd,
Corporation Street, Birmingham
Tel. 021-236 2235

Advice on toys

Toy Libraries Association,
Sunley House, 10 Gunthorpe Street, London, E17 RW
Tel. 01-247 1386
Gives guidance on toys for the handicapped and the setting up of local toy libraries, which often also have facilities for parent consultation or parent groups. Publications include: *Address List* (all affiliated toy libraries throughout the country), *Choosing Toys and Activities for Handicapped Children*, *For Busy Hands*, *Do It Yourself* (advice on making toys for handicapped children), *Why Toys* (the need for play and toys in child development).

Nottingham University Toy Library,
Nottingham University, Nottingham.
Tel. 0602-56101, Ext. 3198
Publications include: *Some Toys Suitable for Handicapped Children* NUTL/7 (list of toys suitable for different age groups and for teaching different skills, with a description of each together with the name and address of supplier). *Suggested Reading List for Parents and Others Concerned with the Care of Handicapped Children* NUTL/5 (titles listed for different handicaps and learning problems as well as general interest titles). *List of Designers, Manufacturers and Suppliers of Toys* NUTL/1. (Toy catalogues can be obtained from manufacturers, many of whom include a special supplement for the handicapped child. Recommended catalogues are starred. Discounts are often available to members of Toy Libraries Association.) *Some Recommended Films* NUTL/8 (films suitable to show to groups of parents on many different aspects of handicap).

Other sources of information on aids, benefits, equipment, etc.

Central Council for the Disabled,
34 Eccleston Square, London SW1.
Tel. 01-834 0747
Information service and useful publications such as *Aids to Independence* and *Holidays for the Physically Handicapped*, etc.

Disability Alliance,
96 Portland Place, London W.1.
Tel. 01-794 1536
Useful pamphlets such as *Disability Rights Handbook for 1977*. An excellent guide to income benefits and certain aids and services for handicapped people of all ages.

Disability Income Group,
Queens House, 180/182a Tottenham Court Road, London W.1.
Tel. 01-636 1946
Many pamplets on benefits; also on information services.

Disabled Living Foundation,
346 Kensington High Street, London W14 8NS.
Tel. 01-602 2491
Permanent exhibition of aids and equipment and an information service on topics such as education facilities for the adult physically handicapped, music for the disabled, physical recreation, etc.

Appendix H

RESIDENTIAL FURTHER EDUCATION AND/OR TRAINING COURSES FOR DISABLED SCHOOL LEAVERS

Derwen Training College and Workshops for the Disabled,
Oswestry, Shropshire.
(Further education and training).

Finchale Training College,
Durham, DH, 5RX.
(Training courses)

Hereward Further Education College,
Branston Crescent, Tile Hill Lane, Coventry.
(Mainly further education; some vocational courses)

Lord Mayor Treloar College,
Froyle, Alton, Hants.
(Further educational and vocational training)

National Star Centre for Disabled Youth,
Ullenwood Manor, Cheltenham, Glos., GL5 39QU.
(Further Education)

Portland Training College for the Disabled,
Harlow Wood, Nottingham Road, Nr. Mansfield, Notts. NG18 4TJ.
(Further education and vocational training)

Queen Elizabeth Foundation for the Disabled,
Leatherhead, Surrey, KT22 0BN.
(Practical, technical and clerical courses)

St. Lloye's College,
Fairfield House, Topsham Road, Exeter, EX2 6EP.
(Further education and vocational training)

Appendix I

USEFULL ADDRESSES (SEE ALSO APPENDIX G)

Association for Spina Bifida and Hydrocephalus,
30 Devonshire Street, London, W1N 2EB
Tel. 01-486 6100

Association of Disabled Professionals,
14 Birch Way, Warlingham, Surrey, CR3 9DA
Tel. 01-820 3801
(An organization of disabled professional men and women.)

Break (Holidays for handicapped or deprived children),
100 First Avenue, Bush Hill Park, Enfield, Middlesex
Tel. 01-366 0253

British Council for Rehabilitation of the Disabled,
Tavistock House (South), Tavistock Square, London, WC1H 9LB
Tel. 01-387 4037/8

Central Council for the Disabled,
34 Eccleston Square, London, SW1
Tel. 01-834 0747
(Co-ordinating body of voluntary associations bringing pressure to improve conditions for the disabled. Publishes information on holidays, aids, etc.)

Centre on the Environment for the Handicapped,
24 Nutford Place, London, W1H 6AN
Tel. 01-262 2641
(Advice and information on the design of the environment for the handicapped.)

The Cheshire Foundation Homes for the Sick,
7 Market Mews, London, W1X 8HP
Tel. 01-499 2665
(Provide permanent care for severely disabled people.)

Disabled Drivers' Association,
Ashwellthorpe Hall, Ashwellthorpe, Norwich
Tel. 0508-41449

Disabled Drivers' Motor Club Limited,
39 Templewood, Cleaveland, Ealing, London, W13 8DV
Tel. 01-998 1226

Disabled Living Foundation, Information Service for the Disabled,
346 Kensington High Street, London, W14 8NS
Tel. 01-602 2491

Disablement Income Group,
Queens House, 180/182a Tottenham Court Road, London, W1P 0BD
Tel. 01-636 1946
(Pressure group aiming to improve conditions, and especially financial provision, for the disabled. Also has information service.)

The Family Fund, Joseph Rowntree Memorial Trust,
Beverley House, Shipton Road, York
Tel. York 29241
(Offers help to families of handicapped children whose needs are not being met under the NHS.)

Handicapped Adventure Playground Association,
2 Paultons Street, London, SW3
Tel. 01-352 6890

Invalid Children's Aid Association,
126 Buckingham Palace Road, London, SW1W 95B
Tel. 01-730 9891
(Provides all kinds of support and help to families with a chronically sick or handicapped child.)

The King's Fund,
24 Nutford Place, London, W1H 6AN
Tel. 01–262 2641

Lady Hoare Trust for Thalidomide and Other Physically Handicapped Children,
7 North St., Midhurst, Sussex
Tel. 073081-3696
(Support and practical help to disabled children and their parents.)

National Association for the Welfare of Children in Hospital,
Exton House, 7 Exton Street, London, SE1 8UE
Tel. 01-261 1738
(Organizes play schemes, transport services; provides information; publishes leaflets etc. to help prepare children for hospital.)

National Bureau for Handicapped Students,
Calcutta House, Old Castle Street, London, E1
Tel. 01-283 1030, Ext. 643

National Fund for Research into Crippling Diseases,
Vincent House, 1 Springfield Road, Horsham, West Sussex, RH12 2PN
Tel. 010-403 64101

National Society for Mentally Handicapped Children,
Pembridge Hall, 17 Pembridge Square, London, W2 4EH
Tel. 01-229 8941

The Open University,
P.O. Box 48, Bletchley, Bucks
(Degree courses: lack of 'O' and 'A' levels does not disqualify. Write to Registrar.)

Physically Handicapped/Able-Bodied Clubs (PHAB),
30 Devonshire Street, London, W1N 2EB
Tel. 01-935 2943
(Runs youth clubs and short residential courses.)

Scottish Council of Social Services, Information for the Disabled,
18/19 Claremont Crescent, Edinburgh, EH7 4HX
Tel. 031-556 3882

Scottish Spina Bifida Association,
190 Queensferry Road, Edinburgh, EH4 2BW
Tel. 031-332 0743

The Shaftesbury Society,
112 Regency Street, London, SW1 4AX
Tel. 01-834 2656
(Provides special residential care and teaching for disabled children, especially those with spina bifida or muscular dystrophy.)

Spina Bifida Association of America,
P.O. Box 266, Newcastle, Delaware, 19720, USA

SPOD Committee on Sexual Problems of the Disabled,
183 Queensway, London, W.2.
Tel. 01-727 4426/7

Toy Libraries Association,
Sunley House, 10 Gunthorpe Street, London, E17
Tel. 01-247 1386
(Promotes understanding of the play needs of handicapped children.)

Author Index

Abercrombie, M. L. M., 130, 141
Adelstein, A. M., 60, 62
Albam, B., 76, 86
Alberman, N. B., 130, 141
Allum, N., 3, 19, 42, 105, 112
Anderson, E. M., 5, 7, 8, 117, 125, 131, 132, 133, 134, 135, 137, 139, 140, 141, 178, 179, 181, 182, 185, 187, 188, 199, 205, 206, 208, 209, 214, 230, 234, 243, 244, 246, 250, 251, 269, 322
Annett, M., 138, 141
Association for Spina Bifida and Hydrocephalus, 232, 234, 236, 291, 292, 297
Ayres, A. J., 41, 42

Badell-Ribera, A., 118, 119, 141
Ball, M., 132, 141, 206, 207, 234
Barclay, A., 183, 199
Barnitt, R., 154, 161, 174, 176, 323
Barrett, M. L., 154, 169, 174, 175
Bayley, M., 71, 72, 75, 85, 102, 109, 112
Bell, W. E., 43
Belmont, L., 137, 142
Benda, C. E., 13
Bengtsson, A., 159, 175
Beresford, A., 287, 297
Bergstrom-Walan, M. B., 266, 268, 269
Birch, H. G., 137, 142
Birchall, D., 87, 113, 274, 298
Bizzi, E., 43
Bleck, E. E., 32, 43
Blomfield, J. M., 41, 43
Bloom, J. L., 267, 269
Boles, G., 183, 199
Boothman, R., 179, 199
Bradshaw, J., 78, 85
Brand, H. L., 161, 176, 323
Brimblecombe, F. S. W., 111, 112
Brimer, M. A., 125, 142
Brock, D. J. H., 53, 62
Brocklehurst, G., 3, 8, 43, 44, 45
Brown, A., 222, 224, 234
Brown, C., 254, 269
Buck, A. R., 63
Buckle, J., 283, 288, 297
Burke, R. E., 43
Burns, R., 118, 142
Burton, L., 76, 80, 81, 86, 91, 103, 112, 202, 234, 240, 248, 264, 269
Butler, N. R., 235

Carter, C. O., 6, 14, 30, 31, 43, 46, 47, 48, 49, 50, 51, 52, 53, 56, 62, 63, 64, 95, 112, 271, 297
Chadwick, O. F. D., 273
Chapman, J., 215, 234, 235
Chard, T., 63
Chilgren, R., 269, 272
Chir, M., 21, 43
Clark, M., 219, 235
Clegg, N., 278, 297
Clements, D. B., 35, 43
Cole, T. M., 266, 269, 272
Connolly, K., 140, 142, 145, 175, 176
Cook, J., 228, 235
Cope, C., 187, 200, 206, 208, 235
Crocker, A. C., 52, 63
Crome, L. C., 35, 43
Crowe, B., 102, 112

Cruickshank, W. M. 43, 200
Cunningham, C. C., 150, 152, 175
Curran, A. P., 96, 112

Daniels, J. C., 215, 235
Davie, R., 87, 113, 203, 235, 274, 298
Delong, M., 43
Department of Education and Science, 142, 183, 192, 194, 200, 222, 232, 233, 234, 235, 290, 297
Department of Health and Social Security, 63 175
Diack, H., 215, 235
Diller, L., 118, 119, 129, 130, 142, 203, 208, 235
Dinnage, R., 239, 269
Dodds, J., 117, 132, 133, 135, 142
Doherty, E. E., 254, 269
Doll, E. A., 251, 271
Dorner, S., 5, 8, 67, 76, 77, 78, 85, 86, 179, 200, 254, 255, 257, 258, 259, 263, 266, 271, 286, 297
Douglas, J. W. B., 41, 43
Dow, R. S., 40, 43
Drake, D. M., 246, 271
Drummond, M., 57, 58, 59, 61, 62, 64
Dunn, L. M., 125, 142

Eckstein, H. B., 21, 26, 29, 43, 44, 61, 63
Ellis, H. L., 60, 63
Emery, J. L., 14, 40, 43, 45
Ericsson, N. O., 44
Errington, J., 271, 297
Evans, K. A., 6, 30, 31, 43, 57, 63, 64, 254, 259, 262, 267, 271, 283, 285, 289, 288, 289, 295, 297
Evarts, E. V., 40, 43

Faulkner, R., 171
Fedrick, J., 52, 63
Feinberg, T., 264, 266, 271
Fiddes, D. O., 72, 86
Findlay, J. A., 198, 200
Finnie, N., 20, 43, 332
Fitzpatrick, W. F., 29, 30, 43
Fleming, C. P., 129, 142
Foltz, E. L., 144
Forbes, G., 332
Forrest, D., 21, 24, 28, 43, 44, 61, 62, 63
Forsythe, W. I., 28, 44, 103, 112
Fox, M., 68, 86, 90, 91, 95, 97, 100, 107, 112
Fraser-Roberts, J. A., 63
Freeman, R. D., 254, 271
Freeston, B. M., 41, 42, 44, 57, 63, 68, 69, 70, 71, 76, 80, 86, 107, 112, 163, 169, 175, 193, 200
Frostig, M., 131, 134, 142, 219, 229, 235
Fulthorpe, D., 249, 251, 258, 271

Gabriel, R. W., 17, 44
Gairdner, D., 63
Galperin, P., 213, 235
Garden, Y. B., 63
Gardiner, P. A., 130, 141
Gibson, E. J., 132, 142
Gibson, J. J., 132, 142
Glanville, R. A., 276, 279, 281, 297
Gilmer, B. V. H., 245, 272
Gleave, J., 63
Goffman, E., 239, 271
Goldberg, J. K., 130, 142
Golding, D., 64
Goldstein, H., 235
Goodman, J., 246, 272
Gordon, B., 41, 44
Gordon, W. A., 142, 235
Grad, J. C., 99, 113
Graham, P. J., 143, 272
Grantham, E., 166, 167, 171, 175
Greaves, M., 285, 288, 289, 297
Griffith, E. R., 30, 44
Gulliford, R., 213, 235, 236

Gullion, M., 150, 152, 175
Guttman, L., 29, 44

Hadenius, A., 128, 142
Hagberg, B., 142
Hall, M. J., 179, 200
Halliday, J., 69, 86
Hare, E. H., 70, 86
Haring, N. G., 185, 200
Haskell, S. H., 130, 142, 209, 229, 235, 331
Hatcher, G., 63
Hedenberg, C. Von, 44
Hellstrom, B., 44
Hendrickson, L. N., 207, 235
Henley, T. E., 76, 86
Hewett, S., 71, 76, 81, 82, 86, 89, 93, 96, 102, 108, 113, 184, 200
Hickman, V., 271, 297
Hicks, J., 251, 271
Hobbs, N., 309, 310
Hodges, D., 247, 271
Holdsworth, L., 231, 232, 235, 236
Holgate, L., 19, 44
Holland, D., 290, 297
Holt, K. S., 176, 323
Horne, D., 229, 235
Hughes, V. A., 130, 142
Hunt, G. M., 61, 63, 69, 74, 80, 86, 148, 175, 197, 200
Hunt, P., 239, 271
Hunt, V. L., 175
Hutchinson, D., 136, 142, 278, 297
Hyttnas-Bensch, K., 142

Ineichen, R., 109, 113, 248, 253, 271
Ingram, T. T. S., 128, 142, 258, 271, 296, 297

Jameson, S., 271, 297
Jebson, R., 144
Jeffree, D. M., 162, 175, 325
Jensen, G. D., 183, 200
Jessel, C., 252, 271
Jeter, K., 271
Johnson, C. A., 150, 175
Johnson, E. G., 136, 140, 143
Johnston, H. A., 64
Johnston-Smith, P., 297
Jones, C. H., 207, 236
Jones, M. H., 154, 174
Jones, M. L., 175

Kagan, J., 143, 246, 271
Karlberg, P., 143
Kastner, S., 142, 235
Katona, F., 29, 44
Katz, R. G., 150, 175
Kaushal, K., 35, 43
Keith, R. A., 183, 200
Kellmer Pringle, M. L., 72, 86, 87, 113, 239, 271, 274, 298
Kershaw, J. D., 191, 200
Kew, S., 80, 81, 86, 109, 111, 113
Kinley, J. C., 28, 44, 103, 112
Kitau, M. J., 63
Knox, E. C., 52, 63
Kogan, K. L., 183, 200
Kogan, N., 246, 271

Laing, A. F., 252, 271
Lancaster-Gaye, D., 265, 269, 271, 272
Langford, W., 271
Large, P., 283, 297
Lattimer, J. K., 271
Laurence, E., 168, 175, 200
Laurence, K. M., 54, 55, 58, 63, 77, 80, 87, 119, 121, 128, 143, 144, 188, 198, 201, 203, 204, 208, 209, 210, 236, 244, 273
Laurence, M., 5, 287, 297
Laurendeau, M., 143
Leck, I., 49, 63
Leek, A. E., 54, 63
Leighton, P. C., 54, 63
Leith, G. N., 236

Lendon, R. G., 14, 43
Levitt, S., 167, 169, 175
Lewis, A., 234
Liedholm, M., 118, 143
Lightfowler, C. R. D., 58, 64
Lonton, A., 138, 143
Lorber, J., 5, 18, 26, 27, 28, 33, 34, 37, 44, 46, 47, 58, 59, 61, 64, 118, 119, 120, 121, 143, 256, 258, 272, 331
Lore, R. K., 246, 272
Lowe, P. B., 279, 297
Lunzer, E. A., 251, 272
Lyle, J. G., 136, 140, 143

McConkey, R., 162, 175, 325
McIntosh, H. T., 57, 64, 68, 70, 71, 81, 86, 89, 92, 95, 96, 100, 107, 113, 180, 200
McMichael, J., 67, 86
MacKenzie, I., 40, 44
MacMahon, B., 50, 64
Mann, L., 229, 236
Markie, G. S., 183, 200
Martin, H. P., 85, 86
Maslow, P., 219, 235
Matson, D. D., 128, 143
Meichenbaum, D., 246, 272
Menkes, J. H., 44
Milhorat, T. A., 33, 35, 44
Miller, E., 35, 44, 117, 132, 143, 154, 175
Mitchell, R. G., 271, 297
Mittler, P., 165, 175
Mooney, T. O., 266, 272
Moore, G., 332
Morgan, M., 254, 257, 272, 281, 283, 297
Moyer, K. E., 245, 272
Muehl, S., 207, 235

Nagel, D. A., 32, 43
Naggan, L., 50, 64
Naughton, J., 128, 142
Neale, M., 203, 205, 236
Nergardh, A., 24, 44
Nettles, O. R., 331
Newson, E., 82, 86
Newson, J., 82, 86
Nordqvist, I., 91, 113, 265, 268, 272
Norris, J., 153, 154, 156, 157, 158, 175

Osser, H. A., 142

Paddock, N., 141
Paine, I., 290, 297
Parfit, J., 98, 108, 110, 113, 171, 172, 175, 181, 200, 298
Parsons, J. G., 117, 125, 136, 143, 284, 285, 297
Patterson, G., 150, 152, 175
Paull, M. E., 229, 235, 331
Payne, H., 87
Pick, A. D., 142
Pilling, D., 239, 272
Pinard, A., 143
Pinkerton, P., 202, 236, 239, 264, 272
Pinsker, E. J., 129, 144
Pless, I. B., 202, 236, 239, 264, 272
Plewis, I., 140, 141
Poznanski, E. O., 78, 86
Presland, J., 228, 236
Purkhiser, C. A., 125, 143

Raikes, A., 173, 176
Rawlings, H. E., 86
Renwick, J. H., 52, 64
Reynell, J., 143
Richards, I. D. G., 57, 64, 68, 70, 71, 76, 81, 86, 89, 92, 95, 96, 100, 107, 113, 180, 200
Richardson, S., 254, 259, 260, 262, 272
Richman, N., 77, 86, 241, 272
Riding, R. J., 208, 236
Roberts, F. R., 95, 112

Roberts, J. A. F., 56, 63
Roberts, M. C. C., 200, 273
Robertson, E., 254, 272
Rosenbaum, P., 161, 162, 176, 323
Rosenberg, P., 269
Rosenbloom, L., 162, 176
Roskies, E., 182, 183, 184, 200
Ross, C. F., 63
Rowland, M., 136, 143, 166, 167, 170, 171, 176
Russell, D. S., 35, 45
Russell, I. T., 87, 113
Rutter, M., 77, 86, 139, 143, 233, 236, 242, 243, 244, 255, 273, 330

Sand, P. L., 144
Sanders, L., 277, 298
Santostephano, S., 246, 273
Schaffer, R., 99, 113
Schloss, A. L., 256, 258, 272
Schonell, F. E., 204, 210, 236
Schonell, F. J., 204, 210, 236
Schutt, W., 41, 45
Schwebel, A. I., 246, 273
Scott, M., 200, 250, 263, 264, 268, 273
Scottish Education Department, 188, 189, 191, 194, 195, 200, 261, 273, 280, 282, 291, 293, 298
Seidel, U. P., 243, 244, 273
Seifert, A., 150, 155, 161, 176
Sella, A., 136, 144
Sen A., 245, 273
Sethi, L., 35, 44, 117, 132, 143, 154, 175
Sharrard, W. J. W., 18, 19, 45
Shearer, A., 265, 267, 273
Sheridan, M., 67, 86
Shore, J. M., 208, 236
Shulman, K., 141
Shurtleff, D. B., 144
Simon, B., 213, 235
Sjogren, I., 142
Slater, E., 63
Smith, E. D., 13, 17, 21, 24, 45, 58, 59, 61, 64
Smith, G. K., 58, 59, 61, 64
Spain, B., 5, 6, 57, 59, 64, 68, 69, 70, 87, 92, 93, 95, 96, 106, 107, 113, 117, 118, 119, 125, 126, 130, 133, 134, 135, 136, 144, 163, 196, 266, 322
Stanworth, A., 35, 45
Stark, G., 57, 58, 59, 61, 62, 64
Stern, G. G., 200
Stern, J., 35, 43
Stevenson, A. C., 64
Stevenson, J. E., 272
Stewart, M. I. P., 64
Stewart, W. F. R., 273
Stollard, J., 210, 236
Stratton, P., 140, 142
Stricker, G., 246, 274
Sutcliffe, R. G., 53, 62
Swann, E., 96, 112
Swinyard, C., 142, 235
Swisher, L. P., 129, 144

Talbot, H., 29, 30, 31, 45
Tansley, E., 228, 236
Taylor, E. M., 123, 124, 139, 144, 241, 273
Taylor, N., 144
Tew, B. J., 5, 58, 63, 76, 77, 80, 87, 117, 118, 119, 121, 128, 131, 132, 143, 144, 183, 198, 200, 201, 203, 204, 208, 209, 210, 236, 244, 250, 251, 267, 273
Thach, W. T., 43
Thomas, D. N., 185, 201, 233, 236
Thomas, M., 87, 113
Timms, R. J., 44
Tizard, J., 5, 8, 86, 99, 111, 113, 236, 273
Tomko, M. A., 44
Tuckett, I., 234, 236
Tuckey, B., 275, 280, 281, 282, 296, 298

Tuckey, L., 275, 280, 281, 282, 296, 298
Turner, A., 138, 141
Turnure, J. E., 245, 274

Variend, S., 40, 45
Vaught, G., 183, 199
Vernon, P. E., 204, 208, 236
Vinken, P. J., 43

Walker, J. H., 68, 69, 70, 71, 76, 81, 85, 87, 92, 93, 94, 95, 96, 107, 113
Wallace, S. J., 41, 45, 136, 144
Walpole, L., 63
Walsh, G., 44, 45
Watson, P., 277, 298
Webster, B., 28, 45, 103, 113, 331
Wedell, K., 215, 228, 234, 235, 236
Welbourn, H., 188, 189, 190, 201, 250, 274
Wessner, G., 143
Whipp, M. A., 86
White, B., 146, 176
Whitmore, K., 86, 231, 232, 235, 236, 273
Wigley, G., 68, 87, 93, 95, 106, 107, 113
Wilson, A. L., 102, 113
Wing, L., 88, 94, 98, 113
Wisbeach, A., 20, 45, 332
Woodburn, M., 5, 8, 41, 42, 45, 70, 73, 74, 75, 79, 81, 87, 89, 92, 93, 96, 97, 99, 100, 103, 108, 110, 113, 124, 144, 164, 165, 166, 167, 170, 171, 176, 180, 181, 188, 198, 201
Wright, B., 239, 256, 274

Younghusband, E., 67, 68, 87, 90, 108, 110, 111, 113, 165, 176, 253, 274, 293, 298

Yule, W., 143

Zucker, J. S., 246, 274

General Index

access, 180, 189–90, 258–9, 260–1, 281, 306
adapted furniture, 20, 147, 152
adolescents, *see also* emotional problems, peer relationships
  anxiety about marriage, children, 256–7, 259, 265, 266–7
  counselling of, 264, 266–70, 307
  dependence on parents, 84, 99, 253–4, 305
  depression in, 254–7, 306
  early puberty in, 105
  feelings about handicaps, 263–5, 307
  fostering independence in, 105, 253–4, 260, 293, 305
  groups for, 262–3, 307
  in institutions, 254, 270
  interest in opposite sex, 256, 259, 307
  sexual development of, 29–31, 256, 265–70
  social isolation of, 199, 253, 257–63, 305
adventure playgrounds, 159, 168
advisers in special education, 226, 232, 304
aids, 19, 20, 23–8, 73, 97, 293, 329–30
alpha-fetoprotein, 53–5
amniocentesis, 53–5
ancillary helpers *see* welfare assistants
anencephaly, 13–14, 46 ff, 313
antibiotics, 1, 23
appliances, *see* aids, urinals
Arnold-Chiari malformation, 12, 39–41, 124–5, 136, 219, 313
arrested hydrocephalus, 33
attendance allowance, 97, 293
attentional problems, 125, 129, 150, 159–60, 161, 210, 211–2, 227–8, 244–5, 303, 304
assessment centres, 111, 173, *see also* school-leavers
Association for Spina Bifida and Hydrocephalus, 92, 105, 110, 222, 286, 291
Association of Disabled Professionals, 179

balance:
  sitting, 138, 146, 147, 148, 153, 160, 223
  standing, 17, 19, 35, 79, 83, 147
behaviour difficulties: *see also* attentional problems, emotional problems, peer relationships
  anti-social disorders, 243, 304
  eating problems, 241
  impulsivity, 133, 246–7
  passivity, 170, 241, 247
  and pre-school children, 167, 240–1
  and primary school children, 241–4
  restlessness, 243
  sleeping problems, 83, 149, 241
  temper tantrums, 84, 241
behaviour modification techniques, 29, 227–8
Bender Visual Motor Gestalt Test, 132

benefits, 293, *see also* attendance allowance, mobility allowance
bifid, 11
bladder expression, 23–4
bladder incontinence, *see* incontinence, urinary diversion
blind children, 150, 174
body image, 154, 222
bowel incontinence, 28–9, 73, 103–4, 110, 189
brothers and sisters, *see* siblings
by-pass operation, *see* urinary diversion

calipers, 19, 74, 314
careers officers, 281, 290–2, 295–6, 308–9, *see also* vocational guideance
catheterization of bladder, 25
central nervous system, development of, 11–13
cerebellar ataxia, 40, 41
cerebellum, 40–1, 145, 314
cerebral palsy, 1, 2, 76, 78, 122, 126, 128, 131–2, 169, 205–6, 209, 220, 234, 243–4, 254, 258, 259, 262, 296
cerebro-spinal fluid, 12, 13, 14, 15, 31–3, 35–9, 314
Chronically Sick and Disabled Persons Act, 293
clubs, *see* leisure activities
'cocktail-party' syndrome, *see* language development
Committee of Enquiry into Special Education, 165, 233
consultants, 70, 100–1, 269
contractures, 18–19, *see also* orthopaedic management, physiotherapists
corpus callosum, 35, 138
cranium, 12, 33, 314
cranium bifidum, 13–14
critical periods, 145
cystic fibrosis, 2, 76, 80, 103, 248–9, 314
cystic sac, 13–14, 15
cystoscopy, 23

Daniels and Diack Standard Reading Test Battery, 215
day centres, 276, 280, 286, 289, 291, 308
day nurseries, 109, 110
deaf children, 150, 174
Department of Education and Science, 184, 192, 194
diet, 191
Disabled Living Foundation, 293
Disablement Income Group, 293
distractability, *see* attentional problems
Down Brothers, 29, 103, 330
driving instruction, 221, 261, 284, 306

educationally subnormal children, 208
education services, *see* services
emotional problems: *see also* adolescents, behaviour difficulties
in adolescence, 253 ff
anxiety, 241, 243, 247–9, 304–5
apathy, 241, 243, 247, 285
dependence, 151–2, 167, 253–4, 305
depression, 254–7
fearfulness, 149, 241, 243, 247–8, 304
feelings about handicaps, 248
immaturity, 151–2, 251, 305
and incontinence, 249–50
in pre-school children, 240–1
in primary school children, 241–4
employment, 276, 280–1, 283–9, 296, 308, *see also* sheltered work
tres, 277, 279–80, 291
Employment Rehabilitation Cen-

Employment Services Agency, 295-6
encephalocele, 14, 53, 121, 124, 135
English Picture Vocabulary Test, 125–6
epileptic children, 231, 232
ethical issues, 60–2
experience, deprivation of, 146–50, 210, 299
extrophy of the bladder, 266, 315
eye-hand co-ordination:
  early training in, 155–8, 161–2
  problems of, 3, 131, 133–6, 139, 146, 210, 221, 223, 300
  special programmes for, 230

families: *see also* father, mother, parents, siblings
  effects of handicap on, 2, 67 ff
  financial assistance, 97, *see also* benefits
  going out together, 73
  help from local community, 74–5, 102–3
  help from professionals, 88 ff
  help from relatives, 74–5, 103
family doctor, *see* general practitioner
Family Fund, 78
family planning, *see* genetic counselling
fathers: *see also* families, parents
  reactions to diagnosis, 68
  involvement in management of child, 90–1, 93, 104, 152, 298
feeding skills, 149
figure-ground discrimination, 131, 141, 207, *see also* visual perception
fluid intake, 24, 28, 191
fontanelle, 33
foramen magnum, 12, 40, 315
fractures, 18
friendships, *see* peer relationships
Frostig Developmental Test of Visual Perception, 131, 132, 133, 229
further education, 275, 276, 277–9, 280–3, 290, 308

games, *see* play activities, physical education
generalization of skills, 212, 229
general practitioners, 57, 59, 71, 94, 96, 192
genetic counselling, 55–7, 94, 95–6, 268, 297
genetic risks, 30, 49, 55–7
Greater London Council (GLC) Study, 6, 42, 69, 73 ff, 91, 119 ff, 147–50, 181, 193, 195–7, 204–5, 214, 230, 240–3, 251
Griffiths Mental Development Scale, 120, 127, 133–4

haemophilia, 2
hand control: *see also* eye-hand co-ordination
  early training, 157–8
  impairment of, 35, 40–1, 79, 133, 135, 136–40, 141, 146, 154, 210, 218, 219–20, 284–5, 300
handedness, 137–8, *see also* left-handers
handicap registers, 174
handwriting, *see* writing
head circumference, 33–4
Health Care Planning Teams, 106, 111, 174
health services, *see* services
health visitors, 71, 94–5, 96, 99, 101, 102, 104, 107–8, 192, 298
hearing, 124–5, 240
higher education, 277
hips, 17–18
holidays:
  day provision, 101, 111–2, 253
  residential care, 104–5, 109, 112

home help service, 101
home tuition, 188
hospitals:
  admissions to, 41–2, 74, 79–80
  difficulties attending, 74
  effects on child, 41–2, 83, 210, 241
housing, 96–7, 108, 284
hydrocephalus: *see also* shunts
  and Arnold-Chiari malformation, 40
  and aptitude tests, 284–5
  causation of, 12, 31–3
  effects on intellectual functioning, 33–4, 117 ff
  effects on physical functioning, 17, 34–5, 41, 136
  and school attainments, 203–10, 303
  treatment of, 36–9
hydronephrosis, 23

ileostomy, 26–7, 315–6
incontinence of bladder: *see also* bowel incontinence, urinals, urinary tract, urinary diversion
  and choice of school, 180, 181 188–9
  and employment, 284, 293
  management, general, 23–8, 73–4, 103–4
  management in schools, 188–9, 250, 305
  and mother's health, 77–81, 104
  nature of problem, 2, 21–3, 73
  social aspects, 249–50, 258, 305
infections, 83, *see also* shunt, urinary tract
integration: *see also* placement, play-groups, schools
  attitudes of disabled children, 178–9
  attitudes of disabled adults, 179
  attitudes of parents, 179–83
  attitudes of teachers, 185–6, 192, 197
  and further education, 282
  in North America, 187, 190
  official policy, 184
  in Scandinavia, 187
intelligence:
  and hydrocephalus, 118–20
  impairment of, 2, 117 ff, 187, 284, 301
  parents' perception of, 183
  and physical handicap, 118, 120
  verbal-performance differences in 118, 122, 135, 187
intravenous pyelogram, 23, 316
Isle of Wight Survey, 77, 139, 233, 242, 244, 255

Joint Consultative Councils, 106, 111, 174

kinaesthetic experience, 212, 226, 316
kidneys, 2, 22–3, 26, 103, 317
kyphosis, 17, 59, 316

language development:
  age of talking, 124
  comprehension skills, 126–8, 212
  fostering language skills, 157, 159–60
  hyperverbal behaviour, 123, 128–30, 300, 320–1
  verbal fluency, 122, 123, 207, 300
  vocabulary skills, 125–6
  syntax, 126
laterality, *see* handedness
learning difficulties, 187–8, 225–30, 232, 303–4, *see also* intelligence, number work, reading, writing
left handers, 25, *see also* handedness
leisure activities, 222, 253, 260–2, 263, 294, 307

limb deformities, 17–19
Link, 28, 329
locomotor function: *see also* mobility
impairment of, 16–18
treatment and management, 18–20

Malaise Inventory, 78
Manchester Scales of Social Adaptation, 251
map-reading, 221, 261, 306
marital relationships, 69, 76, 78, 96
maternity units, 68, 95, 106, 298
Mathematics Attainment Test A (NFER), 209
memory, 123, 125
meninges, 12, 13, 14, 31, 316
meningitis, 16, 32, 316
meningocele, 13–14, 15, 17, 53, 121, 287, 316, *see also* spina bifida
mentally handicapped children, 72, 75, 78, 102
mildly handicapped children, 77, 92, 100, 128, 149, 182, 239
mobility, 19–20, 72–3, 147–8, 167, 189, 190–1, 256, 257–8, 261, 283–4, 305, 306, *see also* driving instruction, locomotor function
mobility allowance, 101, 293
mothers: *see also* families, fathers, parents
advice on management for, 95, 298
anxieties about management, 68–72
anxieties about schooling, 182
daily management problems, 72–5
mental and physical health, 74, 76–7
reaction to diagnosis, 67–9, 91–4
relationship with child, 72, 75, 78, 102
understanding of condition, 68, 70–2
understanding of treatment, 70
multiply-handicapped children, 178
muscular dystrophy, 76, 78, 316
myelomeningocele, 13–15, 17, 21–3, 39–40, 41, 53, 54, 121, 317, *see also* spina bifida

National Fund for Research into Crippling Diseases, 265
Neale Analysis of Reading Ability, 203, 215
neural tube defects, *see* anencephaly, cranium bifidum, spina bifida
neural tube, development of, 11–13
neurological abnormalities: *see also* cerebral palsy, hydrocephalus
and behaviour difficulties, 239, 243–5, 304
and learning difficulties, 209, 210
number work:
difficulties in, 208–12, 303
teaching of, 158, 211–3

occupation centres, *see* day centres
occupational therapists, 19–20, 173, 299
ocular defects, 35, 133, 146, 207, 210, *see also* squint
office work, 284–5, 287–8
operative treatment, *see* surgery
orthopaedic management, 18–20
Oseretsky Test, 139
'over-protectiveness', 81–3, 99, 184–5, 251, 254, 256, 257

parent associations, *see* ASBAH, parents groups
parents, groups, 99–100, 101–2, 108, 110, 111, 298

parents: *see also* families, fathers, mothers, 'over-protectiveness'
advice on fostering child's skills, 150–62, 299, 309
aggression in, 92
consultation about early surgery, 60, 67
consultation about school placement, 192–4
contact with other parents, 94, 99–100, 103, 298
developmental advice, 72, 150–2, 162
feelings about handicap, 84–5, 94, 240
feelings of inadequacy, 69, 72, 89–90, 152
getting out together, 75, 99
increasing confidence of, 89–90, 152, 162, 170, 299, 390
information about condition, 70–1, 93, 100–1, 106, 297
information about management, 70–2, 93–5, 97, 100–1, 297
perception of child's intelligence, 183, 184
reactions to diagnosis, 67–9, 91–4
and teachers, 231–2
peer relationships:
in adolescence, 191, 240, 253, 256, 257–60, 262, 263
explanations to peers, 250, 252
over-protection by peers, 180, 192, 252
in pre-school period, 148, 163, 166–7, 169, 191, 251–2
in primary years, 191, 251–2, 305
teasing, 180, 250, 252, 257
penile urinals, *see* urinals
perception, *see* visual perception
physical education, 191, 221–5, 230
Physically Handicapped and Able-Bodied (Phab) Clubs, 263, 335
physically handicapped children, 2, 3, 150, 183, 209
physicians: *see also* consultants, general practitioners
breaking news of diagnosis, 67–9, 92–4, 106
and information to parents, 100
physiotherapists, 19–20, 70, 173, 180, 189–90, 221
placement: *see also* schools
delays in, 198
procedure, 192–4
reviews of, 178, 194–5
of spina bifida children, 195–8
for trial period, 186, 194
play activities: *see also* playgroups, toys
at home, 153–61, 241, 299
in pre-school groups, 167–9
playgroups: *see also* pre-school education
advantages to child, 101, 166–9, 247, 300
advantages to mother, 169–70, 184
advice for leaders, 111, 172–4, 300
disadvantages, 170
ordinary groups, 171–4, 300
special groups, 109, 166, 168–9, 171, 173
pre-school education, 110, 111, 163–72, 300, *see also* playgroups
Pre-School Playgroups Association, 167, 171–2, 173
pressure sores, 19, 20–1, 42
psychiatric disorder, *see* emotional problems, behaviour difficulties
psychiatrists, 269
psychologists, 184, 192, 226, 299, 304
Pudenz valve, 36, *see also* shunts
pyramidal tract dysfunction, 41, 317

reading:
attainments, 202–8, 303
teaching of, 207–8
reasoning ability, 123
Remploy, 276
renal damage, *see* kidneys
Renfrew Bus Story, 127–8
research, 5, 117, 169
residential care, 104–5, *see also* holidays, schools
Reynell Developmental Language Scale, 125, 126, 127
ribs, 6

sac, *see* cystic sac
Salt and Son, 29, 330
Schonell Spelling Test, 204
school doctors, 192–3, 194, 230–1
school-leavers: *see also* employment further education, vocational training
assessment of, 277, 278, 279, 292
follow-up of, 276, 294–6, 309
with physical handicaps, 280–3
residential courses for, 279, 282, 332
from special schools, 280, 281, 282
with spina bifida, 283–9, 292
supportive services for, 294–6, 309
schools: *see also* placement, teachers
absence from, 188, 210
choice of, 3, 101, 177 ff, 301–2
ordinary schools, 177–82, 185–9, 194–5, 199, 249, 250, 251, 257–8, 290–1, 292, 302
and parents, 105, 321–2, 269
residential schools, 180, 181, 186, 257, 269, 292
special provision in ordinary schools, 177, 179, 181–9, 199, 206, 302–3
special schools, 177, 178, 180–9, 195, 199, 222, 226, 252, 253, 257–8, 259, 261–2, 269, 291–2, 293–4, 302
science lessons, 221
scoliosis, 17, 318
Seebohm Report, 5, 108
sensation, loss of, 20–1, 79, 154, 230, 241, 250, 293
services:
education, 110–2, 173–4, 295–6
health, 106–8, 109, 111–2, 173–4
liaison between, 110–2, 173–4, 300–1
social, 108–9, 111–2, 172, 173–4, 262, 276, 295–6, 309
sexual functioning, 29–31, 268, *see also* adolescents
Sexual Problems of the Disabled (SPOD), 265, 269, 335
sheltered work, 276, 280–1, 286, 289, 291, 308
shunts: *see also* hydrocephalus
blockage of, 2, 38–9, 69, 71
disconnections, 38–9
infections of, 2, 38–9, 42
obstructions to, 38
shunting procedures, 36–9, 317–8
siblings:
symptoms of malfunctioning, 38–9, 69, 83
problems of, 78–81, 98, 241, 298
help for, 97–9
skin care, 21, 28
social development:
and incontinence, 249–50
and pre-school education, 166–7
and restricted experience, 148, 191, 251
social maturity, 251–3, 285
social skills teaching, 123, 251–2
and sport, 222
social education, 282, 293–4
social services, *see* services

social workers:
in the community, 91, 94, 95, 96, 102, 108–9, 192, 269, 296, 298, 309
in hospitals, 93–4, 107–8, 298
South Wales Study, 5, 58, 76, 80, 117–9, 121, 128, 131–2, 183, 198, 203–4, 208–10, 244, 250–1, 267
Spastics Society, 234, 280, 282–3
spatial difficulties, 158, 210, 211, 212, 219, 223, 284–5, 300, *see also* visual perception
spelling, 204
spina bifida: *see also* meningocele, myelomeningocele
and birth order, 51–2, 54, 69
causation, 47 ff
classification of, 13
cystica, 13, 318
development of, 11–14
and dietary factors, 52
ethnic variation in, 48–9
genetic factors in, 12, 48–50, 52–3, *see also* genetic counselling, genetic risks
incidence of, 1, 46–7
and level of lesion, 17
and maternal age, 51
mortality rate in, 46–7
occulta, 11, 318
prevention of, 53
seasonal trends in, 51–2
secular trends in, 51
selection for treatment, 57–62
sex differences in, 48, 118, 121–2, 198
screening for, 53–5
and social class, 51
spinal cord, 11 ff
Spitz-Holter valve, 36–7, *see also* shunts
squint, 33, 35, 130–1, 146, 207, 210
stature, 82
strabismus, *see* squint
stoma, 26–7, 318
surgery:
on back, 15–16, 36
general, 42, 188
orthopaedic, 18–19, 188
selection for, 57–9, 67, 94
shunt surgery, 36–9
on urinary tract, 25–8
Swedish Central Committee for Rehabilitation, 265, 266

tactile development, 154–5, 156–7, 219, 226
talipes, 18, 70, 318
teachers: *see also* schools, teaching techniques
back-up services for, 187, 194, 221–2, 226, 230–3, 234, 303–4
need for information, 185, 192, 196–7, 221–2, 230, 250, 303
and parents, 231–2
and placement decisions, 192–3
training of, 233–4, 269, 303
teaching techniques: *see also* number work, reading, writing, general principles, 225–8
special programmes, 228–30
tendons, 18, 318
Terman-Merrill Test, 120
termination of pregnancy, 54–5
thalidomide children, 182
toys, 20, 146, 153–61, 245, 299, 330, *see also* play activities
training, *see* vocational training
training centres, 280
Training Services Agency, 287, 296
transport: *see also* driving intruction
and leisure, 258–9, 261
and schooling, 180, 188, 189
and work, 261
Tuckey Report, 280, 281–2
typewriting, 220

ultra-sound techniques, 53
Union of the Physically Impaired Against Segregation, 179
ureterostomy, 26–7, 318
ureters, 22, 23, 26
urinals, 24, 103, 189, 223, 249, 258, 259, 319
urinary diversion, *see also* incontinence, urinals
  child's feelings about, 249, 256, 259
  description of, 24–8, 319
  management of, 73, 77–8, 100, 103–4, 189
  parents' understanding of, 70, 100, 264, 267

valve, 36–9, 319, *see also* shunts
ventricles, 12, 31–3, 319
ventriculogram, 33, 319
verbal ability, *see* language development
verbalization, use of, 212, 226–7
Vernon Graded Arithmetic-Mathmatics Test, 208
Vernon Reading Test, 204
Vineland Scale of Social Maturity, 251
visual perception, *see also* eye-hand co-ordination, figure-ground discrimination
  early training of, 153–4, 156
  problems of, 130–3, 135–6, 141, 146, 158, 207, 210, 221, 223–4, 300
  special programmes, 229
visuo-motor ability, *see* eye-hand co-ordination
vocational guidance, 289–92, 296, 308–9, *see also* careers officers
vocational training 275, 278, 279, 280–3, 285, 287, 296, *see also* further education

walking difficulties, *see* locomotor function, mobility
Warnock Committee, *see* Committee of Enquiry into Special Education
Wechsler Intelligence Scale for Children, 122, 126, 133, 134–5, 183, 207, 209
Wechsler Pre-School and Primary Scale of Intelligence, 119, 121, 122, 129, 134–5, 205, 209
welfare assistants, 24, 188, 189, 190–1, 224, 250
work, *see* employment
work experience schemes, 278, 279
writing: *see also* hand control, handedness, left-handers
  alternatives to, 220
  difficulties in, 137, 140, 212, 213–18, 221
  teaching of, 218–20, 230